W9-CPD-720

PEDIATRIC PRIMARY CARE
Well-Child Care

PEDIATRIC PRIMARY CARE
Well-Child Care

Editor

Raymond C. Baker, M.D.

Professor of Clinical Pediatrics
University of Cincinnati College of Medicine
Department of Pediatrics
Associate Director, Division of General and Community Pediatrics
Children's Hospital Medical Center, Cincinnati, Ohio

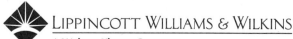

LIPPINCOTT WILLIAMS & WILKINS
A **Wolters Kluwer** Company
Philadelphia · Baltimore · New York · London
Buenos Aires · Hong Kong · Sydney · Tokyo

Acquisitions Editor: Timothy Y. Hiscock
Developmental Editor: Julia Seto
Production Editor: Christiana Sahl
Manufacturing Manager: Benjamin Rivera
Cover Designer: Jeane Norton
Compositor: Circle Graphics
Printer: R.R. Donnelley/Crawfordsville

© 2001 by **LIPPINCOTT WILLIAMS & WILKINS**
530 Walnut Street
Philadelphia, PA 19106 USA
LWW.com

All rights reserved. This book is protected by copyright. No part of this book
may be reproduced in any form or by any means, including photocopying, or
utilized by any information storage and retrieval system without written
permission from the copyright owner, except for brief quotations embodied in
critical articles and reviews. Materials appearing in this book prepared by
individuals as part of their official duties as U.S. government employees are
not covered by the above-mentioned copyright.

Printed in the USA

Library of Congress Cataloging-in-Publication Data

Pediatric primary care : well-child care / edited by Raymond C. Baker.
    p. ; cm.—(Core handbooks in pediatrics)
    Revision, in part, of: Handbook of pediatric primary care. c1996.
    Companion v. has subtitle: Ill-child care
    Includes bibliographical references and index.
    ISBN 0-7817-2889-4
    1. Pediatrics—Handbooks, manuals, etc. I. Title: Well-child care. II. Baker,
Raymond C. III. Handbook of pediatric primary care. IV. Series.
    [DNLM: 1. Pediatrics—methods—Handbooks. 2. Primary Health Care—
Child—Handbooks. WS 39 P37185 2001]
    RJ48 .H343 2001
    618.92—dc21

                                     00-048152

Care has been taken to confirm the accuracy of the information presented
and to describe generally accepted practices. However, the authors, editor,
and publisher are not responsible for errors or omissions or for any consequences from application of the information in this book and make no war-
ranty, expressed or implied, with respect to the currency, completeness, or
accuracy of the contents of the publication. Application of this information in a
particular situation remains the professional responsibility of the practitioner.
    The authors, editor, and publisher have exerted every effort to ensure that
drug selection and dosage set forth in this text are in accordance with current
recommendations and practice at the time of publication. However, in view of
ongoing research, changes in government regulations, and the constant flow of
information relating to drug therapy and drug reactions, the reader is urged
to check the package insert for each drug for any change in indications and
dosage and for added warnings and precautions. This is particularly important when the recommended agent is a new or infrequently employed drug.
    Some drugs and medical devices presented in this publication have Food
and Drug Administration (FDA) clearance for limited use in restricted research
settings. It is the responsibility of the health care provider to ascertain the
FDA status of each drug or device planned for use in their clinical practice.

                                10 9 8 7 6 5 4 3 2 1

To my mother, Ruth Abigail Baker,
who taught me that learning is a lifelong process

🔶 Contents

I. Components of the Well-Child Visit

IV. Miscellaneous Topics in Pediatric Primary Care

V. Appendices

Contributing Authors

Raymond C. Baker, M.D. *Professor of Clinical Pediatrics, University of Cincinnati College of Medicine; Associate Director, Division of General and Community Pediatrics, Children's Hospital Medical Center, Cincinnati, Ohio*

Jeanne L. Ballard, M.D. *Associate Professor of General Pediatrics and Obstetrics and Gynecology, University of Cincinnati College of Medicine; Division of General and Community Pediatrics, Children's Hospital Medical Center, Cincinnati, Ohio*

Paul S. Bellet, M.D. *Professor of Clinical Pediatrics, University of Cincinnati College of Medicine; Director, Generalist Inpatient Service, Division of General and Community Pediatrics, Children's Hospital Medical Center, Cincinnati, Ohio*

Omer G. Berger, M.D. *Professor of Clinical Pediatrics, University of Cincinnati College of Medicine; Director, Lead Clinic, Division of General and Community Pediatrics, Children's Hospital Medical Center, Cincinnati, Ohio*

Barbara W. Boat, Ph.D. *Associate Professor of Psychiatry, Director of The Childhood Trust, University of Cincinnati College of Medicine, Cincinnati, Ohio*

Kathleen Burklow, Ph.D. *Assistant Professor of Pediatrics, University of Cincinnati College of Medicine; Division of Child Psychology, Children's Hospital Medical Center, Cincinnati, Ohio*

Anita Cavallo, M.D. *Professor of Clinical Pediatrics, University of Cincinnati College of Medicine; Division of General and Community Pediatrics, Children's Hospital Medical Center, Cincinnati, Ohio*

Michael A. Gittelman, M.D. *Fellow, Pediatric Emergency Medicine, Division of Pediatric Emergency Medicine, Children's Hospital Medical Center, Cincinnati, Ohio*

Claudia Hoffmann, Ed.D. *Assistant Professor of Clinical Pediatrics, University of Cincinnati College of Medicine; Division of Child Psychology, Children's Hospital Medical Center, Cincinnati, Ohio*

Julie A. Jaskiewicz, M.D. *Assistant Professor of Clinical Pediatrics, University of Cincinnati College of Medicine; Division of General and Community Pediatrics, Children's Hospital Medical Center, Cincinnati, Ohio*

Heidi J. Kalkwarf, Ph.D.   *Assistant Professor of Pediatrics, University of Cincinnati College of Medicine; Division of General and Community Pediatrics, Children's Hospital Medical Center, Cincinnati, Ohio*

Ann W. Kummer, Ph.D.   *Field Service Associate Professor of Pediatrics, University of Cincinnati College of Medicine; Director, Speech Pathology Department, Children's Hospital Medical Center, Cincinnati, Ohio*

Nancy E. Lanphear, M.D.   *Assistant Professor of Pediatrics, University of Cincinnati College of Medicine; Cincinnati Center for Developmental Disorders, Children's Hospital Medical Center, Cincinnati, Ohio*

Nancy D. Leslie, M.D.   *Assistant Professor of Pediatrics, University of Cincinnati College of Medicine; Head, Metabolic Services, Division of Human Genetics, Children's Hospital Medical Center, Cincinnati, Ohio*

Lisa M. Lewis, Ph.D.   *Assistant Professor of Pediatrics, University of Cincinnati College of Medicine; Division of Child Psychology, Children's Hospital Medical Center, Cincinnati, Ohio*

Constance M. McAneney, M.D.   *Associate Professor of Clinical Pediatrics, University of Cincinnati College of Medicine; Division of Emergency Medicine, Children's Hospital Medical Center, Cincinnati, Ohio*

Christine L. McHenry, M.D., M.A.T.S.   *Professor of Clinical Pediatrics, Director, Medical Ethics Program, University of Cincinnati College of Medicine; Director, Medical Ethics Program, Division of General and Community Pediatrics, Children's Hospital Medical Center, Cincinnati, Ohio*

Victoria Meier, M.A.   *Psychology Department, Xavier University, Cincinnati, Ohio*

Janet R. Schultz, Ph.D.   *Professor of Psychology, Xavier University, Cincinnati, Ohio*

Robert M. Siegel, M.D.   *Medical Director, St. Luke Pediatric Center, Bellevue, Kentucky*

James F. Steiner, D.D.S.   *Professor of Clinical Pediatrics, University of Cincinnati College of Medicine; Director, Division of Pediatric Dentistry, Children's Hospital Medical Center, Cincinnati, Ohio*

Lisa M. Vaughn, Ph.D.   *Assistant Professor of Pediatrics, University of Cincinnati College of Medicine; Division of General and Community Pediatrics, Children's Hospital Medical Center, Cincinnati, Ohio*

Jennifer Walker   *Freelance Medical Illustrator, Yellow Springs, Ohio*

Thomas S. Webb, M.D.   *Assistant Professor of Clinical Medicine, Department of Internal Medicine, University of Cincinnati College of Medicine, Cincinnati, Ohio*

Irving L. Wollman, M.A.   *Coordinator, Speech Pathology Services, Speech Pathology Department, Children's Hospital Medical Center, Cincinnati, Ohio*

♣ Preface

The precursor to this book, the *Handbook of Pediatric Primary Care*, was well received. The *Handbook* found a place in the pockets of many medical and nursing students and residents learning how to provide primary care to children as well as young doctors and nurses leaving their formal training to begin careers in pediatric primary care. Because of its utility as a resource, the editor of the handbook series of Lippincott Williams & Wilkins, Timothy Hiscock, asked me to expand the book into two separate volumes covering the well-child visit and the ill-child visit to accommodate more easily additional topics and new information in the field. These books, with others, will be the basis for a new series, the Core Handbooks in Pediatrics.

Pediatric Primary Care: Well-Child Care will concentrate on health maintenance supervision, the foundation of pediatric primary care, and on behavioral and developmental pediatrics, integral components in the provision of well-child care. Several new chapters cover newborn screening, the sports physical, the adolescent visit, and injury prevention. Additional chapters address and expand on age-specific well-child visits. Furthermore, the behavioral and developmental section, significantly expanded, covers common negative behaviors that a primary care provider should be able to help parents manage as well as a chapter on child sexuality. Discussions of developmental topics of importance to the primary care provider include the approach to the developmentally delayed child, school issues, and attention deficit hyperactivity disorder. Finally, other chapters address telephone medicine, medical informatics, cultural competence, and teaching in the primary care setting.

The companion volume, *Pediatric Primary Care: Ill-Child Care,* addresses the common illnesses encountered in primary care sick or problem visits. New topics include common exanthems of childhood, acne, cardiac murmur evaluation, gastrointestinal parasites, gastroesophageal reflux disease, acute abdominal pain, diabetes, and vision and hearing abnormalities.

Medications in this handbook that are written with generic names begin with a lower case first letter. For many drugs, I also give examples of brand names, written with an upper case first letter. The brand names listed do not represent personal preferences and, for most drugs, do not represent all brand names available.

Like the original book, I hope this handbook finds a special place in pediatric and family medicine continuity clinics, now such an important part of the training of primary care physicians in this new age of ambulatory medicine. As with any handbook, my goal of allowing easy access to practical information that can be used *during* the delivery of clinical care required me to undertake the difficult task of compressing large amounts of information into a useable, readable format. I did not intend that this book should definitively describe diseases and disease processes. Therefore, the end of each chapter lists up-to-date references and reviews, including internet sites, for the reader who wishes more information about any of the topics discussed.

Raymond C. Baker, M.D.

I

Components of the Well-Child Visit

1 ♣ Introduction and Overview of the Well-Child Visit

Raymond C. Baker

I. Introduction

Routine health maintenance supervision, or well-child care, is the most rewarding aspect of the health care of infants, children, and adolescents. The opportunity to practice anticipatory and preventive medicine is greatest during routine well-child checkups and is the cornerstone of pediatric medicine. The importance of well-child care to the pediatrician is apparent if one examines the day-to-day activities of pediatric primary care physicians. A survey of Cincinnati community pediatricians in 1993 showed that fully 40% of their time was spent performing well-child examinations, although this varies somewhat with the time of year. Summer and fall commonly are peak times for well-child care, especially of school-aged children, whereas during the winter often the number of ill visits increases, especially in younger children.

Integral to the provision of routine health maintenance supervision is understanding the concept of anticipatory guidance, which is somewhat unique to the field of pediatrics. Although other medical specialties, especially internal medicine, recommend regular health maintenance visits, chronic illness commonly occupies the majority of an internist's time. In pediatrics, on the other hand, the population tends to be healthier, and the routine provision of immunizations provides the opportunity for the physician to interact on a more frequent and regular basis, permitting the formation of a bond with the caregiver. Furthermore, since vaccinations are regulated and required by law, the caregiver must seek the services of the primary care physician. Therefore pediatric medicine has evolved to incorporate extensive counseling of a preventive nature into the routine visits.

The well-child visit in most settings combines the efforts of the physician and nursing or ancillary medical care providers. Growth parameters, vital signs, and the chief complaint are usually obtained prior to the physician's interaction during the initial nursing assessment. With this information the physician can then obtain the history, perform the physical examination, and counsel the parents (and child) regarding anticipatory guidance and behavioral issues. In many physicians' practices some of the routine anticipatory guidance relating to safety, development, and nutrition is provided by nursing and ancillary personnel. Other services that may be performed by ancillary personnel with appropriate training may include developmental testing (e.g., Denver Developmental Screening Test—II) and school visits for children with educational and behavioral problems in the school setting.

Well-child care takes time. How much time is dependent on several factors, including (a) the level of training of the physician, (b) physician interests, (c) space (number of examination rooms

3

and support space) available, (d) number of nursing and ancillary medical providers available, (e) number of ill patients to be seen, and (f) prevalence of chronic illness and psychosocial disorders in the patient population. A lower socioeconomic population tends to have a higher prevalence of chronic medical and psychosocial problems, which require time to evaluate and manage. In a survey of private Cincinnati pediatricians, the average time spent with a well-child encounter was 15 minutes by the physician and 10 minutes by the nurse. This did not include registration time, waiting time, and checkout time. Ill-child care took somewhat less—about 10 minutes per patient by the physician and 5 minutes by the nurse. The average number of patients seen in a typical pediatrician's day (per physician) was about 40 patients.

By contrast, in the pediatric residents' continuity clinic at Cincinnati Children's Hospital, where resident physicians of all levels are seeing patients, four to eight patients per 3- to 4-hour clinic is average, with well-child care requiring about one-half hour and ill-child care taking 15 to 20 minutes. Nursing time is relatively less, because resident physicians are encouraged to address patient education issues themselves rather than to depend on ancillary personnel.

Since the amount of time available for personal, one-to-one counseling of the patient may be limited, the physician must make choices regarding which topics to cover at each visit. In most instances, the history will provide a clue as to which areas require discussion. Sometimes setting another or a later appointment is necessary for patients with complicated psychosocial problems so that a greater amount of time can be spent counseling. One can nearly always accomplish more with a return appointment, scheduled specifically for counseling, rather than with a hurried, one-sided discussion of the problem at the end of a routine visit when a complicated behavioral issue requires counseling. Written educational materials and a suggested reading list are especially helpful in counseling situations such as these.

II. The Well-Child Visit: Components

   A.   Intake visit—first visit to office/clinic. The first visit for well-child care is characteristically an intake visit, at which time extensive historical information is obtained. This should include, in addition to the historical information mentioned in part B of this section ("routine visit"), a detailed maternal/prenatal and birth history, immunization history, dietary history, both medical and surgical illness history, family history, developmental and behavioral history, and psychosocial history. Typically, the first regular office or clinic visit is at 1 to 2 weeks of age. However, the extended intake visit is also appropriate to establish a base of information on infants, children, and adolescents presenting for a first visit, having received previous care elsewhere. A common example of the latter is a parent transferring the care of the child to a new pediatric primary care provider due to a change in insurance carrier.

B. Routine visit. The purpose of the routine well-child visit is to monitor the overall physical growth, psychologic and physical development, and health of the child and to guide the parent or guardian through the complexities of child rearing. The content of each visit is unique to the age of the child and to the circumstances of the child's current state of health. Each element of the encounter is geared toward the expected achievements and problems that may be related to the particular age and developmental stage of the child. (See Part II, "Well-Child Visits by Age and Developmental Stage.")

The history at the **routine well-child visit** represents a chronicle of the child since the last well-child visit. It should include information concerning problems or illnesses, past and present, including immunization-related events, in addition to information about the achievement of developmental milestones and nutrition, including feeding habits as well as content. The physician should elicit the history from the parent in an informal and empathetic way so the parent will be encouraged to share concerns about the child's behavior as well as his health. The use of open-ended questions maximizes the parent's opportunity to discuss problems and concerns. Questionnaires about behavior that the parent or adolescent patient completes in the waiting area before the visit (see Appendices G, H, and I) are used by many primary care physicians to raise behavioral issues that might otherwise be forgotten or overlooked during the encounter. The examiner should actively engage the child in interactive communication by active question and answer in the verbal child or by gesture and imitative speech in the preverbal child. Active participation of the child allows the child some control over the encounter and encourages more cooperation and rapport with the physician.

C. Prenatal visit. The **prenatal visit** commonly occurs during the third trimester of pregnancy, when prospective parents are selecting medical care for their newborn. This visit is the opportunity for future parents to get to know a physician or practice and for the practitioner to advise and discuss with the parents information about breast feeding and nutrition, circumcision, fee schedules, appointment times, on-call services, well-child visit schedule, and general philosophy of medical care delivery. Many practices offer group prenatal classes, supervised either by the physician or by nursing personnel, as well as written materials that provide this information.

D. Postpartum examination. The first examination of the newborn by the primary care physician occurs in the hospital nursery, usually within 24 hours after delivery, barring intrapartum and postpartum complications. This important examination provides the physician with the opportunity to review the birth and maternal history and to evaluate for congenital abnormalities and neonatal problems. It provides new parents with an opportunity to ask questions and the physician with an educational opportunity. Many community pediatricians have nursing personnel who perform much of the educational services needed in the newborn setting.

E.   Postdischarge visit. With the recent move to shorten hospital stays of postpartum mothers and infants, monitoring the first few days at home after discharge from the newborn nursery has become increasingly important. Common problems that may develop during the first few days of life are poor weight gain due to difficulties with feeding, especially breast feeding; hyperbilirubinemia; and infection. Since parents often find coming to the physician's office the first few days following delivery difficult, many hospitals and primary care physicians have initiated programs of routine home visits by nursing personnel. At these visits, the newborn is examined and weighed and may have blood obtained for bilirubin, hematocrit/hemoglobin, or metabolic screening. This is an additional opportunity for new parents to ask questions regarding newborn care. The physician can then determine when the first office or clinic visit will be needed based on these home visits and can address any problems that are reported by the visiting nurse.

F.   Physical examination. The physical examination of the well child should be complete, including growth parameters of height and weight at each visit, head circumference at least until the age of 2 years, and blood pressure beginning at age 3. The child should be undressed for the examination, with gown covering appropriate to age. In the interest of time, some of the history may be obtained during the examination. Time saved in this way can increase the amount of time at the end of the examination for counseling the child and caregivers. During the physical examination, the child's family can be informally observed to determine the appropriateness of interactive skills by the caregiver and the reactions of the child. Such issues as the nurturing and psychologic health of the family are often evaluated better by direct observation from the physician than by sole reliance on information obtained in response to questioning.

G.   Assessment. At the end of the history and physical examination, the child's health can be assessed. This should include assessing the child's physical growth, neuromotor development, and family interactions (psychosocial health). The assessment of the child forms the groundwork for subsequent planning for screening tests and immunizations and for anticipatory guidance for the family.

H.   Screening tests. Routine screening tests are performed in children at different ages according to predetermined standards. These are timed to have the greatest yield of abnormals, to determine abnormalities at critical times in a child's life (such as school and puberty), and to coincide with immunization visits. Routine blood analysis for hemoglobin and hematocrit and lead, along with urinalysis, evaluation of vision and hearing, and tuberculin testing are performed according to standards developed by the American Academy of Pediatrics. Additional screening may be suggested by a number of factors, including family history, ethnic background, socioeconomic background, and geographic considerations.

I. Immunizations. In the United States, children are immunized according to standards set by the Advisory Council on Immunization Practices (ACIP) and the American Academy of Pediatrics (AAP) against diphtheria, tetanus, pertussis, poliomyelitis, *Haemophilus influenzae* type b, pneumococcal disease, rubeola, rubella, mumps, varicella, and hepatitis B. Medical records must be maintained to reflect the date of administration, dose, lot number, educational materials given to caregivers, and possible immunization reactions. Government regulations regarding immunizations and routine well-child care visits vary from state to state but may require the parent or legal guardian to sign written consent for immunizations (as part of overall consent to treat or separately). In addition, documentation that information regarding immunizations and side effects has been given to the parent or guardian verbally, in written form, or both may be required.

J. Anticipatory guidance. At the end of the patient encounter, the physician should sit down with the parent or guardian and discuss the child's health, progress, and suggestions for care appropriate to the age of the child, including information pertinent to the period of time until the next well-child examination. Areas covered should include nutrition, elimination, health habits/hygiene, sleep, sexuality, school, socialization and family, behavior and parenting, discipline, development, and safety issues that relate to the child's age. Most physicians have age-appropriate written materials that are used in conjunction with these discussions to reinforce key points.

K. Closure. At the conclusion of the discussion, arrangements for the next well-child care examination should be made. Any appropriate referrals may also be arranged at this time with pertinent explanation to parents. Nursing discharge procedure should include reviewing by word or brochure the physician's instructions to the patient, setting the follow-up appointment, and giving instructions for reaching the physician when necessary.

ADDITIONAL READING

American Academy of Pediatrics. *Recommendations for preventative pediatric health care* (RE9535). Elk Grove Village, IL: American Academy of Pediatrics; 2000.

American Academy of Pediatrics. *Recommended childhood immunization schedule—United States, January–December 2000* (RE9961). Elk Grove Village, IL: American Academy of Pediatrics; 2000.

American Academy of Pediatrics Committee on Psychosocial Aspects of Child and Family Health. *Guidelines for health supervision III,*

3rd ed. Elk Grove Village, IL: American Academy of Pediatrics; 1997.

American Academy of Pediatrics Committee on Psychosocial Aspects of Child and Family Health. The prenatal visit. *Pediatrics* 1996; 97:141–142.

Fox CE, III. *Put prevention into practice: clinician's handbook of preventive services*, 2nd ed. Washington, DC: U.S. Department of Health and Human Services; 1998.

Green M, Haggerty RJ, Weitzman M, eds. *Ambulatory pediatrics*, 5th ed. Philadelphia: WB Saunders; 1999.

Green M, Palfrey JS, eds. *Bright futures: guidelines for health supervision of infants, children, and adolescents*, 2nd ed. Arlington, VA: National Center for Education in Maternal and Child Health; 2000.

LaBaron CW, Rodewald L, Humiston S. How much time is spent on well-child care and vaccinations? *Arch Pediatr Adolesc Med* 1999; 153:1154–1159.

Neinstein LS. *Adolescent health care: a practical guide*, 3rd ed. Baltimore: Williams & Wilkins; 1996.

Osborn LM. Effective well-child care. *Curr Prob Pediatr* 1994; 24:306–326.

Peter G. 1997 *Red book: report of the Committee on Infectious Diseases*, 24th ed. Elk Grove, IL: American Academy of Pediatrics; 1997.

Sharp L, Pantell RH, Murphy LO, Lewis CC. Psychosocial problems during child health supervision visits: eliciting, then what? *Pediatrics* 1992;89:619–623.

U.S. Preventative Services Task Force. *Guide to clinical preventive services: report of the U.S. Preventative Services Task Force*, 2nd ed. Washington, DC: U.S. Department of Health and Human Services; 1995.

Books for Parents and Caregivers

Greydanus DE, ed. *Caring for your adolescent: ages 12 to 21*. Elk Grove Village, IL: American Academy of Pediatrics; 1991.

Schmitt BD. *Your child's health*, rev. ed. New York: Bantam Books; 1991.

Schor EL, ed. *Caring for your school-age child: ages 5 to 12*. New York: Broadway Books; 1999.

Shelov SP, Hannemann RE, eds. *Your baby's first year*, reprint ed. New York: Bantam Books; 1998.

Shelov SP, Hannemann RE, DeAngelis CD. eds. *Caring for your baby and young child: birth to a°ge 5*, rev. ed. New York: Bantam Books; 1998.

Web Sites

http://www.brightfutures.org/
http://www.aap.org

2 ♣ History

Christine L. McHenry

The pediatric history is the foundation upon which the future physician/patient/parent relationship is built. During the history taking the physician conveys the interest or boredom, concern or annoyance, empathy or lack of understanding that flavors the relationship. It is also a time during which the physician communicates respect for the patient and his or her parent(s). This respect is demonstrated by how the physician greets the patient and the parent(s) (Mr., Mrs., Ms., Mom, Dad), how the physician dresses, and how the physician responds to comments and questions by the patient and/or parent(s).

The goals of the history are (a) to determine why the patient/parent came to see the physician, (b) to determine what the patient/parent is worried about most and why, and (c) to strengthen the physician/patient/parent relationship and thus the therapeutic alliance by observing, listening, and conveying empathy.

I. The Prenatal Interview

The prenatal interview has been popularized over the last 20 years and can be the first step in developing a therapeutic alliance with the parents. Ideally, this interview should take place with both the father and mother. Reasonable goals for the prenatal interview include the following:

A. Identifying problems encountered with previous pregnancies and deliveries that might affect the health of the newborn, such as C-section, preterm labor, jaundice and blood incompatibilities, and diabetes mellitus in the mother.

B. Identifying potential health problems of the newborn, such as hereditary diseases (e.g., cystic fibrosis, metabolic disorders).

C. Acquainting parents with office policies.

D. Informing parents of the birth hospital's procedures for notification of the physician, the physician's involvement in the postpartum care of the infant, and the manner in which complications of newborn care are managed, such as the availability of consulting neonatologists and transfer to outside facilities.

E. Informing parents of the schedule for health maintenance examinations (well-child care).

F. Allowing parents to ask questions and to voice concerns they may have about being a new parent.

G. Discussing issues related to the newborn period, such as breast or formula feeding, choice of formula, circumcision, items needed for taking a newborn home, and items needed in the home nursery.

H. Discussing psychosocial issues that might arise from the pregnancy and delivery, such as family support systems, need for social agency involvement, and nursing care.

II.   The Comprehensive Pediatric Interview

The following is an outline for a comprehensive pediatric interview that occurs as part of the well-child examination at the first office visit to see the physician, either the first regular post-partum visit or the first visit of an older patient transferring to the physician's care. Not meant as an exhaustive list of questions to be asked by the physician, it is a highlight of areas that should be discussed with the patient/parent. Obviously, the interview can be modified according to the age of the patient and the nature of any problems or concerns the parents might have.

Subsequent well-child interviews with established patients remain similar, except that certain unchanging information will not be sought again, such as family history, social and environmental history (unless there are changes, such as a move to a new home), immunization history (which will already be recorded in the medical record), and previous hospitalizations/chronic illnesses (which should already be indicated in the previously recorded past medical history and problem list).

A.   Interim history. A chronologic narrative of the symptom(s) or problem(s), if any are voiced, should be recorded as clearly as possible. Important areas to explore include the symptom(s)' onset, associated symptoms, location, severity, time of day, character, and exacerbating or relieving factors. Asking what the patient or parent thinks is going on and what treatment may already have been tried is equally important. How the patient's symptom is affecting the family is also important. Similarly, behavior problems raised by the parent should be explored, including age of onset, precipitating factors, associated incidents, frequency, the parent's method for dealing with them, and the parent's opinion for the cause of the behavior.

B.   Past medical history

1.   *Prenatal, birth, and neonatal histories.* Prenatal, birth, and neonatal histories are important during the first 2 years of life and when dealing with the patient who is developmentally delayed or neurologically impaired. Prenatal information should include whether or not the mother received prenatal care (and where) as well as the use of cigarettes, alcohol, or drugs (prescription or street drugs) during pregnancy. Intrapartum information should include the mode of birth (vaginal, C-section) and complications during delivery, such as prolonged resuscitation in the delivery suite and low Apgar scores. Complications during the newborn period should be sought, including respiratory problems, feeding problems, formula changes, and jaundice. These details can often be found on the nursery discharge papers.

2.   *Other past medical history:*

a.   Recurrent or chronic illnesses, such as otitis media or asthma.

b.   Childhood illnesses, such as varicella or measles.

  c. Hospitalizations.
  d. Surgeries.
  e. Previous health care, including location, physician or
clinic, immunizations and reactions to immunizations.
  f. Dental care.
  C. Nutritional history. In the breast-fed infant, information on adequacy (satisfaction, crying, urine output, leakage,
"let-down") and maternal complications (nipple soreness,
cracking, bleeding) should be sought. If the infant is 6 months
of age or older, the physician should discuss the need for fluoride supplementation. In the formula-fed infant one should
know the brand name of the formula, the preparation (ready-
to-feed, concentrate, powder) and storage, and the fluoride
content of the available drinking water. If the water is adequately fluoridated, cow's-milk–based formula prepared with
water (powder or concentrate) or the use of soy-based formula
will not require fluoride supplementation. If the infant is on
solid food, the types and amounts should be noted. For the
toddler, exploring how much milk and juice the child drinks
as well as type and quantity of solid foods is important. And
one can never ask too early about "junk food"!
  D. Developmental history. At each visit, information on
the four areas of development should be reviewed, including
gross motor, fine motor, social, and language skills. The level
of skill rather than the age of achievement of that skill is the
most important information that will impact management.
  E. Allergy history. Particular attention should be paid to
reactions to medications. If a patient or parent(s) says he or
she is allergic to a medication, one should ask about the type
of reaction in order to differentiate true allergy from medication effects, such as nausea (e.g., erythromycin) or vomiting
due to bad taste. Allergy information should be prominently
displayed on the medical record and in the problem list.
  F. Medication history. A list of current medications,
doses, and reasons for use should be recorded. Chronic medications should be recorded in the problem list.
  G. Immunization history. The child's complete immunization schedule should be recorded in the medical record in
a standardized location and updated at each well-child visit.
A careful history of reactions to immunizations, with attention to the severity of the reaction (degree of fever; degree of
warmth, swelling, or tenderness at the injection site; timing
of the reaction relative to the injection; and treatment
received for the reaction) should be obtained. Significant reactions, such as those that preclude further immunization with
a particular vaccine, should be recorded in the problem list
and displayed prominently on the medical record.
  H. Family history. The family history includes the age,
height, weight, and health status of the parent(s) and siblings. Many physicians use this opportunity to obtain and
record the names of the siblings, including nicknames, for use

when talking with the child. Significant medical conditions in the family include diabetes, hypertension, renal disease, arthritis, anemia, endocrine disorders, cancer, migraine headache, inflammatory bowel disease, cystic fibrosis, and tuberculosis. The history should be sought on both maternal and paternal sides out to two generations.

I.   Social/environmental history. The social/environmental history develops a sense of the family support system, the environment the patient is living in, and how both might affect the health of the child. Social/environmental issues that should be addressed include the type of dwelling, how many people live in the dwelling, city water versus well (fluoridation issues), type of heat (gas, electric, hot water), pets, parents' occupations, presence of firearms in the home, and religious and cultural beliefs. Baby-sitter and day care information should also be obtained. The parents' support structure, such as grandmothers or other relatives who help with the care of the children, should be explored. The method(s) of discipline used in the family and the method(s) used to resolve disagreements at home should be addressed, either of which may point to an abusive situation. Finally, obtaining some information on family finances and health care coverage is important in order to provide affordable health care services. Frequently this information is obtained at the time of registration. The physician must be aware of the payment mechanisms, as this information may influence certain decisions, such as timing of immunizations or writing a prescription versus suggesting over-the-counter medications.

J.   Review of systems. The review of systems (ROS) includes age-appropriate questions touching on all the major organ systems. Much of the ROS will be included in the interim history. "High-yield" areas for questioning include bowel habits (frequency, consistency, history of encopresis), urinary habits (dysuria, enuresis, frequency, nocturia), and sleeping habits (night waking, crying, sleep walking, sleep talking, nightmares, and night terrors). Behavioral issues that should be addressed might include temper tantrums, sibling rivalry, mealtime behavior, bedtime behavior and ritual, homework behavior, and discipline in general. These all represent areas a parent might not volunteer but that greatly affect the family's overall health. If a concern is uncovered, appropriate counseling and intervention may be initiated before the problem develops crisis proportions.

K.   Interviewing the child. Important information can be obtained from preschool and school-aged children related to friends, activities, school, and family life. With older children asking how they would describe themselves using a weather forecast as the descriptor (e.g., sunny and warm, cloudy, rainy) is helpful. This technique can provide important insight into the emotional well-being of the child. This descriptor, along with asking the child about his or her "three wishes," may point to the source of a problem.

III. Adolescent Interview

A. Autonomy and confidentiality. Adolescence is a time of developing autonomy and independence. As a result, the adolescent patient is entitled to a certain degree of confidentiality in his or her interaction with the physician. At the beginning of the physician/patient encounter, parameters for confidentiality should be established between the physician and the patient and the physician and the parent. Once the parameters are established for the visit, doing some of the interview with both parent(s) and adolescent present is appropriate, followed by separate interviews, especially for sensitive issues.

B. The parent interview. Important information to obtain from the parent(s) includes information about family values and faith tradition, family dynamics and relationships, family history of significant medical or psychiatric illness, and the adolescent's early childhood illnesses and immunizations.

C. The adolescent interview. The adolescent interview obviously includes certain areas that are not a part of the history of the younger child. Most important, the adolescent interview should include questions regarding the following:

1. *Home.* Who is living at home and their relationship with the adolescent, new people at home, family dynamics, recent moves, attempts to run away.

2. *Education and employment.* Grade in school and school performance, favorite and worst subjects, repeated classes, suspensions, future goals, including college or job training, after-school or summer employment, type of job the adolescent enjoys.

3. *Activities.* What the adolescent does for fun with friends, hobbies, clubs, sports, TV, music, religious services/activities, trouble with the law, gun possession.

4. *Drugs.* Drugs/tobacco/alcohol use by the adolescent or a family member, glue sniffing, driving under the influence, drug/alcohol rehabilitation programs.

5. *Sexuality.* Orientation, dating, age of first intercourse, frequency of intercourse, number of partners, contraception, sexually transmitted diseases, pregnancy, menstrual history.

6. *Miscellaneous.* Eating disorders, physical and sexual abuse, feelings of depression, thoughts of suicide, mental health counseling.

IV. The Problem/Ill Visit

The problem visit interview is focused on a particular problem and includes the following:

A. Chief complaint identifying the symptoms or problem.

B. History of the present illness, including pertinent ROS, in which the illness or problem is explored. Including in the history of the present illness what the patient or parent(s) feels is going on, what the patient/parent(s) has already tried in terms of management, and what is most worrisome to the patient/parent(s) is important.

C.   Past medical history, including acute and chronic illnesses, hospitalizations, and surgeries. This is usually necessary only if the physician has not taken care of the patient before or does not have the medical record available.

D.   Current medications, listing both acute and chronic.

E.   Allergies. Including questioning for them should be part of every visit and, when present, should be prominently recorded in the medical record.

F.   Exposures, including family, school, day care, and friends.

G.   Immunizations, including whether the patient is up to date on routine immunizations and the date of the most recent immunization. This history may itself impact the process of the evaluation of an acute illness, such as recent pertussis vaccine in a febrile infant (vaccine reaction) or a recent measles immunization in an infant with a rash (vaccine reaction). Equally important, however, is the opportunity an ill visit may afford the physician to update routine immunizations if the patient has a self-limiting problem.

ADDITIONAL READING

American Academy of Pediatrics. *Guidelines for health supervision III*. Elk Grove Village, IL: American Academy of Pediatrics; 1997.

American Academy of Pediatrics, Committee on Child Abuse and Neglect. The role of the pediatrician in recognizing and intervening on behalf of abused women. *Pediatrics* 1998;101:1091–1092.

Dimond DA. Let's talk about sex. *Contemp Pediatr* 1992;9:19–29.

Goldenring JM, Cohen E. Getting into adolescent heads. *Contemp Pediatr* July 1998:75–90.

Green M, Palfrey JS, eds. *Bright futures: guidelines for health supervision of infants, children, and adolescents*, 2nd ed. Arlington, VA: National Center for Education in Maternal and Child Health; 2000.

Hoekelman RA, ed. *Primary pediatric care,* 3rd ed. St. Louis: CV Mosby; 1997.

Jenkins RR, Sexena SB. Keeping adolescents healthy. *Contemp Pediatr* 1995;12:76–89.

Krugman SD, Wissow LS, Krugman RD. Facing facts: child abuse and pediatric practice. *Contemp Pediatr* 1998;15:131–144.

McMillan JA, DeAngelis CD, Feigin RD, Warshaw JB, eds. *Oski's pediatrics: principles and practice.* Philadelphia: Lippincott Williams & Wilkins; 1999.

3 ♣ Physical Examination

Paul S. Bellet

I. Approach to the Physical Examination

The physical examination of an infant, child, or adolescent must be individualized and purposeful. No examination is routine. The assessment begins as soon as the physician sees the child and parents. For well-child visits, the physician observes the interaction between the child and parents, including displays of affection, amount of separation tolerance, and response to discipline, and the child's language, nutrition, and developmental skills. For ill-child visits, the acuity and severity of the illness must be assessed quickly, as this determines the speed of the examination and the management of the child. The physician should note the child's degree of illness, mood, cry, respiratory pattern, and activity.

During the interview, the examiner should try to form a relationship with the child to instill trust and confidence. This involves talking to the child and sometimes playing together. Children usually respond to a physician who is kind and who genuinely likes them. The physician should be firm but friendly and should give the child instructions about what to do. When two or more siblings are to be examined, the older one should be examined before the others. Usually the older child will be more cooperative and will set a good example for the younger children. If older children request that younger children or parents leave the room during the examination, these wishes should be respected. Even with young children, the physician should explain in simple terms what he or she is going to do during the examination, so the child will be less anxious or will at least understand. Children should have the opportunity to touch and hold some of the instruments, such as the stethoscope, reflex hammer, otoscope, and ophthalmoscope. This gives them a sense of control and participation rather than the feeling that the physician is doing something against their will. The health care provider should not say that potentially painful procedures will not hurt. This deceives children and compromises any confidence or trust that has been established.

Before examining a child, physicians should wash their hands in view of the parents. This not only models appropriate hygienic measures but also warms the examiner's hands, making the examination more comfortable. The physician's gentle manner in talking, handling, and holding an infant or young child presents a model of interaction to the parents. Infants and young children may be examined in the parent's arms or lap, which gives the young patient a sense of reassurance. The examination should begin with observation before any touching, holding, or manipulation. When a complete examination must be performed, the physician may only need to expose that part of the body that is examined at that time so that the child does not need to be totally undressed during the entire examination. Modesty should be respected regardless of age.

In infants and young children, the physician should examine the lungs, heart, and abdomen first and then move distally before the child tires or becomes restless. The head, including the tympanic membranes and pharynx, should be examined last because this often requires some holding and infants often cry. If the mother can hold the child's head against her shoulder with one hand and restrain the child's arms with her other hand, the ears, eyes, nose, mouth, and throat may be examined. If this proves unsuccessful, the child may be placed on the examination table, and the mother can hold the forearms while leaning on the legs, so that the physician can control the head while performing the examination. Some parents have difficulty holding their children properly, and a nurse may be necessary. In the older child the examination can proceed from head to toe, as in an adult. Areas of pain should be examined near the end of the examination. In older children, the genitalia and anus are examined last. One of the most difficult challenges is completing an examination without producing a physical struggle, a crying child, or an upset parent. This requires all of a physician's skill in gaining the confidence and trust of the child and parents.

II. Outline of the Physical Examination

The order of the physical examination depends on the child's age and behavioral characteristics and on the reason for the visit (e.g., a well-child examination versus a focused, problem visit). The proper method of recording the examination is often not the order in which the examination is performed, especially in infants and toddlers. The physical examination includes the following:

A. General description of the patient—well or ill appearing, acutely or chronically ill appearing, degree of distress.

B. Vital signs—pulse rate; respiratory rate; blood pressure; height, weight, and head circumference, including percentiles.

C. Skin, hair, and nails—rashes, lesions, hydration, color, jaundice, cyanosis, abnormalities of hair and nails.

D. Lymphatic system—size, consistency, mobility, tenderness, and location of lymph nodes.

E. Head—size, shape, fontanelles, sutures, masses, tenderness.

F. Face—asymmetry, weakness, tenderness, edema.

G. Eyes—extraocular movements, nystagmus, visual fields, lids (ptosis, lid lag, edema), conjunctivae (color, lesions, discharge), sclerae (color, pigmentation, lesions), pupils (size, equality, response to light and accommodation), cornea, fundi, visual acuity.

H. Ears—external ear, canal (inflammation, discharge, tenderness), tympanic membranes (color, architecture, perforation, mobility), middle ear effusion, mastoid (tenderness), hearing.

I. Nose—mucous membranes (color, discharge, edema, lesions), patency, septum deviation, perforation, turbinates (color, edema), sinuses (tenderness), masses, foreign body.

J. Mouth and pharynx—breath; lips (color, lesions); tongue (size, papillae, movement, lesions, masses); teeth (caries, gums, staining, plaque); buccal mucosa, palate, tonsillar area, and pharynx (color, movement, pigmentation, masses, lesions); tonsils (size, color, exudate, peritonsillar tissue).

K.   Neck—mobility, tenderness, masses, thyroid (size, tenderness, nodules), torticollis.

L.   Breasts—sexual maturity rating, symmetry, tenderness, glandular tissue, masses, nipples (discharge, retraction, ulceration).

M.   Thorax and lungs—shape, symmetry, masses, scars, position of the trachea; tenderness of skin, muscle, ribs, sternum; expansion, retraction, or abnormal movement of the chest; presence and location of wheezes, rhonchi, crackles, or rubs; location of abnormalities by changes in tactile fremitus, whispered or spoken sounds, resonance, breath sounds, or percussion.

N.   Cardiovascular system:
  1.   *Heart.* Character and location of apical pulse, right ventricular impulse, pulsations, thrills, heart sounds (rate and rhythm, intensity and splitting of first and second heart sounds), clicks, rubs, gallops, murmurs (location, timing, intensity [grade 1 to 6], duration, quality, pitch, and radiation).
  2.   *Peripheral vascular system:*
  a.   ***Jugular veins.*** Distention and pulsation, noting the patient's position and distention in centimeters above the sternal angle.
  b.   ***Arterial pulses.*** Including carotid, radial, femoral, popliteal, posterior tibial, and dorsalis pedis: amplitude and contour of the pulse, strength of pulses (grade 0 = absent, grade 1 = decreased, grade 2 = normal, grade 3 = increased, and grade 4 = full and bounding).
  c.   ***Extremities.*** Edema, color, temperature, capillary refill.

O.   Abdomen—size, contour, symmetry, scars, distention, visible movements, peristalsis, tenderness, edema, bowel sounds; palpable organs (liver, spleen, kidneys, bladder, uterus); masses (location, size, consistency, tenderness, mobility, pulsations); hernias; umbilicus; peritoneal fluid.

P.   Genital examination:
  1.   *Male.* Penis—circumcision, prepuce, urethral meatus, discharge, inflammation, lesions; scrotum—testes, epididymis; perineum, sexual maturity rating.
  2.   *Female.* External genitalia—labia, clitoris, introitus, urethral orifice, perineum. Pelvic examination—vagina, cervix, fundus, adnexal areas, and cul de sac (inflammation, discharge, tenderness, masses, erosions), sexual maturity rating.

Q.   Anal and rectal examination—perianal area (fissure, hemorrhoids, fistula, sphincter tone, anal canal), rectum (masses, tenderness, blood), prostate (size, masses, consistency, tenderness).

R.   Skeletal system. Back—scoliosis; upper and lower extremities—bones (tenderness, deformity); joints (range of motion, deformity, swelling, redness, warmth, tenderness, crepitation); ligaments, bursae, tendons (swelling, redness, warmth, tenderness, tendon contracture).

S.   Neurologic examination:

1.   *General status.* Appearance, behavior, speech, posture, gait, gross coordination.

2.   *Cranial nerves.* I through XII.

3.   *Motor system.* Handedness—muscle bulk, contracture, and tenderness; tremor; involuntary movements; muscle fasciculation, strength, and tone; coordination (cerebellar signs).

4.   *Sensory system.* Light touch, pain and temperature, position and vibration sense; stereognosis; tactile localization; two-point discrimination; higher cortical function (aphasia, agnosia, apraxia).

5.   *Reflexes.* Triceps, biceps, radial, knee, ankle, plantar, abdominal, cremasteric, and anal reflexes; jaw jerk, grasp reflex, abnormal reflexes. Strength of reflexes may be described as follows: grade 0 = absent; grade 1 = decreased; grade 2 = normal; grade 3 = increased; grade 4 = with clonus.

6.   *Spinal nerve irritation.* Meningeal signs, sciatic pain (straight leg raising).

T.   Mental status examination. The patient's general behavior and psychologic status are usually included in the general description of the patient. When a mental status examination is performed, the following should be included:

1.   *Behavior.* Unusual or bizarre conduct, mannerisms.

2.   *Cognitive function.* Orientation to time and place, attention, recent and past memory, serial subtraction of 3s or 7s, general information, judgment.

3.   *Thought content.* Illogical, bizarre, depersonalized; feelings of unreality or persecution; delusions; compulsive, phobic, or obsessive thoughts.

4.   *Perception.* Illusions and hallucinations (auditory, visual, tactile, gustatory, olfactory).

5.   *Affect and mood.* Appropriate, anxious, depressed, helpless, hopeless, suicidal, euphoric, manic, guilty, ashamed, panicked, hostile, irritable.

III.   Newborn

The physical examination of the newborn should include an initial assessment in the delivery room, including inspection and Apgar scoring, followed by a complete examination in the nursery. In the nursery, specifics to observe include the following:

A.   General appearance—dysmorphic features.

B.   Vital signs—including appropriateness of weight for gestational age.

C.   Skin—jaundice, cyanosis, rashes.

D.   Head, ears, eyes, nose, and mouth—fontanelles; sutures; signs of birth trauma; ear shape and position; red reflex, abnormal eye movements, and cataract; nasal patency; natal teeth, tongue, and palate.

E.   Neck—masses, torticollis.

F.   Breasts—neonatal hypertrophy.

G.   Thorax and lungs—configuration, clavicles, respirations, breath sounds.

H.   Heart—impulses, heart sounds, murmurs, peripheral pulses, especially femoral pulses.

I.   Abdomen—distention, hepatosplenomegaly, masses, palpation of kidneys, bowel sounds, umbilicus.

J.   Genitalia.

    1.   *Male.* Phallus length, testes, meatal opening.

    2.   *Female.* Clitoral size, introitus, virilization.

K.   Anus and rectum—patency and position of anus.

L.   Skeletal system—extremities (anomalies, movement, *in utero* positional deformity versus a fixed deformity), hips (dislocation or instability), spine (defects, sinuses).

M.   Neurologic—overall state of alertness, vigor of cry, tone, weakness, reflexes (deep tendon and primitive), response to light and voice, symmetry of movement.

N.   Behavioral—alertness; response to holding, feeding, and voice; overall degree of activity.

IV.   Subsequent Visits

    A complete examination should be performed at each well-child visit with particular attention given to parental concerns and risk factors (based on the history). Gross and fine motor development, language, and personal social interaction should be assessed at each visit (discussed elsewhere). Hearing and vision also should be assessed at each well-child visit. This can be done subjectively in a young child and then objectively as the child grows older.

V.   Other Comments

    Examination of the breasts should become a regular part of the physical assessment, starting from the time of breast budding, usually between 9 and 12 years of age. Inspecting the genitalia and determining the Tanner stage of sexual development is likewise important at similar ages. A rectal examination for either a male or female is not part of the routine physical examination but depends on the clinical circumstances.

ADDITIONAL READING

Athreya BH, Silverman BK. *Pediatric physical diagnosis.* Norwalk, CT: Appleton-Century-Crofts; 1985.

Avery ME, First LR, eds. *Pediatric medicine,* 2nd ed. Baltimore: Williams & Wilkins; 1994.

Barness LA. *Manual of pediatric physical diagnosis,* 6th ed. St. Louis: Mosby Year Book; 1991.

Green M. *Pediatric diagnosis,* 6th ed. Philadelphia: WB Saunders; 1998.

Gundy JH. The pediatric physical examination. In: Hoekelman RA, ed. *Primary pediatric care,* 3rd ed. St. Louis: Mosby Year Book; 1997:55–97.

Hoekelman RA. The physical examination of infants and children. In: Bickley LS, Hoekelman RA. *Bates' guide to physical examination and history taking,* 7th ed. New York: Lippincott Williams & Wilkins; 1999:621–703.

McAnarney ER, Kreipe RE, Orr DP, Comerci GD, eds. *Textbook of adolescent medicine.* Philadelphia: WB Saunders; 1992.

Morgan WL, Engel GL. *The clinical approach to the patient.* Philadelphia: WB Saunders; 1969.

Rudolph AM, ed. *Rudolph's pediatrics,* 20th ed. Stamford, CT: Appleton & Lange; 1996.

4 ♣ Newborn Screening

Nancy D. Leslie

The role of newborn screening for phenylketonuria (PKU) as part of pediatric care was established in the 1960s; since then universal newborn screening has expanded to include a variety of conditions. Because each state has specific rules prescribing the diseases for which screening is performed and the manner in which this screening will be accomplished, the panel of diseases for which screening is required varies widely.

I. Principles of Screening

To justify screening large numbers of normal newborns, the following principles are applied:

A. A test must exist that is easily performed on large numbers of specimens. This test must be optimized to detect all (or nearly all) affected newborns; the false-positive rate must be acceptably low.

B. The test results must be available within an appropriate time window, and an intervention must be available. Originally, screening was limited to those conditions where clinical diagnosis was ineffective in preventing morbidity (see Sections II ["Phenylketonuria"] and III ["Congenital Hypothyroidism"]). More recent additions have involved conditions where clinical diagnosis is possible but perhaps would be delayed or unlikely.

C. A system must be in place to find and initiate treatment in all diagnosed infants.

D. Appropriate attention must be paid to confidentiality and the possibility of stigmatization.

E. The benefit of the program should outweigh the cost.

To illustrate the application of the preceding principles, PKU will be discussed in detail. Other applications of newborn screening will be compared with the PKU example.

II. Phenylketonuria

Untreated phenylketonuria causes mental retardation. In PKU, the conversion of phenylalanine to tyrosine is impaired, and excessive phenylalanine builds up in blood, and consequently, in the brain. Although high phenylalanine levels impair brain function at any age, the period of susceptibility for irreversible damage is during the first months and years of life. However, PKU is clinically silent during this critical period. A treatment for PKU was devised in the 1950s and was demonstrated to be successful in preventing mental retardation in subsequent siblings of diagnosed patients. This treatment severely limits (but does not remove) dietary phenylalanine and replaces the other nutrients in high-phenylalanine foods with a special-purpose amino acid mixture (referred to as formula). Until Guthrie devised the bacterial inhibition assay, this successful treatment could not be implemented in families with no previous history of PKU. His method utilizing blood collected on filter paper allowed screening of all newborns before discharge from the birth hospital.

The incidence of PKU is about one in 10,000, and the Guthrie test costs about $1 per test. So the cost to detect one case is about $10,000. Treatment, now continued for life, costs only $5,000 to $10,000 per year—minimal when compared to the cost of special education, the inability to live independently, and poor contribution to the economy—a loss of millions of dollars per case.

The Guthrie test is still used in some state labs, but other tests are gradually taking its place. Shorter newborn hospital stays have mandated that another methodology be adopted to optimize the number of newborns evaluated before hospital discharge. With evolving technology physicians must follow the guidelines set out by the states where they practice, since cutoffs and time constraints will not necessarily translate from one lab to another.

Following are some key facts about phenylketonuria (PKU):

- Incidence: One in 10,000
- Cause: Genetic deficiency in phenylalanine hydroxylase
- Screening method: Blood phenylalanine
- Screening limits: Phenylalanine is normal at birth and rises with age (not amount of food), so early discharge risks missing cases.
- Symptoms:
  - Early—none
  - Late—mental retardation
- Treatment: Special diet
- Prognosis with treatment: Normal IQ
- Method for evaluating abnormal screen: Serum phenylalanine
- Urgency: Days

III. Congenital Hypothyroidism

Untreated congenital hypothyroidism (CH) leads to irreversible mental retardation. Eventually, the growth retardation and clinical features of cretinism lead to a clinical diagnosis, but cognitive abilities do not return to normal when thyroid replacement therapy is initiated late. However, the low thyroxine (T4) and high thyroid stimulating hormone (TSH) levels found in primary hypothyroidism are present long before clinical diagnosis is possible. Treatment consists of oral replacement of thyroid hormone (usually L-thyroxine). Medication is inexpensive, and the costs of specialty care and laboratory monitoring are reasonable. Congenital hypothyroidism is about three times more common than PKU (1:3,000). Testing costs a little more (about $2 per sample), so the detection costs are similar to those of PKU.

Following are some key facts about congenital hypothyroidism:

- Incidence: 1:3,000
- Cause: Malformation of thyroid gland, usually not genetic
- Screening method: Immunoassay for TSH and/or T4

- Screening limits: Very early screens (<24 hours) show false positives with the physiologic TSH surge; prematures have delayed rise and lower T4 levels.
- Symptoms:
  - Early: usually none, occasional jaundice
  - Late: mental retardation (MR), short stature, puffy skin, big tongue (cretinism)
- Treatment: Oral thyroxine
- Prognosis with treatment: Near normal IQ
- Evaluation of abnormal screen: Serum TSH, free or total T4
- Urgency: Days

IV. Galactosemia

Most states currently screen for galactosemia, specifically the form in which galactose-1-phosphate uridyl transferase (GALT) is deficient. Various testing algorithms are used, including testing only the GALT enzyme activity, testing for galactose metabolites, or a combination of both. Unlike PKU and CH testing, GALT testing is insensitive to time after birth, but transfusion of whole blood or packed red blood cells may cause false negatives. False-positive GALT levels are more common when specimens are exposed to heat, as may occur during the summer months.

Galactosemia screening illustrates some of the exceptions to the screening principles. Many infants with classical galactosemia are symptomatic in the first week of life, before the screen returns. However, the clinical presentation may be masked by removal of galactose from the diet. Furthermore, the clinical presentation may not be recognized, since galactosemia is uncommon (1:50,000) compared with the conditions which it mimics (neonatal sepsis). Most disturbing is the fact that early detection and treatment do not prevent long term problems with learning and female fertility. For screening to be a benefit, screens must be collected as early as possible, shipped in a way so as to minimize false positives, and collected before transfusion if at all possible. Clinicians must be aware that screening does not excuse them from exercising clinical judgment.

Following are some key facts about galactosemia:

- Incidence: 1:50,000 (variant form 10 times more common)
- Cause: Genetic deficiency of galactose-1-phosphate uridyl transferase
- Screening methods: Enzyme assay + assay of galactose metabolites
- Limits:
  - Transfusions—false-negative results
  - Heat—false-positive GALT level
  - Delayed feeding—false-negative galactose metabolites
- Symptoms:
  - Early: Poor feeding, failure to thrive (FTT), jaundice, coagulopathy, sepsis
  - Late: Cataracts, MR or learning problems, ovarian failure
- Treatment: Withdraw galactose/lactose from diet (empiric treatment if panic value or clinical symptoms)

- Prognosis: Acute symptoms improve; late symptoms are not prevented.
- Evaluation of screen: Clinical evaluation, GALT level with electrophoretic genotype, galactose-1-phosphate
- Urgency: Hours, if ill or panic value

V.   Hemoglobinopathy

Sickling disorders do not produce obvious vasoocclusive symptoms until fetal hemoglobin levels have decreased, usually after 6 months of age. However, serious bacterial infection with encapsulated organisms may precede clinical ascertainment of sickle cell disease. With the demonstration that oral penicillin may prevent morbidity and mortality from sepsis, screening for hemoglobinopathy meets many of the criteria for widespread screening. As with GALT testing, transfusion of red cells interferes with testing, but time after birth is not critical.

Hemoglobinopathy screening brings up the issues of confidentiality and stigmatization. Although the incidence of hemoglobinopathy justifies screening of African-Americans, logistics preclude stratification of testing by race, so practicality dictates universal screening, regardless of race. In addition, most testing methods identify sickle heterozygotes. The primary purpose of newborn screening is not to identify newborns who are trait positive, but the information is there to be transmitted in a sensitive and confidential manner.

Following are key facts about sickle cell anemia:

- Incidence: 1:100 African-Americans
- Cause: Genetic mutation in beta chain of hemoglobin
- Screening method: Electrophoresis or HPLC
- Screening limits: Red cell transfusion interferes
- Symptoms:
  - Early—none
  - Late—sepsis, vasoocclusive crises, anemia
- Treatment: Penicillin prevents bacteremia; supportive care; transfusions
- Prognosis with treatment: Chronic illness with variable morbidity
- Evaluation of screen: Hemoglobin electrophoresis
- Urgency: Weeks

VI.   Congenital Adrenal Hyperplasia

Congenital adrenal hyperplasia (CAH) due to 21-hydroxylase deficiency may lead to virilization of female infants and salt wasting crisis in both males and females. Classically, all females should be ascertained at birth because of ambiguous genitalia, whereas phenotypically normal males are discharged, presenting with shock in 10 to 14 days. Elevated 17-hydroxyprogesterone levels identifies infants at risk and may allow earlier diagnosis and treatment with replacement glucocorticoids and mineralocorticoids. Therefore the benefit of screening is to prevent critical illness and possible death, and the rare case of missed sex assignment. The pitfalls of CAH screening are that (a) the results must be returned to the clinician quickly, and (b) false positives are common, particularly in low-birth-weight infants.

Following are some key facts about CAH:

- Incidence: 1:30,000
- Cause: Genetic deficiency of 21-hydroxylase
- Screening method: Immunoassay for 17-hydroxyprogesterone
- Limits: High false-positive rate, especially in prematures. Screen may not pick up variants
- Symptoms:
  - Early: Girls—ambiguous genitalia at birth, then same as boys if untreated; boys—vomiting, shock in second week of life
  - Late: Early virilization, growth acceleration
- Treatment: Glucocorticoid and mineralocorticoid replacement
- Prognosis with treatment: Normal growth and development
- Evaluation for positive screen: Clinical evaluation, serum electrolytes, 17-hydroxyprogesterone level, consider empiric treatment if clinical or electrolytes abnormal
- Urgency: Hours

VII.   Maple Syrup Urine Disease (MSUD)

Maple syrup urine disease is a disorder of branch chain amino acid metabolism. It is much less common than PKU but occurs at increased frequency in Mennonite populations. It can be identified by bacterial inhibition testing for increased blood leucine. The classic presentation of MSUD is coma and apnea at about 8 days of age. Treatment includes supportive care and special-purpose amino acid formulations. Unlike PKU, treated patients with MSUD may have periodic decompensation and crisis. MSUD screening is controversial because of the low incidence, the high false-positive rate, and the high rate of clinical presentation before screen availability.

Following are some key facts about MSUD:

- Incidence: 1:80,000 or less
- Cause: Genetic defect in branch chain ketoacid dehydrogenase
- Screening method: Bacterial inhibition for leucine
- Limits: Levels rise with age, high false positive with bacterial inhibition assay (BIA)
- Symptoms:
  - Early—poor feeding, abnormal tone, apnea, coma
  - Late—spasticity, mental retardation, recurrent crises
- Treatment: Special diet, supportive care
- Prognosis with treatment: Variable
- Evaluation for positive screen: Clinical evaluation, serum amino acids, consider empiric treatment if symptoms
- Urgency: Hours

VIII.   Homocystinuria

Screening for homocystinuria specially targets infants with cystathionine beta synthase deficiency. The disorder of sulfur amino acid metabolism results in mental retardation, thrombosis, and eye and skeletal problems. Treatment involves a methionine-restricted, special medical purpose food, pyridoxine, and betaine. Detection is accomplished by bacterial inhibition assay for methionine (not homocystine). Homocystinuria screening is controversial: early discharge has made detection of cases difficult, the incidence is probably in the 1;100,000 to 1:300,000 range, and newborn screening misses the 30% of cases which are pyridoxine responsive. False positives are frequent in premature infants.

Following are some key facts about homocystinuria:

- Incidence: 1:100,000 or less
- Cause: Genetic deficiency of cystathionine beta synthase
- Screening method: Bacterial inhibition for methionine
- Limits: High false positive with prematures, all pyridoxine responders are false negative, high false negative with early screens
- Symptoms:
  - Early—none
  - Late—MR, lens dislocation, thromboses
- Treatment: Special diet, pyridoxine
- Prognosis with treatment: MR prevented, other problems delayed
- Evaluation of screen: Serum amino acids (evaluate with pediatric ranges)
- Urgency: Days

IX.   Biotinidase Deficiency

Biotinidase is an enzyme that enhances absorption and recycling of the vitamin biotin from its protein-bound form. Biotin deficiency impairs the catalytic activity of several carboxylase enzymes, resulting in mental retardation, seizures, and skin rash, usually beginning after 1 month of age. The screen tests the biotinidase enzyme activity of serum. Treatment consists of large oral doses of free biotin. This treatment is well tolerated, is inexpensive, and prevents most of the symptoms. The test is inexpensive, sensitive, and specific. Its major drawback is incidence (about one case of profound biotinidase deficiency per 120,000 births).

Following are some key facts about biotinidase deficiency:

- Incidence: 1:120,000 profound, 1:120,000 partial
- Cause: Genetic defect in biotinidase
- Screening methods: Colorimetric assay for biotinidase activity
- Symptoms:
  - Early—none
  - Late—seizures, mental retardation, skin rash, sparse hair
- Treatment: Oral biotin
- Prognosis with treatment: Normal growth and development
- Evaluation of screen: Serum biotinidase level
- Urgency: Days

X.   Medium-Chain Acyl Co-enzyme A (COA) Dehydrogenase Deficiency (MCAD) and Tandem Mass Spectrometry (TMS) Screening

MCAD is a relatively frequent disorder of fatty acid oxidation, with an incidence of about 1:10,000. MCAD interferes with adaptation to fasting and may cause symptomatic hypo-glycemia, a Reye syndrome–like picture, or unexplained infant death. The peak age of presentation is in the second year of life, although younger infants may have serious or lethal illnesses. The treatment for MCAD is education: Don't fast! Infants under 1 year of age should be fed every 4 hours, and an 8-hour overnight fast is allowed for older infants. Intercurrent illness is treated with aggressive management of intake, with intravenous fluids if necessary.

MCAD meets the incidence and treatment guidelines for screening. A sensitive and specific test is available. The problem is technological. Screening for MCAD requires highly sophisti-cated tandem mass spectrometry screening. Instruments capable of high-throughput, low-cost screening of blood spot samples are available, and programs in a few states have demonstrated feasi-bility; but implementation of this technology requires large capi-tal investments and acquisition of expertise.

Tandem mass spectrometry screening is attractive for other reasons. The same instrument can screen for a variety of organic and fatty acid metabolism disorders that may not sepa-rately qualify for screening because of incidence but that could be detected in a combined screen. In addition, the same tech-nology may replace bacterial inhibition or other testing for amino acids, making early testing for PKU more sensitive and specific and making MSUD and homocystinuria screening prac-tical from a cost/benefit standpoint. Clearly, the potential advantages of this technology suggest a greater role in future newborn screening programs.

XI. Other Conditions

Although genetic, metabolic, and endocrine diseases have occupied a prominent place in screening programs, infectious con-ditions such as toxoplasmosis and HIV are detectable by newborn screening. Cystic fibrosis testing is in place in a few states and is an example of two-tier testing with a "simple" analyte (immuno-reactive trypsinogen) followed by limited DNA-based testing. Large-scale DNA-based testing is still not practical for most con-ditions described previously because the mutations are too het-erogeneous and the technology is too labor intensive, but "chip" readers (high-tech instruments capable of high-throughput muta-tion screening) may bring such technology into the realm of wide-spread newborn screening in the future.

XII. Practical Considerations

Some radical differences exist between widespread new-born screening and clinically based testing. By its very nature, newborn screening cards are sent to a centralized laboratory, and the results will return after the infant has left the point of origin, the birth hospital. Between the time the blood specimen is obtained and the time the results return, the infant may have changed names, telephone number, address, or primary care source; and the results may be normal, unsatisfactory (a specimen card that is unusable), inconclusive (because of timing, transfusion, antibiotics), or frankly abnormal. Moreover, no clinical judgment will sort the affected baby from the normal for many conditions.

XIII. Record Keeping

Thirty years ago, newborn screening was a one-way conduit. A specimen was sent, and "no news was good news." Early discharge and expansion of screening panels have changed that, and current recommendations are to make sure that a hard copy of the newborn screening results is part of the child's primary medical record, along with notes of any abnormal testing and what diagnostic testing was done. This requires some expenditure of energy on the part of the physician's office, because the hard copy may be delayed or may have gone to a different physician. Physicians who see newborns in the hospital only should similarly adhere to a compulsive protocol. Documentation of normal screening results is insufficient for infants with clinically suspicious symptoms. Screening is for low-risk populations. An infant with growth retardation, umbilical hernia, and dry skin should have diagnostic studies for hypothyroidism, not a note in the chart that *"the newborn screen was normal."*

XIV. False Positives/False Negatives

Although an ideal screen should have no false negatives and few false positives, no such thing exists. False positives are built into the system as a cost of doing business. Certain screens are notorious for generating false positives (see CAH, earlier); others have a minimal rate. In some labs, the report differentiates panic values from abnormal values. Although all reports require action, some require emergency action and empiric treatment while waiting for results; others do not. Although normal reports are part of routine pediatric care, handling abnormal reports is a rare event for most offices, and seeking advice from a local or regional consultant may be helpful before calling a parent.

False negatives occur when a normal screen is documented in an affected child. Some have biologic causes (a slowly failing thyroid remnant), some are clerical (wrong specimen), and some are due to known test interference (transfusion, antibiotics, specimen drawn at 12 hours of age).

XV. Variants

Universal screening is a great tool for demonstrating biologic variability. Within groups of infants with abnormal screens are individuals with mildly elevated phenylalanine levels (benign hyperphenylalaninemia), variant galactosemia (Duarte-galactosemia compound heterozygotes), transient hypothyroidism, partial biotinidase deficiency, and nonclassic 21-hydroxylase deficiency. Since these cases may be more difficult to evaluate and manage than their counterparts with classic disease, the help of a consultant may be beneficial, even if the only management necessary is reassurance.

XVI. Guidelines for Primary Care

A. Learn the rules in your state and adhere to them. If a specimen is required before discharge, make sure it is drawn. (It is not worthless. Nobody would mandate hundreds of thousands of worthless tests!) If a repeat specimen is required, encourage parents to have it done.

B.   Track the results of all infants in office and hospital care. Find out how to get hard copies back to charts. Make sure no abnormal results are filed without action.

C.   Watch infants who change practices between hospital and office because they are at risk for disaster. Avoid fumbles.

D.   Have a protocol in place for dealing with abnormal results.

E.   Remember that abnormal newborn screens are very stressful to parents. Find out what the results mean and what action will be necessary before calling them.

F.   Try to get at least one screen before transfusion for sick babies. Don't wait too long to draw a screen.

G.   Observe proper technique if screens are drawn in the office. Training videos are available.

ADDITIONAL READING

Brosnan PG, Brosnan CA, Kemp SF, et al. Effect of newborn screening for congenital adrenal hyperplasia. *Arch Pediatr Adolesc Med* 1999;153:1272–1278.

Chace DH, Hillman SL, Van Hove JL, et al. Rapid diagnosis of MCAD deficiency: quantitatively analysis of octanoylcarnitine and other acylcarnitines in newborn blood spots by tandem mass spectrometry. *Clin Chem* 1997;43:2106–2113.

Daliva AL, Linder B, Di Martino-Nardi J, et al. Three-year follow-up of borderline congenital hypothyroidism [see comments]. *J Pediatr* 2000;136:53–56.

Farrell PM, Kosorok MR, Laxova A, et al. Nutritional benefits of neonatal screening for cystic fibrosis. Wisconsin Cystic Fibrosis Neonatal Screening Study Group [see comments]. *N Engl J Med* 1997;337:963–969.

Gudmundsson K, Majzoub JA, Bradwin G, et al. Virilising 21-hydroxylase deficiency: timing of newborn screening and confirmatory tests can be crucial. *J Pediatr Endocrinol Metab* 1999;12:895–901.

Korson MS. Advances in newborn screening for metabolic disorders: what the pediatrician needs to know. *Pediatr Ann* 2000;29:294–301.

LaFranchi S. Congenital hypothyroidism: etiologies, diagnosis, and management. *Thyroid* 1999;9:735–740.

Levy HL. Newborn screening by tandem mass spectrometry: a new era [editorial; comment]. *Clin Chem* 1998;44:2401–2402.

Lord J, Thomason MJ, Littlejohns P, et al. Secondary analysis of economic data: a review of cost-benefit studies of neonatal screening for phenylketonuria. *J Epidemiol Community Health* 1999;53:179–186.

Paul D. Contesting consent: the challenge to compulsory neonatal screening for PKU. *Perspect Biol Med* 1999;42:207–219.

Peterschmitt MJ, Simmons JR, Levy HL. Reduction of false negative results in screening of newborns for homocystinuria. *N Engl J Med* 1999;341:1572–1576.

Reed W, Lane PA, Lorey F, et al. Sickle-cell disease not identified by newborn screening because of prior transfusion. *J Pediatr* 2000;136:248–250.

Rovet JF. Long-term neuropsychological sequelae of early-treated congenital hypothyroidism: effects in adolescence. *Acta Paediatr Suppl* 1999;88:88–95.

Schweitzer S. Newborn mass screening for galactosemia. *Eur J Pediatr* 1995;154:S37–S39.

Scriver CC. A simple phenylalanine method for detecting phenylketonuria in large populations of newborn infants by Robert Guthrie and Ada Susi. *Pediatrics* 1963;32:318–343.

Sinai LN, Kim SC, Casey R, et al. Phenylketonuria screening: effect of early newborn discharge. *Pediatrics* 1995;96(4 Pt 1):605–608.

Yap S, Naughten E. Homocystinuria due to cystathionine beta-synthase deficiency in Ireland: 25 years' experience of a newborn screened and treated population with reference to clinical outcome and biochemical control. *J Inherit Metab Dis* 1998;21:738–747.

Web Sites

http://www.slh.wisc.edu/newborn/guide4.html (Collection technique for newborn screens)

http://www.AAP.ORG/policy/01565.html (Newborn Screening fact sheets)

Many state laboratories and newborn screening programs have web sites. They provide a good review of current guidelines in your state.

5 ♣ Screening Tests in Well-Child Care

Omer G. Berger

Screening tests are performed to identify occult disease or risk factors for disease in childhood. Before deciding to implement a routine screening test, a cost-versus-benefit assessment should be undertaken. Benefits considered include the possibility of prevention of disease, early diagnosis before permanent disability, and effective treatment. Costs extend beyond monetary considerations, including psychologic trauma and stigmatization. Parents must be informed of the benefits and risks of all screening tests.

I. Newborn Metabolic Disorders

All states require newborn blood sampling for various metabolic and genetic disorders, including phenylketonuria (PKU), congenital hypothyroidism, galactosemia, and homocystinuria. Early discharge may dictate the need for repeat testing to screen accurately for PKU and homocystinuria. Recently, the National Institutes of Health has recommended universal screening for hemoglobinopathies; this has been implemented in many states. See Chapter 4 for further details.

II. Hypertension

Routine screening for hypertension should begin at 3 years of age, when the child is able to cooperate with the procedure. Blood pressure should be taken with the child in the sitting position and the arm at the level of the heart with an appropriate-sized cuff. The current recommendation for cuff size is that the cuff bladder width should be approximately 40% of the mid–upper arm circumference. In practice, this is a cuff height that is 80% to 100% of the circumference of the mid–upper arm or approximately two-thirds of the length of the upper arm. For diastolic pressure, the fourth Korotkoff sound (muffling) should be used until 12 years of age; the fifth Korotkoff sound (disappearance) should be used after age 12. Appendix B contains normative values for blood pressure according to age, sex, and height. Hypertension is defined as readings equal to or greater than the 95th percentile, found on three separate visits.

III. Urinalysis

Morning specimens of urine for dipstick testing for protein, glucose, and blood cells should be obtained in 4- to 5-year-old children at the preschool visit. If abnormal results are found, a careful microscopic examination is indicated. Several historical and clinical aspects of routine care may also suggest the need for complete urinalysis and/or urine culture. These include enuresis, dysuria, polyuria, urgency, pollakiuria, and a family or personal history of hematuria, urinary tract infection, proteinuria, or diabetes mellitus. The American Academy of Pediatrics (AAP) also recommends screening dipstick urinalysis for leukocytes in sexually active adolescents.

IV.   Tuberculosis

Although routine skin testing for tuberculosis (TB) is not indicated, all children must be assessed for TB risk factors. Immediate TB (Mantoux) skin testing is necessary for children who are contacts of persons with infectious TB or who have been in prison during the past 5 years. Immediate testing is also indicated for children who have been in endemic countries. Annual TB testing is indicated for children with HIV and for adolescents in detention centers. Periodic retesting is recommended for incarcerated adults or adolescents and children exposed to the homeless, drug users, and elderly in nursing homes. Complete recommendations for TB skin testing and interpretation of test results may be found in the *2000 red book: report of the Committee on Infectious Diseases,* 25th edition.

V.   Iron Deficiency

The incidence of iron deficiency in the United States has decreased but remains the most important deficiency state in children. Because anemia is a late sign of iron deficiency, physicians must utilize the tests that assist in early identification of iron deficiency before the development of anemia. Most primary care physicians screen with a complete blood count (CBC) with red cell indices. If this is suggestive of iron deficiency (low mean corpuscular volume [MCV], elevated red cell distribution width [RDW]), a trial of iron supplementation is usually begun with repeat CBC in a few weeks. The optimal age of screening is 12 to 24 months, as the toddler diet tends to be low in iron because of the change from iron-fortified formula or breast milk to cow's milk. Infants especially at risk are those more than 12 months of age with prolonged bottle feeding with cow's milk. Periodic rescreening for iron deficiency should be considered in children with evidence of inadequate nutrition and chronic illness as well as in menstruating adolescents.

VI.   Vision

Formal visual acuity determination using the Snellen charts or Allen cards should be initiated at 3 to 4 years of age. Children with decreased acuity (less than 20/60) or those with more than two lines of disparity between eyes should be referred for specialized eye examination. One of the goals of screening is to identify children with unilateral refractive errors so that amblyopia can be detected and treated. Routine vision screening should be carried out at all health supervision visits since 20% of children will require eyeglasses before the late teenage years.

VII.   Hearing

The incidence of hearing loss in newborns is three in 1,000, about 20 times greater than the incidence of phenylketonuria. Universal screening at birth is necessary to confirm the diagnosis by 3 months of age because language development is significantly better when intervention begins before 6 months of age. To achieve this goal, most medical centers are moving from "paper" screening to electrophysiologic measures—auditory brainstem response (ABR) or otoacoustic emissions (OAE).

Clinicians must be aware of risk factors for delayed-onset hearing loss, especially prenatal infection and chronic otitis media with effusion. Infants at risk require audiologic evaluation every 3 to 6 months until 3 years of age and later, as needed.

In the office, hearing should be assessed before 3 months of age by history and examination as described earlier. Hearing can be screened in the school-aged child by pure tone audiometry.

VIII. Cholesterol

For children more than 2 years of age whose parents or grandparents have a history of coronary disease before 55 years of age, the AAP recommends a fasting lipid profile. For children with a parent who has an elevated total cholesterol (>240 mg/dL), a test of total cholesterol level is recommended. If the child's level is >200 mg/dL, the physician should obtain a fasting lipid profile. In one large study, 38% of all children in whom adequate history was available satisfied criteria for testing. However, histories are often incomplete or not available. In such instances, the presence of other factors (e.g., obesity or hypertension) may assist in identifying those in need of screening

ADDITIONAL READING

American Academy of Pediatrics. Tuberculosis. In: Pickering LK, ed. *2000 red book: report of the Committee on Infectious Diseases,* 25th ed. Elk Grove Village, IL: American Academy of Pediatrics; 2000.

American Academy of Pediatrics, Committee on Children with Disabilities. Screening infants and young children for developmental disabilities. *Pediatrics* 1994:93:863–865.

American Academy of Pediatrics, Committee on Nutrition. Cholesterol in childhood. *Pediatrics* 1998;101:141–147.

American Academy of Pediatrics, Committee on Practice and Ambulatory Medicine, Section on Ophthalmology. Eye examination and vision screening in infants, children and young adults. *Pediatrics* 1996;98:153–157.

American Academy of Pediatrics, Task Force on Newborn and Infant Hearing. Newborn and infant hearing loss: detection and intervention. *Pediatrics* 1999;103:527.

Daniels SR. The diagnosis of hypertension in children: an update. *Pediatr Rev* 1997;18:131–135.

6 ♣ Immunizations

Robert M. Siegel

Active immunization by inoculating the host with all or part of a microorganism has been used for centuries. The first attempts at active immunization were made in the Middle East and China by taking residue of healing smallpox scars and introducing it to a host by intranasal or dermal inoculation. The English physician Jenner, observing that milkmaids who were exposed to cowpox were immune to smallpox, developed the first safe and effective vaccine using cowpox virus. With the advent of routine immunization, smallpox has been totally eradicated, and the incidence of several other illnesses has been significantly reduced. Vaccines have now been developed against many infectious agents, and currently more than 30 vaccines are available in the United States.

I. Routine Childhood Immunizations

Vaccination against childhood illness clearly has been one of the most cost-effective responses to illness to date. Over the past 50 years physicians have seen remarkable declines in polio, measles, mumps, rubella, diphtheria, tetanus, and pertussis. Unfortunately, immunization rates have fallen in preschool children. Experts estimate that for every dollar spent on immunizations, 10 are saved in treatment costs. In this age of medical reform and cost containment, every effort at every opportunity available must be made to immunize appropriately every child that comes into contact with the medical system. The routine immunization schedule of healthy children is shown in Table 6.1 and in Appendix L.

II. General Principles of Childhood Vaccination

A. Live vaccines, unless given simultaneously, should not be given within a month of each other. Recent oral polio vaccine (OPV), however, does not contraindicate giving measles/mumps/rubella (MMR) at the appropriate time.

B. In general, vaccines should not be given within 3 months of receiving a gamma globulin product with the exception of hepatitis, rabies, respiratory syncytial virus (RSV), or tetanus prophylaxis.

C. Premature infants should be kept on the same schedule as full-term infants; split doses of vaccine are unnecessary.

D. Lapsed immunizations do not require reinstitution of an entire vaccine series; immunizations should be given as though the proper interval has elapsed.

E. Children whose vaccination status is uncertain should be considered unimmunized and should be given appropriate vaccines.

F. A child's immunization status should be reviewed at every physician or medical caregiver visit in order to update immunizations. Even at ill or problem visits, immunization status should be reviewed, since this may represent an opportunity to update immunizations (provided the degree of illness does not preclude administration of vaccines).

Table 6.1. Recommended childhood immunization schedule

Vaccine	Recommended Schedule	Comments
Hepatitis B (HBV)	Birth; 1–2 months; 6 months or 2 months; 4 months; 6–12 months	Second dose at least 1 month after first dose; third dose at least 4 months after first dose *and* 2 months after second dose
H. influenzae type b (Hib)	2 months; 4 months; 6 months; 12–15 months	If PRP-OMP (PedVaxHIB or ComVax) is used, 6-month dose unnecessary. Minimum 6 weeks between doses of primary series.
Diphtheria, tetanus, pertussis (acellular) (combined DTaP)	2 months; 4 months; 6 months; 12–18 months; 4–6 years Td at 11–16 years and every 10 years thereafter	Fourth dose of DTaP must be given at least 6 months after the third dose of the primary series. Minimum 4 weeks between doses of primary series.
Poliomyelitis (inactivated) (IPV)	2 months; 4 months; 6–18 months; 4–6 years	Oral polio vaccine no longer recommended. Minimum 4 weeks between doses of primary series.
S. pneumoniae (Spn) (conjugate vaccine)	2 months; 4 months; 6 months; 12–15 months	Minimum 6 weeks between doses in primary series.
Measles, mumps, rubella (combined MMR)	12–15 months; 4–6 years	Minimum 4 weeks between first and second doses.
Varicella (Var)	12–18 months	If child not immunized until age 13 years or older, two doses at least 4 weeks apart required.
Hepatitis A (HAV)	2–12 years in selected areas	See text.

Adapted from American Academy of Pediatrics. Active and passive immunization. In: Pickering LK, ed. *2000 red book: report of the Committee on Infectious Diseases,* 25th ed. Elk Grove Village, IL: American Academy of Pediatrics; 2000.

G.   **A pamphlet of patient immunization education materials listing common adverse reactions of each vaccine should be given to parents, and informed consent should be obtained at each immunization visit.**
H.   **There are no contraindications to simultaneous administration of multiple vaccines, which are routinely recommended for infants and children.**
III. **Immunizations in Those Who Are Not Up to Date**
   A.   **Table 6.2 contains guidelines for immunization of children who are behind on immunizations.**
   B.   **Although most children generally have been fully immunized by the time they enter school, many American preschool children are behind in their immunization status.** Some studies suggest that as many as 50% of inner-city children under 2 years of age are underimmunized. Many of these children have multiple missed opportunities

Table 6.2.   Suggested vaccine schedule for children in the United States not immunized during the first year of life

Recommended Time/Age	Immunizations	Comments
Younger Than Age 7 Years		
First visit	DTaP, Hib, HBV, MMR, IPV	TB testing if indicated. If child >5 years of age, Hib is generally not indicated.
1 month later	DTaP, HBV, Var	
2 months later	DTaP, Hib, IPV	Second dose of Hib is indicated only if first dose received at <15 months of age.
≥8 months later	DTaP, HBV, IPV	
Age 4 to 6 years	DTaP, MMR, IPV	DTaP not necessary if fourth dose given after fourth birthday. IPV not necessary if third dose was given after fourth birthday.
Age 11–14 years	See Table 6.1.	
Age 7 to 12 Years		
First visit	HBV, MMR, Td, IPV	
2 months later	HBV, MMR, Var, Td, IPV	
8–14 months later	HBV, Td, IPV	
Ages 11–14 years	See Table 6.1.	

Adapted from American Academy of Pediatrics. Active and passive immunization. In: Pickering LK, ed. *2000 red book: report of the Committee on Infectious Diseases,* 25th ed. Elk Grove Village, IL: American Academy of Pediatrics; 2000.

by health care workers to immunize them. Common causes of missed opportunities include physicians' misunderstanding of contraindications of vaccination and the mindset that immunization issues are appropriate only during routine well-child visits. If a child is behind in immunizations, every effort should be made to vaccinate the child at every medical encounter.

IV. Misconceptions About Immunizations

There are many misconceptions among health care providers about what constitutes contraindications to vaccination. True contraindications are discussed in individual vaccine sections. Table 6.3 lists conditions that are commonly mistaken for contraindications to vaccination but *which are not true contraindications*.

V. Special Considerations

A. DTaP. This vaccine, because of the pertussis component, is the most common vaccine to cause side effects in children and is the one most often responsible for litigation. For the two most catastrophic associations of DTaP, encephalopathy and sudden infant death, no scientific evidence suggests causation; these complications should no longer be thought to be side effects of DTaP. The acellular pertussis vaccine is now recommended over the whole-cell pertussis vaccine, as the rates of local and systemic reactions are lower

Table 6.3. False contraindications to vaccination

Mild acute illness with low-grade fever or mild diarrhea
Current antimicrobial therapy
Reaction to DTP or DTaP that involved only soreness, redness, or swelling at the site of vaccination or temperature <105°F.
Prematurity
Pregnancy of mother or household contact
Breast feeding
A history of nonspecific allergies
Allergies to penicillin or any other antibiotic except anaphylactic reaction to neomycin or streptomycin
Allergies to duck meat or duck feathers
Family history of convulsions in a child considered for pertussis or measles vaccination
Family history of sudden infant death syndrome in a child considered for DTP (DTaP) vaccination
Family history of an adverse event unrelated to immunosuppression after vaccination
Malnutrition

Adapted from American Academy of Pediatrics. Active and passive immunization. In: Pickering LK, ed. *2000 red book: report of the Committee on Infectious Diseases,* 25th ed. Elk Grove Village, IL: American Academy of Pediatrics; 2000.

with the acellular vaccine. Whether the rarer and more significant reactions seen with the whole-cell vaccine are reduced with the acellular pertussis vaccine is still unknown.

Parents should be made aware of all these possible side effects and should be encouraged to report any adverse events. The pertussis component should be withheld if encephalopathy occurs within 7 days or if an immediate allergic reaction to vaccine occurs.

Although in the past the following events, if temporally related to a previous pertussis immunization, were considered contraindications, they are now considered *precautions* against immunization:

1. *Persistent inconsolable screaming for 3 or more hours* with high-pitched cry within 48 hours of the immunization.

2. *A convulsion with or without fever* within 3 days of the immunization.

3. *Collapse or shocklike state* within 48 hours of the immunization.

The decision to give pertussis vaccine following any of the precautionary events must be made on a case-by-case basis. Parents should always be questioned carefully about previous reactions to the pertussis vaccine.

B.   Poliomyelitis. The trivalent oral polio vaccine (Sabin) on very rare occasions has been associated with paralysis (vaccine-associated paralytic poliomyelitis). The American Academy of Pediatrics (AAP) and the Advisory Committee on Immunization Practices (ACIP) of the Communicable Disease Center (CDC) now recommend the use of inactivated polio vaccine (Salk) except under special circumstances, such as travel to a poliomyelitis endemic area.

C.   Measles/mumps/rubella (MMR). Measles, mumps, and rubella vaccine is indicated in all healthy children and should be given in two doses before 12 years of age. Some confusion exists regarding the appropriate age to give the second booster dose. The AAP initially chose 12 years of age or secondary school entry for the second dose, and the CDC recommended age 6 or primary school entry. The latter recommendation proved to be more feasible, as most states mandate school systems to monitor immunizations and exclude from school those children not appropriately immunized at primary school entry.

The most common adverse reaction to MMR is fever in 5% to 15% of recipients about 1 week after vaccination. A morbilliform rash occurs in 5% of children receiving vaccine. Febrile seizures can occur, but no evidence of any permanent sequelae exists. Subacute sclerosing panencephalitis (SSPE), a known devastating effect of measles virus, has been described in patients with no history of natural measles infection but with a history of measles vaccination. Although SSPE may be a very rare adverse reaction to MMR, the incidence of SSPE has drastically declined since the introduction

Table 6.4. Contraindications to MMR vaccination

Condition	Comments
Pregnancy	Theoretical risk of fetal damage
Anaphylactic allergy to neomycin	Vaccine contains neomycin
Immune globulin within 3 months	Blunts immune response
Immunocompromised except HIV (includes chronic steroids)*	Possibility of severe symptomatic infection

Adapted from American Academy of Pediatrics. Measles. In: Pickering LK, ed. *2000 red book: report of the Committee on Infectious Diseases,* 25th ed. Elk Grove Village, IL: American Academy of Pediatrics; 2000.
*MMR: administration should be delayed for one month after discontinuing steroid therapy.

of measles vaccine. Thrombocytopenia is an uncommon adverse reaction to MMR administration but is generally transient and benign. Preexisting thrombocytopenia is considered a precaution to vaccination. Table 6.4 lists contraindications to the MMR vaccine.

D. Haemophilus influenzae type b. Since the introduction of the first *Haemophilus influenzae* type b (Hib) vaccine in 1985 and the conjugate vaccine in 1990, Hib infection in the United States has declined dramatically. Now several Hib conjugate vaccines, including one combined with hepatitis B vaccine (ComVax—Merck), exist. Side effects from the vaccines are very unusual. All the available conjugate vaccines will give immunity with one dose when given at the age of more than 15 months. Most of the conjugate Hib vaccines are given routinely at 2, 4, and 6 months of age simultaneously with the DTaP primary series to achieve immunity at a younger age. A booster dose is recommended between 12 and 15 months of age. Table 6.5 summarizes the Hib immunization schedule. The minimum interval between vaccinations given before 15 months of age is 2 months.

E. Hepatitis A vaccine (HAV). Two vaccines licensed in the United States for use in children 2 to 18 years of age include (a) Havrix dosed at 720 EL units given at the initial visit and again 6 to 12 months later and (b) Vaqta dosed at 25 units of hepatitis A virus antigen given at the initial visit and again 6 to 18 months later. HAV is recommended for children at increased risk for hepatitis A and includes those traveling to endemic areas and those who live in the following high-prevalence states: Arizona, Alaska, California, Idaho, Nevada, New Mexico, Oklahoma, Oregon, South Dakota, Utah, and Washington. Vaccination should also be considered for children living in the following moderate-prevalence states: Missouri, Texas, Colorado, Arkansas, Montana, and Wyoming. Each pediatric practitioner should consult the

**Table 6.5. *Haemophilus influenzae*
conjugate vaccine recommendations**

Age of First Dose	Required Number of Doses
2–6 months	4*
7–11 months	3
12–14 months	2
15–59 months	1†
60 months and older‡	1 or 2†

Adapted from American Academy of Pediatrics. Active and passive immunization. In: Pickering LK, ed. *2000 red book: report of the Committee on Infectious Diseases,* 25th ed. Elk Grove Village, IL: American Academy of Pediatrics; 2000.
* If PRP-OMP (PedvaxHIB, ComVax) is used, only three doses are required at 2, 4, and 12 months of age.
† Some experts recommend two doses separated by 2 months for children at risk for impaired antibody response to the Hib.
‡ Only for children with chronic diseases known to be at increased risk for *Haemophilus influenzae* infections.

local health authority to determine the risks in his/her own community.

F. Hepatitis B vaccine (HBV). In 1992 the AAP made the recommendation to immunize all infants and high-risk children and adolescents with HBV. Immunization of healthy adolescents was recommended when feasible. The standard regimens of vaccination are at 0, 1, and 6 months of age or 2, 4, and 6 months of age as well as various other intervals (Table 6.1). All infants born after April 1, 1992, should be given HBV along with their other childhood immunizations. Those born before then should receive their HBV series as young adolescents. There are no recommendations on HBV booster doses at this time.

G. Pneumococcal vaccine (Spn). A heptavalent conjugate pneumococcal vaccine (Prevnar) has been extensively field-tested and was recently approved for use in children. The AAP recommends immunizing all infants under 24 months of age as well as children more than 23 months of age who are at high risk of invasive pneumococcal infection (Table 6.6). The vaccine is given at 2, 4, and 6 months of age with a booster dose at 12 to 15 months. If the series is begun between 7 and 11 months of age, two doses, 6 to 8 weeks apart, are given with a booster dose at 12 to 15 months of age. If the series is begun between 12 and 23 months of age, two doses 6 to 8 weeks apart are given with no booster. If given to children more than 23 months of age, a single dose is effective. The administration of the conjugate pneumococcal vaccine should lower the incidence of invasive disease and otitis media caused by the most common serotypes of pneumococcus (contained in the vaccine).

Table 6.6.   High-risk factors
for invasive pneumococcal disease

Sickle cell disease, congenital or acquired asplenia, splenic
 dysfunction
HIV infection
Congenital immune deficiency (including some B-cell and T-cell
 deficiencies and complement deficiencies)
Chronic cardiac disease, especially cyanotic coronary heart disease
 and patients with cardiac failure
Chronic pulmonary disease including asthma with high-dose oral
 corticosteroids
Cerebrospinal fluid leaks
Chronic renal failure, including nephrotic syndrome
Patients receiving immunosuppressive therapy or radiation therapy
 and organ transplant patients
Diabetes mellitus

Adapted from American Academy of Pediatrics, Committee on Infectious Diseases. Policy statement. Recommendations for the prevention of pneumococcal infections, including the use of pneumococcal conjugate vaccine (Prevnar), pneumococcal polysaccharide vaccine, and antibiotic prophylaxis. June 2000.

   For children at high risk of invasive pneumococcal disease who are more than 23 months of age, the heptavalent conjugated vaccine is recommended in addition to the older 23-valent polysaccharide pneumococcal vaccine. If the 23-valent vaccine has already been given, the heptavalent vaccine is given in two doses, 6 to 8 weeks apart at least 6 to 8 weeks after the last dose of the 23-valent vaccine. The 23-valent vaccine is used for subsequent booster doses at 3- to 5-year intervals. If the child has received no previous pneumococcal vaccine, two doses of heptavalent vaccine are given 6 to 8 weeks apart followed by one dose of the 23-valent vaccine (with boosters as indicated earlier).
   H.   Lyme disease. A Lyme disease vaccine is licensed for adolescents 15 years of age or more and adults. This vaccine should be considered for those who live, work, or travel extensively in areas of high or moderate risk. The recommended vaccine schedule is three doses of vaccine given at 0, 1, and 12 months. The decision to vaccinate individuals traveling to a Lyme-endemic area depends on the timing of the travel and on their length of stay in the endemic area.

ADDITIONAL READING
Advisory Committee on Immunization Practices. Prevention of hepatitis A active or passive immunization. *MMWR* 1999;48(RR-12).
Advisory Committee on Immunization Practices. Recommendations for the use of Lyme disease vaccine. *MMWR* 1999;48(RR-07).

American Academy of Pediatrics. Recommended childhood immunization schedule—United States, January–December 2000. *Pediatrics* 1999;105:148.

American Academy of Pediatrics, Committee on Infectious Diseases. Policy statement: recommendations for the prevention of pneumococcal infections, including the use of pneumococcal conjugate vaccine (Prevnar), pneumococcal polysaccharide vaccine, and antibiotic prophylaxis. June 2000. AAP Web site (http:/www.aap.org).

Edwards KM. Pediatric immunizations. *Curr Prob Pediatr* 1993; 23:186–216.

Garber MR, Mortimer EA. Immunizations: beyond the basics. *Pediatr Rev* 1992;13:98–106.

Peters G. Childhood immunizations. *N Engl J Med* 1992;327: 1794–1800.

Pickering LK, ed. *2000 red book: report of the Committee on Infectious Diseases,* 25th ed. Elk Grove Village, IL: American Academy of Pediatrics; 2000.

Shinefield HR, Black S, Ray P, et al. Safety and immunogenicity of heptavalent pneumococcal CRM197 conjugate vaccine in infants and toddlers. *Pediatr Infect Dis J* 1999;18:757–763.

7 ♣ Nutrition

Heidi J. Kalkwarf and Anita Cavallo

Appropriate nutritional intake is essential for optimal physical growth, cognitive development, and physical and cognitive performance. Development of good nutritional practices in childhood fosters the development of good eating patterns for life. Pediatricians' efforts to help establish good eating patterns in childhood will help ensure the good health of their patients in adulthood. Many of the chronic diseases of adulthood are related to poor dietary practices adopted during childhood.

I. **Dietary Assessment**
   Each well-child visit should include a dietary history and nutritional anticipatory guidance, even when growth is adequate. The dietary history involves a review of the infant's or child's diet, including information on the different types and amount of foods consumed regularly, meal and snacking patterns, intake of nutritional supplements (e.g., vitamins, iron, and fluoride), appetite, and behavioral issues around feeding. Information on the number of servings of food from the different food groups, the variety of foods within the food groups, serving sizes, and feeding frequency should be evaluated in relation to expectations for the child's age and growth, as described later. This information helps with the formulation of plans for dietary management and with anticipatory guidance for the period between well-child visits.

II. **Growth**
   Length (or height) and weight should be measured and plotted on growth charts at each well-child visit. Head circumference also should be measured and evaluated during the first 2 years of life, when brain growth velocity is highest. Height and weight and variations in the rate of growth should be analyzed carefully. Significant changes in growth warrant further in-depth probing of dietary intake and physical activity.

III. **The First Year of Life**
   A. **Nutritional goals for infants**
      1. *To support the high rate of growth.*
      2. *To maintain hydration*, especially in the first weeks of life.
      3. *To introduce and develop acceptance of solid foods* in the second half of the first year of life.
   B. **Nutritional guidance**
      1. *Breast milk and infant formula.* Breast milk or infant formulas are the main sources of nutrition in the first year of life. The American Academy of Pediatrics recommends that all infants, including sick and premature infants, be breast-fed for the first year of life with exclusive breast feeding for approximately the first 6 months of life. Breast milk provides the appropriate balance of nutrients in an easily digestible form, protection against some infections, and apparent reductions in the risk of development of certain illnesses, such as diabetes mellitus, Crohn disease,

and atopic disease. Specific information on establishing and maintaining breast feeding is discussed in Chapter 8 of this handbook. Alternatively, the nutritional needs of infants during the first year of life may be met by infant formulas based on cow's milk or soy and fortified with iron.

2. *Feeding frequency.* Newborn infants may need to be fed 8 to 10 times a day; the frequency of feeding will slowly decrease to about 6 times a day by 5 to 6 months of age. Parents should learn to distinguish crying cues indicating hunger from other causes of crying in the young infant. The recommended nutritional intake for the normal infant during the first year of life is summarized in Table 7.1. Bottles containing infant formula or breast milk should not be put in the microwave because of uneven heating and the risk of overheating.

3. *Introduction of solid foods.* Both breast-fed and formula-fed infants should begin solid foods around 4 to 6 months of age. Solid foods are needed at this time to provide adequate nutrition, to introduce different textures and flavors, and to promote the development of swallowing independently from sucking (4 to 6 months of age) and of chewing (8 to 12 months of age). The infant should have the following developmental skills for the safe introduction of solid foods: (a) sits with support, (b) displays good head and neck control, (c) displays no extrusion reflex, and (d) can indicate interest (leaning forward, opening mouth) and disinterest (leaning backward, turning head) in foods. Iron-fortified cereal is generally the first solid food introduced, though other solid foods are equally acceptable. Cereals should only be offered from a spoon and should not be given in a bottle with formula. Vegetables and fruits may be introduced around 5 to 8 months of age. Both commercially prepared and homemade, strained foods are acceptable. Homemade baby foods should be cooked without added salt. Foods should be introduced one at a time, and a 1-week interval should be allowed between introduction of new foods to ascertain tolerance. Commercially prepared or home-cooked and strained beef, chicken, veal, lamb, beans, tofu, split peas, yogurt (plain), cottage cheese, and egg yolk can be introduced gradually between 7 and 9 months of age. Egg white is not recommended before 1 year of age to reduce risk of allergies. Honey should not be given until the child is 1 year of age because of the risk of botulism.

4. *Supplemental fluids.* Breast milk and infant formulas provide the normal fluid requirements during the first 4 to 6 months of life. Other fluids may be given with caution as follows:

a. *Water* may be needed if the infant is exposed to high environmental temperatures. Care should be taken to avoid excess water intake, particularly in the first 2 months of life. Up to 4 ounces of water (without added

Table 7.1. Feeding guidelines for the first year of life

| Age | Breast milk or infant formula | | | Cereal* | Vegetables | Fruits | Meats | Egg yolk† | Starch‡ and breads |
	Feedings/ day	Each feed (ounces)	Total/24 hr. (ounces)						
1–2 wk.	8–10	2–3	22	—	—	—	—	—	—
2–8 wk.	6–9	3–5	28	—	—	—	—	—	—
2–4 mo.	5–8	4–6	30	—	—	—	—	—	—
4–6 mo.	5–7	5–7	32	2 T × 2§	—	—	—	—	—
6–8 mo.‖	3–5	6–8	28	⅓ c × 1	2–4 T × 2	2–4 T × 2	1 T × 2	1 T	—
8–12 mo.¶	3–4	6–8	24	½ c × 1	4 T × 3	2–4 T × 2	2–4 T × 2	1 T	2 T

Abbreviations: T tablespoon; c cup.
*Cereal prepared with breast milk or infant formula is given by spoon, not in a bottle.
† Egg yolk may be given two or three times per week; egg whites should not be given until 1 year of age.
‡ Examples are mashed potatoes, pasta.
§ Serving size and number of servings per day.
‖ Begins to use cup; strained solid foods, one new food/week.
¶ Learns to chew. Mashed or chopped solid foods; avoid hot dogs, grapes, nuts, raisins.

substances) may be offered in a day between 2 and 6 months of life, and more liberal amounts thereafter, provided the infant's breast milk or formula intake is maintained to meet nutritional needs.

b.   *Juices* should be introduced when the infant can drink from a cup. Juices provide little nutritional advantage. Although no harm results from giving juice in a bottle before teeth erupt, this practice may lead to nursing bottle caries after teeth erupt. Fruit juice should be limited to 4 to 6 ounces/day; excessive amounts of fruit juices may cause diarrhea and gastrointestinal symptoms.

5.   *Vitamin and mineral supplements.* Supplements containing vitamin D, iron, and fluoride (e.g., Tri-Vi-Flor with iron infant drops) are commonly recommended for breast-fed infants in the first year of life, although the practice is controversial. Breast milk and iron-fortified formulas provide adequate iron. Supplementation is needed only if the infant is receiving a formula without iron, which is not recommended. Premature infants fed exclusively breast milk also require iron supplementation. Beyond infancy, a well-balanced diet provides sufficient iron. Supplemental fluoride (250 µg/day for infants 6 months to 3 years of age) should be given if the infant receives ready-to-use formula or if the water used to prepare the formula contains less than 0.3 ppm of fluoride. Note that although the city water may be fluoridated, the family may be using bottled water, which is not fluoridated, for preparation of infant formula. Vitamin D supplementation is not needed for formula-fed infants. Vitamin D supplementation (400 IU/day) of breast-fed infants is needed only if the mother is vitamin D deficient or the infant is not exposed to adequate sunlight (e.g., cold weather months).

IV.   The Second Year of Life
A.   Nutritional goals for toddlers
1.   *To achieve adequate intake to support growth.*
2.   *To transition to the toddler diet composed of table foods.*
3.   *To achieve acceptance of a wide variety of new foods.*
4.   *To develop skills for self-feeding.*

B.   Nutritional Guidance
1.   *Food intake.* The rate of growth and weight gain decreases during the second year of life compared with infancy, and energy requirements relative to weight also decrease. Toddlers usually receive three meals and two or three snacks per day, primarily composed of table foods. The source of protein now is more varied than in early infancy and includes milk, meats, and eggs. Whole milk enriched with vitamin D should be used in place of infant formula. Low-fat milk is not recommended, and there should be no restriction on total fat or cholesterol intake during the second year of life because growth is still rapid.

Yogurt and cheese may substitute for milk. Excessive milk intake is often accompanied by reduced intake of the wider variety of foods required to meet the nutritional needs of the toddler, including iron. Some infants will continue to breast-feed into the second year of life. Breast feeding at this age is less for nutritional value and more for comfort and bonding between mother and child.

2. *Self-feeding.* Toddlers master the art of self-feeding. Toddlers will first explore the texture of foods and feed themselves with their hands. Over the course of the year they develop the skills to feed themselves with a spoon and cup. At this stage letting the child set the pace on how much he or she consumes and not allowing feeding to become a power struggle between parents and toddlers is important. This stage of feeding must be approached with humor and patience by parents since the toddler may appear to treat feeding more as an art form and medium of expression than as a nutritional event!

3. *Food acceptance.* Sporadic eating and food jags are common among toddlers. Energy requirements are considerably lower in the second year than in the first year of life, and often parents worry unnecessarily about the child's decreased appetite. Many toddlers are reluctant to accept new foods, so parents frequently describe their toddler as being a "picky eater." Neophobia is a normal adaptive response, though it often frustrates caregivers. Food acceptance patterns develop as a result of predisposition and the context in which different foods are offered. Children learn to associate foods within certain contexts and consequences, and these in turn affect their food preferences. Caregivers should be cautioned not to resort to coercive feeding practices, as these may be counterproductive and set up a conflicting environment that predisposes to rejection of the food. Furthermore, coercive feeding results in loss of innate satiety signals. Continuing to offer an initially rejected food a few times a week in an unpressured manner generally leads to food acceptance after eight to 10 exposures. Use of sweet foods, such as candy and cookies, as a reward for eating vegetables may also set up a preference for sweet food and a rejection of the "bad" food that has to be eaten first.

4. *Iron intake.* The switch from iron-fortified formula and iron-fortified cereals after the first year of life may result in greater risk of iron deficiency in toddlers, especially when milk intake is excessive. Iron stores become depleted after 6 months of age, and the diet must contain adequate iron to meet ongoing nutritional needs. Iron deficiency is greatest in toddlers due to the changeover from iron-sufficient formula or breast milk to cow's milk and increases again during adolescence due to rapid growth. Because iron deficiency (even without anemia) has been

shown to affect cognitive development adversely, parents should ensure that their child is provided a variety of iron-rich foods (e.g., meats, egg, iron-fortified breakfast cereal, legumes) daily.

5.   *Choking.* Choking is a concern for this age group. Parents should avoid giving nuts, grapes, raw carrots, popcorn, hot dogs, and round candies. Running with food in the mouth increases the likelihood of choking.

V.   Preschool Children: Ages 2 to 5 Years

A.   Nutritional goals for preschool children

1.   *To achieve adequate intake to support continued growth.*

2.   *To achieve acceptance of a wide variety of new foods.*

3.   *To promote the development of healthful eating patterns.*

4.   *To promote self-regulation of food intake and prevent obesity.*

B.   Nutritional guidance

1.   *Food intake.* Most preschool children need one or two snacks each day in addition to three regular meals. Grain products and starches should form the base of the diet and should be complemented with vegetables, fruits, protein-rich foods, and low-fat milk. Children should be offered a wide variety of foods from each of the food groups. The recommended number of servings from each of the food groups and the typical serving sizes for this age group are given in Table 7.2. Children will have an increasing list of accepted foods. Parents can encourage their children to get involved with planning and can make eating fun to encourage acceptance of new foods. The transition to an adult diet should occur gradually during this time period. By 5 years of age, children should have a diet that contains 30% fat.

2.   *Development of healthful eating patterns.* Preschool children should begin to establish healthful eating patterns that, over a lifetime, will prevent the development of nutrition-related chronic diseases in adulthood. One of the best things parents can do to improve their children's diets is to set a good example. Parents have a major role in their children's eating patterns, and children's patterns often reflect their parents' eating patterns. Reminding the parent that the child's appetites may fluctuate from day to day is important. Parents should serve a variety of healthful foods and let their children decide what and how much to eat. Children cannot select a balanced diet unless nutritious choices are offered to them; sweet snacks and other high-calorie snacks without nutritional value should be offered sparingly. Counseling for parents must be individualized; some parents are too restrictive, and others are too permissive.

3.   *Obesity prevention.* An increase in the proportion of overweight children more than 3 years of age has been

Table 7.2. Recommended number of servings per day and typical serving sizes from each of the food groups for children of different ages

Food Group	Age (Years)			
	2–3	4–5	6–10	12–18
Milk				
Servings/day	2	2–3	2–3	2–3
Serving size				
Milk, yogurt	1 cup	1 cup	1 cup	1 cup
Cheese	2 oz.	2 oz.	2 oz.	2 oz.
Meats				
Servings/day	2	2	2–3	2–3
Serving size				
Meat, poultry, fish	1 oz.	2 oz.	3 oz.	3 oz.
Beans	5 tbsp.	½ cup	½ cup	½ cup
Eggs	1	1	1	1
Vegetables				
Servings/day	3	3	4	4–5
Serving size	5 tbsp.	½ cup	½ cup	½ cup
Fruits				
Servings/day	2	2	2–3	2–4
Serving size	1 piece	1 piece	1 peace	1 piece
	½ cup	½ cup	½ cup	½ cup
Grains				
Servings/day	6	6	6–11	6–11
Serving size				
Bread	½ slice	1 slice	1 slice	1 slice
Rice, pasta, cereal	5 tbsp.	½ cup	½ cup	½ cup

observed. In most cases obesity is a result of excess energy intake relative to physical activity level. Limited success has been achieved with weight loss programs for children. Emphasis should be placed on prevention of obesity by avoiding overfeeding in infancy and the preschool years, letting the child self-regulate food intake, avoiding of the use of food treats for behavioral management, and encouraging regular exercise. Extra attention to obesity prevention should be given for children whose parents are overweight, as these children are at the greatest risk for becoming obese.

VI. School-Aged Children: 6 to 11 Years
A. Nutritional goals for school-aged children
1. *To support appropriate growth.*
2. *To support optimal school performance.*

  3. *To develop healthy eating patterns.*

  4. *To develop skills in planning and selecting a well-balanced diet.*

  5. *To prevent obesity.*

 B. Nutritional guidance

  1. *Food intake.* School-aged children should be consuming a diet that is 30% fat, with less than 10% of total calories from saturated fatty acids and less than 300 mg/day of cholesterol. Recommendations for fat intake can be achieved by using lean meats and low-fat dairy products; limiting the amount of fried foods, prepared snacks, and desserts; and limiting fast foods. The number of meals and snacks is usually reduced to four or five per day. Grain products and starches should form the base of the diet and should be complimented with vegetables, fruits, protein-rich foods, and low-fat milk. Children should be offered a wide variety of foods from each of the food groups. Table 7.2 lists the recommended number of servings from each of the food groups and the typical serving sizes for this age group. Children in this age group often do not eat the recommended numbers of servings of fruits and vegetables; therefore emphasis should be placed on developing healthy eating patterns. Children should begin to learn the foundations of a healthful diet and the process for selecting nutritious food choices. The media and friends will have increasing influence on food choices at this age and should be taken into consideration when counseling about nutrition.

  2. *Breakfast.* Breakfast is an important meal for growing children and enhances attention in school and overall school performance. Skipping breakfast may occur because of early school starting times or because school-aged children have increased responsibility to get themselves dressed and out the door. Therefore breakfast may require specific attention when counseling parents and children about nutrition. For like reasons, children require a balanced lunch at school to facilitate classroom attention in the afternoon.

  3. *Energy needs.* Physical activity is an important determinant of the child's energy needs. Children should be encouraged to engage in physical activities daily to promote optimal overall health and to prevent obesity.

VII. Adolescents: 12 to 18 years

 A. Nutritional goals for adolescents

  1. *To achieve adequate intake to support the pubertal growth spurt.*

  2. *To eat a diet that includes a wide variety of nutritious foods.*

  3. *To take increasing responsibility for selecting a well-balanced diet.*

  4. *To achieve and maintain appropriate weight.*

 B. Nutritional guidance

  1. *Food intake.* Physical growth and pubertal maturation are accompanied by greater nutritional requirements

for energy, protein, calcium, iron, and zinc. The increased nutrient needs can be met by an overall increase in the amount of foods consumed. Grain products and starches should continue to form the base of the diet and should be complemented with vegetables, fruits, protein-rich foods, and low-fat milk. Table 7.2 lists the recommended number of servings from each of the food groups and the typical serving sizes for this age group.

2. *Behavioral changes.* Common behavior patterns during adolescence include skipping meals, eating more outside the home, increasing intake of fast foods, snacking, dieting, adopting fad diets, and replacing milk and juice with soft drinks. As a consequence, adolescents' diets are often low in calcium, iron, and vitamins A and C. Adolescents should be encouraged to select a wide variety of foods from each of the food groups (Table 7.2) and to limit snacking on sweets and high-fat foods.

3. *Weight control.* Obesity and eating disorders are more common in this age group. Adolescents should be encouraged to eat three meals a day and nutritious snacks. Furthermore, they should be encouraged to achieve and maintain a healthy weight through appropriate eating habits and regular exercise. Regular physical activity should be encouraged for all children and adolescents.

VIII. Special Topics

   A. Food allergies. Adverse reactions to food may occur because of food intolerance or food allergy. Food allergies or food hypersensitivity occurs when an immune mechanism elicits clinical symptoms. The reported incidence of food allergies varies from 0.3% to 20% in infants and declines with age. Genetic predisposition and early introduction of certain foods in the infant diet are the main factors in the development of food allergies. Breast feeding reduces but does not eliminate this risk. The dominant food allergies in infants are eggs, cow's milk, peanuts, and soy; and in children, tree nuts, fish and other seafood, and wheat and other cereal grains. Most children outgrow cow's milk and egg allergies by 3 or 4 years of age, but other food allergies tend to persist longer, sometimes for life. Children are unlikely to outgrow food allergies that develop after the age of 3 years. Food allergies must be treated by strict avoidance of the allergen. When multiple food allergies are suspect or present, their avoidance may have a significant deleterious impact on the child's nutrition; referral to a registered dietitian should be made for adequate nutritional planning and education.

   B. Vegetarian diets. Some individuals and families may choose to consume a vegetarian diet for religious, health, ecologic, or other personal reasons. Vegetarian diets are classified as semivegetarian (excludes red meat), lactoovovegetarian, lactovegetarian, and vegan (or strictly vegetarian, which means no animal products). Plant-based diets supplemented with milk or milk and eggs are nutritionally similar to diets that contain meat. Vegan, or pure vegetarian, diets also can be nutritionally adequate but require more careful planning. Cereal grains combined with legumes, nuts and seeds, fortified soy, or nut beverages should be included. Vitamin B-12 is found naturally only in animal products; some plant-based products are fortified with vitamin B-12. Growth is normal among children consuming a vegan diet that is based on a sound food pattern that provides adequate amounts of amino acids, calcium, riboflavin, iron, vitamin D, and vitamin B-12. In general, a dietitian should be consulted to help the parent formulate an adequate vegetarian diet. Adequate energy intake is a significant concern for weaning infants and toddlers, as they have the highest energy needs and are least able to tolerate large amounts of foods that are high in bulk. Severely restrictive vegetarian diets, such as macrobiotic diets, may be associated with stunted growth and should be discouraged.

C. Sports. Some children and adolescents engage in competitive sports, and the duration, frequency, and intensity of training increase during adolescence. Generally, an overall increase in food and fluid intake without significant alterations in the proportions of dietary constituents is sufficient. This can be achieved by inclusion of additional snacks and carbohydrate-containing drinks. No evidence suggests that athletes need additional vitamin supplements. An iron supplement may be needed to compensate for exercise-induced iron losses that occur with high-intensity training. Maintenance of hydration is essential, and water intake should be encouraged during and after exercise. Beverages with glucose, chloride, sodium, and potassium may be beneficial, particularly in hot climates, but they should be hypotonic. Inappropriate food restriction, periodic fasting, vomiting, and laxative or diuretic use are areas of concern in adolescents participating in sports that encourage thinness or sports that encourage "making weight," such as wrestling, ballet, gymnastics, and figure skating.

D. Cholesterol screening. Cholesterol screening and, if appropriate, dietary adjustments need to be considered for children whose parent(s) has a cholesterol concentration of greater than 240 mg/dL or for children whose parent(s) or grandparent(s) had one of the following under the age of 55 years: documented atherosclerosis, myocardial infarction, angina pectoris, cerebrovascular disease, peripheral vascular disease, or sudden cardiac death. Growing children with elevated serum cholesterol concentrations and a strong family history of atherosclerosis should be referred to a dietitian for assistance in selecting a lipid-lowering diet that is well-balanced and meets the needs for growth.

ADDITIONAL READING

The Food Guide Pyramid. United States Department of Agriculture, Center for Nutrition Policy and Promotion, *Home and Garden Bulletin*, No. 252.

Kleinman RE, ed. *Pediatric nutrition handbook,* 4th ed. Elk Grove Village, IL: American Academy of Pediatrics; 1998.

Web Site

www.usda.gov/KidsPyra/index.htm (United States Department of Agriculture. The Food Guide Pyramid for Young Children)

8 ♣ Breast Feeding

Jeanne L. Ballard

I. Prenatal Counseling: Benefits of Breast Feeding

A. Maternal benefits—now and later. Early in pregnancy, prospective parents will benefit from a discussion regarding their child's expected method of feeding and source of nutrition. Emphasizing at this time that human milk is the standard recommended nutrient for human infants is important. Proprietary formulas are artificial feedings and should be considered human milk substitutes.

The benefits of breast feeding extend to both mother and child. Mothers recover their uterine tone more rapidly than with bottle-feeding because of the secretion of oxytocin from their posterior pituitary gland, and they experience a sense of relaxation and well-being, as prolactin is secreted from their anterior pituitary gland. These women also enjoy early infant attachment to themselves and are rewarded by a healthy psychosocial interaction between themselves and their infants. Later in the puerperium, lactating women resume their prepregnant weight more rapidly because of increased caloric utilization. Long-term benefits include a decreased incidence of premenopausal breast cancer, ovarian cancer, and osteoporosis.

B. Benefits in infancy, childhood, and beyond. In infancy breast feeding lowers the incidence of sudden infant death syndrome (SIDS), gastrointestinal illnesses, urinary tract infections, colic, and milk allergy. Childhood illnesses, such as otitis media, upper respiratory infections, bronchiolitis, pneumonia, and asthma, are less frequent. Older children are at decreased risk of leukemia, diabetes mellitus, Crohn disease, obesity, and food and other allergies. Recent studies also show that the IQ of breast-fed infants is approximately 10 points higher than that of infants fed artificially. This intellectual advantage extends beyond childhood and into adolescence and adulthood, as seen in enhanced high school achievement test scores. Infants nurtured at the breast tend to have improved psychosocial behavior, usually have better communicating skills, and are more confident and self-reliant as adults.

II. Self-assessment

A. General health. To anticipate a successful breast-feeding experience, a prospective mother is advised to review her own general health. Conditions that may impede lactation include hypothyroidism, previous breast surgery, or chronic malnutrition. Few conditions categorically preclude breast feeding.

B. Motivation. The mother's motivation to breast-feed should be explored as well. Self-motivated mothers are far more likely to succeed than are those whose decision is forced by a relative, spouse, friend, or health care worker. Research has shown, however, that pediatricians can exert a powerful influence on the method of feeding of a newborn. This is best accomplished through appropriate and timely prenatal education.

C. Breasts. The mother should be encouraged to examine her own breasts for size, shape, symmetry, and appropriate enlargement since the time of conception. Inadequate glandular tissue or failure of glandular proliferation in pregnancy may impede sufficient milk production during lactation.

D. Nipples. The mother would do well to assess her nipples at some time during the pregnancy, since all women are not endowed with nipples that protrude just the right amount and are just the right diameter to fit precisely into a newborn infant's mouth. Nipples that are short, flat, inverted, or retractile may present a significant challenge to the breast-feeding dyad.

Helpful devices called shells can be applied to the flat or inverted nipple during the latter part of pregnancy. These help to stretch the fibrous bands that extend into the areola, allowing the nipple to protrude in preparation for the suckling infant. These shells are ventilated, hard plastic cups fitted with a smooth, round central rim through which the nipple can protrude. They may also be worn inside the bra after delivery, between feedings. Care must be taken to keep the shells very clean so as to avoid bacterial or fungal contamination of the nipples and also to place these shells concentrically on the areola to avoid trauma to the nipple. One common complaint is that the shells may cause excessive leakage of breast milk due to compression of the areola. One solution to this problem is to place sterile cotton balls inside the lower portion of the shells to absorb the milk and to change these frequently. The use of a breast pump, set on low suction, just before offering the breast may be as successful as wearing the shells, and is less uncomfortable for the mother.

Another device, the nipple shield, which is a soft silicon cover with a perforated tip, may be worn over the mother's breast while feeding and may help the baby to latch onto a retractile or inverted nipple. Caution should be used with the nipple shield, however, since these have been shown to diminish the milk transfer, and hence supply, if used over a prolonged period of time, possibly because of incomplete breast emptying. Furthermore, the infant may become accustomed to the shield and is reluctant to accept the breast without it. In some mothers, gentle compression of the nipple will cause it to protrude long enough for a hungry infant to accomplish a latch successfully. These issues may be introduced and discussed, as appropriate, during prenatal counseling, but their implementation is best reserved for early lactation.

E. Diet. Whether the mother plans to breast-feed or not, certain helpful dietary recommendations may foster good health for both mother and baby. These include the food pyramid established by the American Dietary Association, in which grains and fiber, fresh fruits and vegetables, proteins, and complex carbohydrates play an important role in the diet. Current caloric recommendations during lactation are that women take in about 100 additional kilocalories (as opposed to 500 extra kilocalories previously recommended for lactating women). Prenatal vitamins containing added vitamin D, folic acid, calcium, and the B complex should be taken daily and continued during lactation. Current recommendations for calcium intake during pregnancy and lactation are 1,000 mg/day, no more than any other woman in the child-bearing age, as lactation itself induces a calcium-conserving state in the maternal metabolism.

Although some lay pamphlets advocate a high intake of dairy products during pregnancy and lactation, excessive dairy intake may result in bovine whey sensitization of some fetuses. The infant may present with severe abdominal discomfort after breast feeding, variably accompanied by flushing, hematochesia, or an elevated serum IgE or IgM. This has been shown to be related to bovine beta-lactoglobulin secreted into human milk. Breast-feeding mothers may be required to eliminate dairy products from their diets for 3 to 5 weeks before the infant's symptoms subside. Other less common allergens include eggs, peanuts, and chocolate. Most foods, taken in moderation, are compatible with breast feeding.

III.   Birth Plan

A.   Type of delivery. The prospective mother may wish to discuss her anticipated type of delivery with her pediatrician or primary caregiver. This may range from a normal vaginal delivery to a scheduled cesarean section or a vaginal birth after C-section. At this time, unanticipated eventualities can be introduced, such as fetal distress or failure to progress, which may result in emergency C-section. The physician should stress that none of these factors preclude breast feeding. The mother should be encouraged to request assistance with breast feeding from hospital personnel as her medical condition warrants.

B.   Analgesics. The decision to accept or request analgesics during labor may impact the success of breast feeding in the first several hours after birth. Narcotic analgesics do cross the placenta into fetal circulation and may impair the infant's ability to suck vigorously at the breast when administered within 1 to 4 hours before delivery. Typically, these infants are active at birth and may even go to breast immediately, but within 3 to 4 hours they become sleepy and unable to sustain a nutritive suck for more than 3 or 4 minutes. Even when feedings are attempted by bottle, they exhibit poor coordination of their suck/swallow reflex. This suppressed feeding ability may persist for as long as 24 to 48 hours. During this time avoid formula supplementation by bottle, and encourage the mother to pump her breasts to stimulate her milk production. Pumped colostrum or mature milk mixed with a low-iron milk substitute may be fed to the infant by syringe, dropper, or cup, or using the finger-feeding method.

C. Anesthesia. Currently, the most popular local anesthetic is the epidural. This modality affords most mothers adequate relief from the painful contractions of active labor. The local anesthetic in the epidural does not affect the infant. If a narcotic analgesic is added, however, the drug may cross over into fetal circulation, resulting in a sleepy baby who is unable to suck effectively at the breast. This effect may also last several hours. General anesthesia in labor may cause early neonatal depression, which will likely interfere with the sensitive period immediately after birth. It also may cause temporary anorexia in the infant, but both of these effects usually dissipate within a few hours of birth.

D. Postdelivery pain management. Whether the delivery is spontaneous or operative, usually some postdelivery pain must be managed. Anticipating this postpartum pain can be advantageous so that the mother can be prepared to assist in her own pain management. She may wish to know that the patient-controlled anesthesia (PCA) pump, containing morphine sulfate, will probably not affect her infant, as the drug is very short acting and the dose in colostrum will be so low as to be homeopathic. The pain relief to the mother, however, will enable her to breast-feed more comfortably and therefore more successfully. Oral analgesics that contain synthetic narcotic agents may seriously affect the infant's ability to breast-feed, depending on the maternal dose, frequency of administration, and timing between dosing and breast feeding. The mother should be advised to ingest only the minimal effective dose at the longest tolerable intervals and to try to breast-feed before, rather than after, taking the medication.

IV. The First Feed

A. Early contact. The most conducive approach to successful breast feeding is to assess the infant's health and stability immediately following birth and in as close proximity to the mother as possible (e.g., on her abdomen). The infant should be dried thoroughly, examined for physical and physiologic abnormalities, and placed quickly onto the mother's abdomen in the prone position. An overhead heat source helps with neonatal thermoregulation, as does a warm coverlet laid over the infant's back.

B. Self-attachment. The mother's body heat will provide adequate warmth for the infant as he or she begins to search for the mother's breast, eventually self-attaching to the mother's nipple. This sequence is most likely to occur in nonmedicated births but is not impossible in lightly medicated births. Even simple contact of the infant's lips with the mother's nipple is adequate stimulation to the efferent nerves from the nipple to the hypothalamus to induce prolactin and oxytocin secretion by the anterior and posterior pituitary, respectively. This early contact is certainly more conducive to the onset of timely lactation than is taking the infant away to a distant nursery for the performance of the myriad of interventions that are frequently unnecessary and counter-productive to breast feeding: nasopharyngeal and gastric suctioning, injections, bath, nursing assessment, vital sign recording, weighing on a cold scale, and a "trial feeding" of water using a rubber nipple.

C. Imprinting. Oral imprinting at the breast rather than at the bottle is thought to be one of the most important indicators of a successful breast-feeding experience and of duration of lactation. Physicians have a perfect and powerful opportunity to influence not only the feeding choice of the mother, but also the likelihood of success of the new dyad's breast-feeding experience, its duration, and hence the long-term health of both the current and new generations.

V. Infant Assessment

A. Physical and neurologic exam. In occasional instances, the infant's physical and/or neurologic examinations may reveal a finding that impedes the ideal situation described earlier. For example, self-attachment may be difficult or impossible if the infant has significant micrognathia, cleft lip or palate, a short or tight lingual frenulum, or other orofacial abnormalities. The neurologic examination may reveal a floppy or lethargic infant with poor tone, inability to suck and swallow in a coordinated fashion, or inability to sustain a nutritive sucking pattern long enough to obtain adequate nutrition at the breast. None of these situations need necessarily preclude infants from receiving breast milk as their major nutrient, however. Most infants with micrognathia will outgrow their recessed chin in several weeks or months, unless it is part of a true Pierre-Robin sequence. Some infants with a cleft of the lip or palate may have difficulty maintaining good suction at the breast, rendering it difficult to accomplish adequate drainage. Others may nurse quite comfortably at the breast. When infants cannot obtain the breast milk on their own, mothers should be advised to pump their breasts for proper stimulation and drainage. The breast milk thus obtained may be fed to the infant by dropper or syringe or with a cleft palate feeder until surgical correction is accomplished.

If the infant is floppy or lethargic, the physician must determine the reason for the decreased tone or altered level of consciousness. Depending upon the cause, the solution may be temporary or permanent. For example, the infant with traumatic Erb or Bell palsy will likely recover within a day or two; the infant affected by maternal narcotic or magnesium sulfate administration in labor will become more alert and responsive within several hours. In contrast, the infant who suffered profound perinatal asphyxia or who has a primary neurologic or muscular disorder will likely have a persistent inability to extract milk from the breast. Each situation must be addressed individually, and the mother counseled accordingly. Temporary problems will require that the mother pump her milk and feed it to the infant in a manner that is conducive to eventual nursing at the breast (e.g., syringe, dropper, or finger feeding), while remaining watchful to introduce the breast as soon as oral tone and function have returned. When the infant has a static, permanent, or progressive disability, the mother may still be encouraged to pump while being advised that her milk may be fed to the infant by bottle or orogastric tube and while being reassured that her milk is still the best nutrient for her infant.

B. Assessment of latch. To assess the latch, every maternal/infant dyad should be observed while breast feeding. The *LATCH score* is used in some hospitals to help the professional address specific problem areas with the latch.

1. *L* is for *latch*. The infant should be securely attached to the breast so that the lips are splayed outward about 140 degrees and cover a significant portion of the areola. The infant's nose and chin should touch the breast and the infant's hips should be rotated toward the mother's body. It is most conducive to lactation if the infant's naked chest is in direct contact with the mother's naked breast.

2. *A* is for *audible* swallowing. On the first day post partum, the mother may expect to hear occasional swallowing (one for every five to seven sucks), increasing to frequent (one for every three to four sucks) and consistent swallowing (one for every one or two sucks) by days 2 and 3, respectively.

3. *T* is for *type* of nipple. As mentioned earlier, if the nipples are short, flat, retractile, or truly inverted, this may present an increasing challenge for the breast-feeding dyad.

4. *C* is for *comfort* of the mother (i.e., freedom from pain). Ascertain the level of a mother's pain using the 0 to 10 pain scale. Nipple pain is most commonly associated with a distal or incorrect latch.

5. *H* is for *hold*. How a mother holds her infant during a feed may affect pain, latch, and audible swallowing. A close, well-aligned, and relaxed but secure hold of the baby, without help from professionals, is likely to be accompanied by pain-free milk transfer, a contented infant, and a successful breast-feeding experience.

C. Oral assessment. As with any infant, oral assessment is important. In the breast-feeding infant, the oral cavity—its size, shape, and depth—is crucial to the infant's ability to obtain milk from the mother's breast. Some characteristics that may present challenges to successful breast feeding are a recessed chin, a high-arched palate, a short tongue, and a tight lingual frenulum. These findings may be isolated or found in various combinations in the same infant. If lingual function is impeded by the tight frenulum, the breast-feeding experience may be salvaged by performing a frenuloplasty. The remaining oral characteristics frequently improve over time once the tongue is released, as the tongue can then grow to its normal length, protrude to the lips and beyond, reach the hard palate, and keep the gums properly aligned. Early release of the tongue can also prevent future speech and orthodontic problems.

D.   Body language. Observing the mother and baby during a breast-feeding session affords an opportunity to see how they interact and communicate through body language without any verbal interchange. When healthy communication is established, the baby's mouthing movements elicit a feeding response from the mother. Her skin warms to the baby's touch, bringing an increased blood supply to the breast. This increases her milk production and induces her to pull the baby close so that a large portion of the areola can enter the baby's mouth. As the baby's lips massage the areola, the let-down reflex is stimulated, and both mother and baby relax with satisfaction.

E.   Nutritive and nonnutritive suck. Differentiating between nutritive and nonnutritive sucking patterns is important. When the baby is obtaining nutrition, the jaw drops rhythmically with each suck, the pace is relatively slow, and the lips are widely separated. A nonnutritive suck is characterized by lack of jaw movement, rapid sucking bursts, and pursed lips. Only nutritive sucking should be counted as time spent breast feeding. Nonnutritive sucking at the breast should be kept to a minimum, since it may fatigue the mother and usurp her time for her own self-care. In addition, nipple stimulation without breast drainage may lead to breast engorgement, difficulty latching, decreasing milk supply, and poor infant weight gain.

VI.   Early Days

A.   Intake. Many new mothers worry that their infant is not receiving adequate nutrition on the first 2 or 3 days of life. Some express the concern that the baby is "not getting anything" or that their milk is "not in yet." These fears and misconceptions are often difficult to dispel, but a brief explanation of the physiology of early lactation may be helpful. *In utero,* the fetus has been swallowing amniotic fluid in very small amounts, as if sipping almost continually. The newborn stomach is therefore quite small and can comfortably hold only 10 to 15 mL initially. The early milk, colostrum, is secreted in small quantities initially, until the baby's stomach can accommodate larger volumes. Meanwhile, the infant will want to feed at frequent intervals, typically every 1 or 2 hours on the first day of life. As the transitional, then mature milk is produced, it mixes with the colostrum and increases in volume. This provides progressively greater quantities of milk per feeding, so that the infant begins to space the feedings at longer intervals. If the infant cannot adequately drain the breast consistently, the breast may become firm, tender, and edematous. This is called *engorgement* and is not considered a normal phenomenon. Indeed, engorgement can be prevented by frequent and adequate breast drainage.

B. Output. Neonatal urinary and stool output are important parameters to follow during the first few days of breast feeding. Adequate intake of colostrum stimulates bowel motility so that the passage of meconium usually follows the first or second successful breast feeding. Meconium is usually passed after each feeding or at least three or four times in a 24-hour period. By the second or third day, the color of the stools should be growing lighter and should become soft and light yellow by the fourth day. This is one indication that the infant is receiving an adequate amount of milk. The infant's urine should be pale yellow and should be passed at least six times per day. A tea- or coral-colored urine may indicate inadequate fluid intake and heralds early or impending dehydration. In this case, the mother may be asked to breastfeed more frequently; or her latch, milk production, or feeding technique may need to be assessed.

C. Neonatal response. The newborn's behavior at the breast and after the feeding is also an important observation. This neonatal response may vary from contentment to frustration to agitation or irritability to apathy, lethargy, or somnolence. Contentment is the only appropriate neonatal response to a successful breast-feeding session. All other responses warrant a thorough investigation.

D. Weight curve. The infant's weight curve in the early days is one of the most informative elements in determining adequate milk intake. A loss of 3% to 4% of the birth weight in the first 3 to 4 days of life is probably physiologically normal. When an infant loses 7% or 8%, however, the adequacy of milk production and transfer needs to be evaluated; and measures need to be taken to correct the problem. By the fourth or fifth day after birth, the infant should gain about 1 ounce each day, regaining to birth weight by 2 weeks of age.

E. Milk transfer. Feeding test weights are helpful in assessing the infant's milk intake at the breast. The baby is weighed wearing a diaper just before a feeding and again immediately afterward with the same diaper. A gram of weight gain is roughly equivalent to 1 mL of milk; thus the physician can estimate the amount of milk consumed at that particular feeding. Between 2 weeks and 2 months of age the infant should consume about 1 ounce each hour. One must remember that milk production and supply may vary according to the time of day. The most abundant volume is produced in the early morning, and the lowest supply is available in the late afternoon and early evening. When the milk supply is clearly inadequate, measures should be taken promptly to improve the mother's milk production, delivery, or both, thus ensuring the infant's well-being and optimal health. This can be accomplished through improvement of the latch, increasing the frequency of feeds, instituting pumping sessions, implementing relaxation techniques to facilitate the milk ejection reflex, and possibly using galactogogues.

VII.   Early Weeks

   A.   Infant weight gain. The breast-fed baby normally gains 1.5 to 2 ounces each day in the first 2 months. This rapid growth tapers off between 3 and 12 months, so that one need not be concerned regarding obesity in the breast-fed infant. Weight curves in the first year of life traditionally have been based on formula-fed infants. Recently, weight curves based on infants who were exclusively breast-fed have become available. Breast-fed infants may double their birth weight well before 6 months but may level off during the latter half of the first year, as the fat content of the milk declines and the protein content increases. Breast-fed infants tend to be leaner, to have normal or accelerated development, and to have fewer infectious illnesses than their bottle-fed counterparts. Length measurements do not differ significantly; hence breast-fed infants have lower weight-to-length ratios and are less likely to be categorized as obese. Head growth in breast-fed infants is comparable to that of formula-fed infants, despite the lower protein content of breast milk.

   B.   Overproduction/foremilk–hindmilk imbalance. Some mothers may actually produce greater quantities of milk than their infant needs to grow appropriately. This may be a result of overstimulation of the breasts or may occur spontaneously. Milk overproduction, or hyperlactation, may be accompanied by an overactive milk ejection, or "letdown," reflex. Typically, the infant consistently coughs and arches away at the beginning of the feed, satiates early, and demands another feed within an hour or two. The mother's breasts refill very rapidly and become uncomfortably full. The infant gains weight more rapidly than expected and may develop watery diarrhea and gaseous distention. The latter may be explained by an imbalance between the ingestion of foremilk, which is high in lactose, and that of hindmilk, which is high in fat. The high lactose load may overwhelm the infant's metabolic capacity, resulting in excessive bacterial breakdown of lactose, osmotic diarrhea, and acid irritation of the perianal skin.

      Management consists of asking the mother to drain one breast as thoroughly as possible before offering the second breast (i.e., a feeding session within 2 hours of the previous one should be on the same breast as before). The baby will thus obtain hindmilk and sleep longer and more comfortably, and the unstimulated breast will begin to suppress milk production because of the milk-inhibiting factor in breast milk. This down-regulation of milk production gradually adjusts the mother's milk supply to the infant's needs. If the overactive letdown reflex persists, the mother may manually express a small amount of milk just before offering the breast to the infant. This usually relieves the initial high pressure in the lactiferous sinuses so that the infant is not overwhelmed by the initial rapid outpouring of milk.

 C.   **Underproduction/delayed lactogenesis.** Underproduction of milk occurs in a small percentage of women. The causes may be anatomic, physiologic, hormonal, or iatrogenic. Approximately 1% of women suffer from underdevelopment of their mammary glandular tissue. These women may experience little or no breast enlargement during pregnancy, may produce little or no colostrum after delivery, and do not become engorged or feel a surge in milk production, despite adequate stimulation by a nursing baby or a breast pump. These women may still feed their babies at the breast with the help of a supplemental nursing system, thereby experiencing the closeness and nurturing sensation of breast feeding.

 Physiologic causes of delayed lactogenesis include significant blood loss at delivery, cesarean section, fever, fatigue, and anxiety. Hormonal causes include thyroid hypofunction and oral contraceptives. Iatrogenic causes are probably the most frequently encountered. These include the use of sedative or pain medication in labor, separation of the baby from the mother after birth, the use of bottles and rubber nipples for supplementation, and interruption or postponement of breast-feeding sessions for procedures and examinations. In addition to avoiding the preceding impediments, physicians can further promote, support, and protect the breast-feeding dyad by offering encouragement, breast pumps, shells, supplemental nursing systems, and other equipment to help sustain or salvage the breast-feeding experience.

 D.   **Supplementation.** Occasional medical reasons for supplementing the breast-fed infant arise. These can be divided into maternal and infant indications. Maternal conditions include fatigue and/or anxiety, flat or inverted nipples, nonelastic or engorged areolae, sore or traumatized nipples, illness, and short-term use of a contraindicated medication. Infant conditions include hypoglycemia, lethargy or irritability after breast feeding, weight loss beyond 7% to 10% of birth weight, inadequate stool and/or urine output, and breast-feeding-associated jaundice.

 Supplemental nutrition, in order of preference, may include fresh-pumped breast milk, breast milk mixed with formula, formula whenever breast milk is not available, and frozen breast milk (thawed and warmed).

 Preferred routes of delivery include a supplemental nursing system attached to the breast, finger feeding using the feeding device attached to a caretaker's finger, syringe, cup, dropper, or bottle with silicone or orthodontic nipple.

VIII.   Working Moms

 A.   **Pumping milk.** One of the challenges of breast feeding is coordinating returning to work with maintaining an adequate milk supply. Some places of employment provide a private, quiet, sanitary facility where a mother may pump her breasts so that she can leave an appropriate amount of milk for her baby for the next day. Portable breast pumps can be both effective and comfortable. Pumping should occur at about the same frequency as the baby's feeding schedule (i.e., every 3 to 4 hours), and sessions should last 15 to 20 minutes. The mother needs to be relaxed and comfortable during these sessions to be able to maintain her milk-ejection reflex. To maintain an adequate milk supply for her infant, she will also need to be encouraged to maintain her rest, nutrition, and hydration after returning to work.

B.   Storing milk. Pumping milk for future use requires clean equipment and storage containers. These may be made of glass or food-quality plastic and should be sealed and labeled with the date and time of milk collection. Freshly pumped milk may be held at room temperature for 7 or 8 hours; kept refrigerated for 6 to 7 days; kept frozen in a self-defrosting freezer for 5 to 6 months; or kept frozen in a deep-freezer indefinitely. Fresh breast milk is superior to frozen because of the preservation of many biologically active substances that may be destroyed by freezing. Fresh breast milk contains antiinfective properties that reduce and eventually eliminate bacterial contamination when refrigerated for prolonged periods (e.g., up to 1 month). Partial freezing and thawing, as may occur in some self-defrosting freezers, can convert the palmitic acids in breast milk to palmitates, which are poorly absorbed by the infant gut. This phenomenon has been implicated in some cases of failure to thrive in infants fed exclusively thawed, conventionally frozen breast milk.

C.   Alternate feeding methods. When babies must be separated from their mothers, methods other than feeding directly from the breast must be implemented. These include syringe, cup, dropper, finger feeding, and bottle feeding. During the first 3 to 5 weeks, the preferance is to avoid bottle feeding because of the risk of causing nipple confusion or preference. Until the mother's milk supply is well established, the infant's preference will be to suck wherever milk is most easily obtained (i.e., at the bottle). However, once the infant has mastered the technique of efficiently obtaining milk from the breast, he or she will likely move from breast to bottle and back to breast with ease. Since this usually occurs well before the mother returns to work, most infants may be fed by the alternate caretaker, who uses a bottle containing breast milk pumped the previous day. The mother may still prefer to breast-feed the infant during nonworking hours. Thus the breast-feeding experience can be prolonged and enjoyed as long as mother and infant desire.

IX.   Breast Milk Nutrients

A.   Proteins, fats, and carbohydrates. Human colostrum contains approximately 2.3% protein, whereas mature milk contains about 1.0%. The fat content of colostrum is roughly

3.0%, whereas that of mature milk averages 3.9%. Lactose, the major carbohydrate in breast milk, increases from 5.5% in colostrum to 6.8% in mature milk.

Human milk proteins may be subdivided into the whey and casein fractions. The whey component consists of alpha-lactalbumin, IgA, lysozyme, and serum albumin, and accounts for approximately 60% of the total protein in milk. The caseins beta and kappa, linked to calcium phosphate, account for 20% to 30% of the total protein content. The remaining are the proteins, glycoproteins, and lipoproteins of the fat globule membrane, and the peptides, nucleotides, nucleosides, and free amino acids.

Human milk fat is secreted in the form of milk fat globules. The fat content of human milk changes with the volume of milk secreted, increasing markedly from the start to the finish of a given feeding. The milk secreted during the last two-thirds of the feeding or milk expression may contain up to two or three times as much fat as that secreted at the beginning of the feeding. Awareness of this phenomenon may help the pediatrician manage failure to thrive, breast milk diarrhea, infant sleeplessness, and gastrointestinal discomfort in the breast-fed infant. The fat globule contains triacylglycerols and sterol esters. The milk fat globule membrane contains proteins, phospholipids, cholesterol, enzymes, trace minerals, and fat-soluble vitamins.

Lactose and oligosaccharides remain relatively constant throughout the feeding, and the content varies little from mother to mother. The only real change is the increase in lactose and decrease in oligosaccharides from colostrum to mature milk. This gradual increase in lactose parallels the infant's gastrointestinal increase in lactase over the first week of life.

B.   Minerals. The calcium/phosphorus ratio of human milk is higher during the colostrum phase (2.8 : 1) than during the mature milk phase (2.3 : 1). Sodium and potassium are higher in colostrum than in mature milk, as are zinc, iron, copper, and sulfur. Magnesium remains stable or increases minimally in the mature milk.

C.   Water. A common belief among parents and nursery professionals is that newborn infants must be fed sterile water as their first feed and that infants should be given water in addition to breast milk on a daily basis. Neither tenet is true. The first feed should be at the breast to establish imprinting at the breast and not at the bottle. The misconception that the newborn's anatomy must be "tested" before the breast is offered is a carry-over from the realization that bottle feeding is not always tolerated by sick infants; therefore one should begin with water in the event that the baby would vomit or aspirate the feeding. One should remember that to obtain colostrum from the breast, the infant must have a relatively strong suck, as opposed to the bottle, which is largely a passive feed. Breast milk contains the proper amount of water, even in hot, dry climates. When the mother is well hydrated and breast feeding is well established, taking the infant to the breast more often is more beneficial than introducing a bottle after the breast if the infant is still hungry. The common practice of suggesting a postbreast bottle is often the first step toward lactation failure. Even water will fill the infant's stomach so that nursing will be less frequent, leading to poor infant weight gain and a decrease in maternal milk production.

D.   Water-soluble vitamins. Human milk contains all the water-soluble vitamins. These include vitamins C, B-1, B-2, niacin, B-6, folate and B-12, pantothenic acid, and biotin. All increase from colostrum to mature milk except for B-12, which is dependent on maternal intake. Infants of totally vegetarian mothers may be at risk of vitamin B-12 deficiency with resultant neurologic damage; therefore these mothers should receive a B-12 supplement. In general, the recommendation is that breast-feeding mothers continue taking their prenatal vitamins, although only niacin and B-12 can be increased in breast milk by increased maternal intake when the mother's status is already adequate.

E.   Fat-soluble vitamins. The fat-soluble vitamins contained in human milk include vitamin A, beta-carotene, and vitamins D, E, and K. Vitamins A and E and beta-carotene are found in higher amounts in colostrum than in mature milk. Vitamin D increases slightly, and vitamin K remains about the same as colostrum is replaced by mature milk. An increase in the mother's diet increases all the fat-soluble vitamins except for vitamin E, which remains unchanged, unless relatively large amounts are ingested by the mother. The vitamin D content of human milk is lower than the recommended dietary intake and is influenced by degree of sunlight exposure and skin pigmentation. Thus, although the bone mineral densities of term, healthy, breast-fed, unsupplemented babies have been reported to be normal, the current recommendation is that breast-fed infants in Europe and northern regions of the United States be given 400 IU of vitamin D daily. Newborn infants have low concentrations of vitamin K, and breast-fed babies who do not receive vitamin K at birth are at higher risk of developing hemorrhagic disease than are bottle-fed babies. Thus vitamin K supplementation at birth in term infants and daily in small, preterm infants is the current recommendation.

F.   Micronutrients. Iron, zinc, copper, and selenium are higher in colostrum than in mature milk. Iodine and fluorine appear to be present only in mature milk, and manganese is the same in colostrum and mature milk.

X.   Bioactive Substances in Human Milk: Defense Agents

A.   Antimicrobials. In general, the antimicrobial factors in breast milk are highest in quantity in colostrum and decrease as lactation progresses. These include secretory IgA, lactoferrin, lysozyme, oligosaccharides, glycoconjugates, complement C3, fibronectin, and mucins. In concert these substances protect the breast-fed infant against a number of respiratory and enteric pathogens by blocking their adhesion to mucosal surfaces, neutralizing toxins, and preventing bacterial translocation, thereby protecting the infant against sepsis.

B.   Antiinflammatory agents. Certain breast milk antimicrobials possess antiinflammatory properties. These include lactoferrin, secretory IgA, and lysozyme. Other antiinflammatory agents include the antioxidants, such as vitamins E and C, beta-carotene, and cysteine. The enzymes catalase and glutathione peroxidase, as well as epithelial growth factors, also assist in reducing inflammation by protecting and enhancing the maturation of the intestinal mucosa and by decreasing immune stimulation in the infant. The platelet activating factor acetylhydrolase, the antiproteases alpha-1-antichymotrypsin and alpha-1-antitrypsin, and prostaglandins are also present in breast milk.

C.   Immunomodulators. These substances promote the development of the infant's own immune system. Breast-fed infants are capable of making their own IgA and exhibit increased responsiveness to their immunizations. In addition to vitamin E, these include nucleotides, cytokines, and anti-idiotypic antibodies. Some of the long-term benefits of breast feeding are illustrations of the enhancement of these infants' immune systems: the lower incidence of insulin-dependent diabetes, Crohn disease, and atopic disease in later life.

D.   Leukocytes. Human milk leukocytes are most abundant in colostrum and decrease in number over time during lactation. Neutrophils and macrophages account for about 90% of total leukocytes, with the remainder being primarily T-cell lymphocytes. The neutrophils and macrophages possess chemotactic, bactericidal, and fungicidal antibody-dependent activity. They have also demonstrated a degree of antiinflammatory activity *in vitro*. The lymphocytes are capable of generating lymphokines, IgA, and growth factors. They maintain function and viability in the infant gastrointestinal tract and adhere to the intestinal mucosa, or enter into the infant's circulatory and lymphatic systems, imparting both local and systemic immunocompetence to the infant.

XI.   Introducing Solids
    The most recent recommendations regarding the introduction of solids to breast-fed infants were offered by the World Health Organization. These are based on the finding that solid food does not increase the energy intake of breast-fed babies but rather displaces the energy intake from human milk. On the other hand, children who go beyond 6 months without receiving complementary foods do not maintain adequate growth. At about 6 months therefore, the infant should be offered solid foods, other beverages, and breast milk, with the intent of broadening the child's eating

experiences but not of decreasing the intake of breast milk. First solids are often called weaning foods. With the addition of solids, the infant may begin to request the breast less frequently, leading to a gradual decrease in milk production or to a plateau in milk supply that can be maintained for 2 to 4 years or more.

XII.   Weaning

Each breast-feeding dyad has individual needs and circumstances. Some may wish to continue nursing well beyond the second or third year, whereas others may want to return to work or to be free from the breast-feeding experience after just a few weeks. The major emphasis should be placed on the physical comfort and psychologic ease of both mother and child during the weaning process. Ideally, weaning should be gradual enough for the infant to adjust to other foods and feeding methods in a positive manner and for the mother's breasts to down-regulate milk production without incident. The primary care physician may need to support some mothers through physical pain as well as feelings of sadness, loss, guilt, or depression if weaning has been forced, abrupt, or premature in the mother's estimation.

ADDITIONAL READING

Auerbach KG. The effect of nipple shields on maternal milk volume. *J Obstet Gynecol Neonatal Nurs* 1990:19:419–427.

Baker B:Weight of infant helps assess adequacy of breast milk intake. *Pediatric News* September 1997:31.

Balmer SE, Wharton BA. Diet and faecal flora in the newborn: iron. *Arch Dis Child* 1991:66:1390–1394.

Benjamin JT, Shariat H. Overcoming impediments to breastfeeding: how pediatricians can help. *Contemp Pediatr* 1999;16:73–83.

Calhoun DA, Lunoe M, Du Y, Christensen RD. Granulocyte colony-stimulating factor is present in human milk and its receptor is present in human fetal intestine. *Pediatrics* 2000:105(1):e7.

Evans K, Evans R, Simmer K. Effect of the method of breast feeding on breast engorgement, mastitis and infantile colic. *Acta Pediatr* 1995;84:849–852.

Haldeman W. Can magnesium sulfate therapy impact lactogenesis? *J Hum Lact* 1993:9:249–252.

Hale TW. Anesthetic medications in breastfeeding mothers. *J Hum Lact* 1999:15:185–194.

Hamosh M, Peterson JA, Henderson TR, et al. Protective function of human milk: the milk fat globule. *Semin Perinatol* 1999;23: 248–249.

Heineg MJ, Francis J, Pappagianis D. Mammary candidosis in lactating women. *J Hum Lact* 1999:15:281–287.

Hildebrandt HM. Maternal perception of lactogenesis time: a clinical report. *J Hum Lact* 1999:15:317–323.

Howard CR, deBliek EA, ten Hoopen CB, Howard FM, Lanphear BP, Lawrence RA. Physiologic stability of newborns during cup and bottle feeding. *Pediatrics* 1999;104:1204–1206.

Lawrence RA, Lawrence RM. *Breastfeeding: a guide for the medical profession,* 5th ed. St. Louis: Mosby; 1999.

Lonnerdal B, Hernell O. Iron, zinc, copper and selenium status of breast-fed infants and infants fed trace element fortified milk-based infant formula. *Acta Paediatr* 1994:83:367–373.

Niefert M. Early assessment of the breastfeeding infant. *Contemp Pediatr* 1996:2–15.

Rodriguez-Palmero M, Koletzko B, Kunz C, Jensen R. Nutritional and biochemical properties of human milk I, II. *Clin Perinatol* 1999; 26:307–359.

Sosa R, Barness L. Bacterial growth in refrigerated human milk. *Amer J Dis Child* 1987:141:11–112.

Von Kries R, Koletzko B, Sauerwald T, et al. Breastfeeding and obesity: cross sectional study. *Br Med J* 1999;319:147–150.

Walker M. Mastitis in lactating women. *LaLeche League Int* 1999: 298:2–16.

WHO Working Group on the Growth Reference Protocol and WHO Task Force on Methods for the Natural Regulation of Fertility. Growth patterns of breastfed infants in seven countries. *Acta Pediatr* 2000:89:215–222.

Working Group on Breastfeeding, AAP. Breastfeeding and the use of human milk. *Pediatrics* 1997:100:1035–1039.

Web Site

http://www.breastfeedingbasics.org/ (Web-based breast feeding curriculum)

9 ♣ Anticipatory Guidance

Julie A. Jaskiewicz

Every health supervision visit is an opportunity for the primary care physician to share information and suggestions for parenting that enhance good parent/child interactions and facilitate health promotion. This process is called *anticipatory guidance,* and it allows the physician to anticipate for parents the child's development, behavior, and issues that arise at various ages. The health care provider makes parents aware of the changes that occur in their children over time and offers suggestions for adapting to those changes. Every physician will develop his or her own style for guiding individual families. The primary goal is to help parents relate positively to their children and enjoy them.

I. Principles of Anticipatory Guidance

A. **Partnership.** Ideally, physicians and parents work as partners to provide the best possible nurturing environment for their child. Parents should be encouraged to see themselves as the best caregivers and teachers of their children, with the physician as a guide and support. When parents view themselves as competent caregivers, their self-esteem and self-confidence are enhanced, which may in turn improve compliance with preventive health maintenance.

B. **Parents' agenda.** The physician should ask parents about their specific concerns, questions, or problems with the child rather than present them with a laundry list of predetermined topics. Discussing all issues at each health maintenance visit is impossible. Carefully listening to parents' concerns enables the physician to determine which information needs to be shared at that visit and which information can wait until a later time. A few minutes of specific advice for a parent's most pressing concern is usually more meaningful than a long discussion of issues that may seem insignificant at that moment to an overwhelmed parent. The physician should try to avoid a judgmental or dogmatic approach. When a problem with the child exists, the physician should ask parents what they already have tried and incorporate that information into subsequent counseling.

C. **Anticipate normal development.** A key principle of anticipatory guidance is to enlighten parents ahead of time about normal development and expected changes in routine (e.g., starting solid foods) or potential problems (e.g., nighttime awakening). Discussing potential problems with parents before they occur is preferable. If parents are made aware that certain behaviors can be expected and are normal (e.g., temper tantrums in toddlers), they will be more equipped to handle them and less likely to develop the misconception that their child's behavior is bad or a result of their failure as parents.

D. **Timing.** The timing of anticipatory guidance within the health maintenance visit varies among physicians and from one visit to another. Issues may be discussed at the end of the visit, or some issues may be raised as the physical examination proceeds. Many physicians provide written materials about these issues to supplement office discussion. The smart physician also takes advantage of unique opportunities. For example, if an infant is left unattended on the examination table by a parent who is across the room, the physician can use that opportunity to discuss safety issues for infants with the parent and can model more appropriate care.

II. Components of Anticipatory Guidance

  A. Development. Many anticipatory guidance issues relate to the child's developmental stage and projected development over time. At each visit, the physician should update the parents on the child's developmental progress (cognitive, somatic, motor, and psychosocial milestones) and advise them about what the child should be capable of doing by the time of the next health maintenance visit. At the same time, the child's developmental stage and expected advances (by the next visit) will influence other topics for discussion. For example, the infant's motor development determines which safety issues require discussion (the infant's newfound ability to crawl necessitates attention to stairs and electrical outlets), and the development of pincer grasp suggests introducing finger foods as part of nutrition counseling.

  B. Nutrition. The physician should discuss diet and caloric requirements at different ages, the variability in appetite among individual children, and the normal development of feeding skills. Parents often are concerned more about the feeding behaviors of their child than about the nutritional aspects of food. Some parents use their child's feeding success as proof of their success or failure as a caregiver. Some children learn quickly that they exert tremendous control over the family by their behavior at mealtime. The physician should anticipate for parents the different psychosocial/developmental issues that relate to a child's feeding behavior, such as the usual decrease in appetite during the toddler years and the need for self-feeding in spite of the mess it creates. By discussing these issues with parents before the child is developmentally capable of the behaviors, parents will feel more in control, less anxious, and less responsible for their child's normal, though often challenging, feeding behavior.

  C. Injury prevention. The dangerous situations children get into are directly related to their developmental capabilities. Parents often do not anticipate these dangers because they are unaware of their child's abilities. Parents should be prepared early about what to expect and how to ready themselves and the child's environment by relating their child's developmental stage to potential common hazards. Specific hazards in a child's environment, such as living next to a busy four-lane highway, merit specific discussion. The physician should be sure to emphasize seasonal safety (discuss water safety beginning in the spring) and to stress the need for appropriate supervision.

D.   Behavior and discipline. Some of the most challenging behaviors exhibited by children, such as temper tantrums, are actually the result of the child's developmentally appropriate expression of normal feelings. When parents understand that these new feelings and expressions are normal and necessary for their child's successful maturation, they may be more able to tolerate the behavior and to set age-appropriate limits. The physician should talk to parents about the normal yet challenging behaviors their children are likely to demonstrate before they actually do; thus parents will feel empowered to manage their child before he or she gets out of control. Setting consistent limits, praising good behavior, and ignoring bad behavior (within reason) are the hallmarks of good discipline. When discussing behavior problems with parents, the physician's exploration with them of their feelings of frustration at the child's behavior is helpful. Acknowledging these feelings to the empathetic and understanding ear of the physician in the safe environment of the office setting is often an important first step towards successful management of the child's behavior. Occasionally, a group meeting between parents with children of similar ages can be helpful for sharing ideas and helping parents realize that their experience is not unique.

E.   Sexuality. The appropriate time to begin discussing the concept of sexuality as a normal, lifelong developmental process (much like sleeping, feeding, or elimination) is early in infancy with parents first and then with the child once he or she is old enough. Adolescence is too late to bring up sexuality issues for the first time. A teenager may be uncomfortable talking about these issues with a physician who has never mentioned the subject before. By starting these discussions in infancy and continuing them throughout childhood, parents will feel more knowledgeable and comfortable as sexuality educators of their children.

F.   Parenting. This component of anticipatory guidance includes the central theme of good parenting—namely, the mutual enjoyment of parent and child. Physicians can help parents view child rearing as rewarding and enjoyable by remaining sensitive to the extreme challenges some parents may experience, especially single or medically or emotionally limited parents. The physician should give parents practical and age-appropriate tips to enhance interaction with their children and should compliment their good parenting skills. They should be encouraged to keep a sense of humor too. Many parents easily get so bogged down in the routine of day-to-day child care that the joy is overlooked, and the environment may then hold the potential for neglect or even abuse. Each health maintenance visit is an opportunity for the physician to reassess the parent/child interaction, to identify potential problems, and to intervene as necessary. The physician may also recommend a favorite book on parenting to supplement in-office counseling.

ADDITIONAL READING

American Academy of Pediatrics. *Guidelines for health supervision III,* 3rd ed. Elk Grove Village, IL: American Academy of Pediatrics; 1997.

Green M, Palfrey JS, eds. *Bright futures: guidelines for health supervision of infants, children, and adolescents,* 2nd ed. Arlington, VA: National Center for Education in Maternal and Child Health; 2000.

Kreipe RE, McAnarney ER. Psychosocial aspects of adolescent medicine. *Semin Adol Med* 1985;1:33–45.

Rudolph AM. Counseling and anticipatory guidance. In: Rudolph AM, ed. *Rudolph's pediatrics.* Norwalk, CT: Appleton & Lange; 1991.

Schulman JL, Hanley KK. *Anticipatory guidance: an idea whose time has come.* Baltimore: Williams & Wilkins; 1987.

Books for parents

Christophersen ER. *Beyond discipline: parenting that lasts a lifetime.* Kansas City: Westport Publishing Group; 1990.

Christophersen ER. *Little people: guidelines for commonsense child rearing,* 3rd ed. Kansas City: Westport Publishing Group; 1988.

Schmitt B. *Your child's health,* rev. ed. New York: Bantam Books; 1991.

Web Sites

http://www.brightfutures.org/
http://www.aap.org

10 ♣ Injury Prevention: A Guide for Pediatricians

Michael A. Gittelman
and Constance M. McAneney

If a disease were killing our children in the same proportions as injury, we would be outraged and demand this killer be stopped.
—C. Everett Koop, former surgeon general of the United States.

As indicated by Dr. Koop's quote, injuries are one of the most serious health problems facing our society. They are the leading cause of disability and death among the pediatric population and a major contributor to health care costs. In the past, injuries were overshadowed by other causes of illness. However, with the introduction of vaccines and antibiotics, many of these diseases have been controlled, but injuries continue to take a heavy toll on our children's lives. Today the health care community has become more involved in trying to control these injuries. The development of both the National Center for Injury Prevention and Control and the Centers for Disease Control and Prevention (CDC) has been instrumental in funding research and preventive programs to combat this problem. As advocates within our community, pediatricians must also be aware of common pediatric injuries, successful prevention techniques, and methods for educating their families to prevent these occurrences, ultimately reducing injuries among children.

I. Magnitude of the Problem

Well known is the fact that injuries are the leading cause of death for persons 1 to 44 years of age. They account for approximately 82,000 deaths per year for individuals within this age range in the United States. For children between 1 and 19 years of age, injuries cause more death than all other diseases combined. However, mortality is only a small portion of the problem. The amount of morbidity and disability cost among this population, as well as the health care costs forced upon the community as a result of injuries, is enormous. Each year 16 million children who are less than 20 years of age visit an emergency department in the United States because of an injury, resulting in approximately 600,000 hospital admissions and 30,000 permanent disabilities. This means that nearly one out of every four children receives medical attention for an injury. As a result, the annual direct and indirect cost of injuries within the United States has been estimated to exceed $260 billion. This makes injuries the second largest source of medical expenditures in the United States (exceeded only by circulatory diseases).

In reviewing the data on injuries, the *National Vital Statistics Reports,* compiled by the CDC, categorizes injury mortality by mechanism (e.g., drowning or falls) with subcategories showing intent (e.g., unintentional, homicidal) (Table 10.1). Unintentional injuries make up most injury deaths, accounting for 92,353 (63%)

Table 10.1.   Number of deaths by mechanism of injury for children <24 years of age

Cause	Unintentional	Homicides	Suicides	Other	Total
Motor vehicle	12,708	—	25	6	12,739
Occupant					7,951
Pedestrian					1,280
Motorcyclist					396
Bicyclist					324
Firearm	442	5,456	2,714	191	8,803
Drowning	1,630	39	35	37	1,741
Poisoning	811	26	338	174	1,349
Fall	361	10	82	20	473
Fire/scald	884	74	25	15	998
Other	2,524	1,626	1,274	126	5,550
Total	19,360	7,231	4,493	569	31,653

Source: Mortality files of the National Vital Statistics Reports, 1999.

out of the 146,400 deaths, for all ages, from the 1997 data. In the pediatric population (age <24 years), 31,653 children died due to injury. Motor vehicle collisions and firearm deaths were the major contributors, with falls, poisonings, and drowning as the next most prevalent causes.

II.   Epidemiologic View of Injury

Recently, as injuries have been shown to be the leading cause of death for our children in the United States, the idea of preventing injuries has become an important goal; however, this concept is not a novel one. In the first portion of the twentieth century, people involved in an injury event were believed to be reckless and indifferent. In an attempt to eradicate these behaviors, several educational programs were implemented within various communities (e.g., 1920, traffic safety; 1950, home safety). However, in 1942, Hugh DeHaven, a pilot and researcher, showed that structural revisions and biomechanical changes, as opposed to attitude adjustments, could actually decrease the damage that occurred during an injury event. These changes could "modify injuries and enhance survival within accidents."

In the late 1940s, John Gordon added to Hugh DeHaven's concepts and began to model injury epidemiology after a similar framework used by infectious disease specialists. He introduced the concept of an "epidemiologic triangle," where an injury event was due to the interaction of the host, the agent (vector), and the environment. By preventing any of these parts or intersecting any section of the triangle, the injury could be limited. William Haddon, Jr, considered by many to be the father of injury prevention, applied Gordon's model in developing interventions to control injuries. Haddon later adapted the theory and added his

**Table 10.2.   Matrix framework for injury cause
and prevention for motor vehicle collisions**

Phases	Host	Agent/ Vehicle	Physical Environment	Socioeconomic Environment
Preevent	Age of the child; driver's ability	Appropriate car seat; car brakes, lights	Weather conditions; road conditions	Traffic; over-crowding; speed limits.
Event	Wearing safety belts	Car in good condition; bumpers, air bags	Driving surface; shoulder lanes	Seat belt laws; attitudes about belting
Postevent	Child's health status, age		EMS systems; trauma centers	Funding for EMS; training EMS personnel

Adapted from Haddon's model.

concept of a phase-factor matrix. This model united the host/agent/ environment model with the preevent, event, and postevent phases for preventing injuries (Table 10.2). These phases also help to differentiate between the types of prevention strategies sought (i.e., primary, secondary, or tertiary). For example, primary prevention (preevent) deals with reforms that prevent the injury; secondary prevention (event) involves techniques that minimize any injury that does occur, and tertiary prevention (postevent) employs mechanisms to reduce disability if a child is injured.

III.   Approach to Prevention

Today Haddon's matrix is still utilized in injury prevention models. However, to apply his techniques, one must first begin with accurate and available data sources. This information is necessary to identify specific individuals at risk for childhood injuries. Once the target population has been determined, injury control strategies geared to the high-risk children can be implemented. As more advanced technology and data banks become developed (e.g., trauma registries and national surveillance systems), more information is obtainable for identifying and targeting specific populations at risk. Thus more research can be established, and more appropriate intervention programs can be originated. Finally, after a particular intervention is under way, it must be evaluated. If an injury control measure is unsuccessful, then it should be discontinued so that resources may be utilized for more effective programs.

The most successful prevention strategies are usually passive techniques (i.e., work automatically). Child safety caps on medications, safer roadways, and automatic safety belts exemplify passive preventive concepts. In contrast, active strategies—ones that require action by an individual to prevent an injury (e.g., putting on a bicycle helmet or placing a battery in a smoke alarm)—are usually not as successful. In reality, most prevention ideas have a combination of both active and passive techniques; yet the more emphasis on passive measures, the more successful the program is in decreasing injuries.

IV. Pediatrician's Role

Most prevention strategies today involve one or more of the following three ideas: product modification, enforcement of safety regulations, and education. Pediatricians are the primary educators for parents and their children. Thus they play a crucial role in curbing injuries within their communities. Table 10.3 provides pediatricians with a suggested list to guide them in discussions with parents at each age level. The goal of these discussions is to determine what motor and cognitive milestones a child has achieved and will achieve by the next health maintenance visit and to anticipate the injuries they are most likely to encounter. If parents are aware of these potential injuries, they may be more successful in preventing them. For many topics repetitive counseling to parents of specific prevention strategies is encouraged to remind parents and their children continually. Of course, discussing all pediatric injuries in detail is beyond the scope of this chapter; however, potential injuries common for each developmental age will be presented. A more complete listing of the most lethal and common injuries and the successful prevention techniques will follow.

V. Specific Injury Prevention Topics

When counseling parents on injury prevention at well-child checks or ill visits, specificity is crucial. Vague generalities, such as "watch your child" or "be careful," are usually not helpful in educating caretakers on injury prevention. The following are specific techniques and questions to ask when counseling families about common pediatric injuries.

A. Injuries involving motor vehicles. Injuries from motor vehicle crashes are the leading cause of unintentional injury-related deaths in children under 14 years of age. The three-point lap/shoulder restraints are thought to reduce the risk of death or serious injury by 45%, and car seats for children reduce the risks by 70%. Most motor vehicle collisions occur close to home, so proper restraint should be used whenever traveling, no matter how short the distance. The rate of use of car seats is about 75% for infants but drops to 29% for children older than 3 years. Current estimations indicate that 85% of car seats are used improperly. Front seat air bags are estimated to reduce risk of death by an additional 9% among belted drivers and by 20% among unbelted front seat passengers. Air bags have caused deaths in some collisions; occupants at risk are infants in rear-facing car seats, children under 13 years of age, and adults shorter than 62 inches. All but two of the reported deaths were of children in rear-facing

Table 10.3.   Injury Prevention topics to be discussed with families during their well-child care visits

Development Age	Injury Topic—Specific Concerns
Prenatal/newborn	**Crib safety**—slat distance, firm mattress, "back to sleep," raised sides **Hot water heaters**—heater thermostat <120°F, check water temperature with wrist **Car safety seats**—read owner's manual, securely fasten, place in back seat **Smoke detectors**—change batteries yearly and *Smoking should be prohibited in the house* **Sun exposure**—avoid overexposure to sun, sunscreen in older infants
Early infancy (2 wks. to 6 mo.)	**Toy safety**—avoid sharp objects and small objects (object is too small for children <3 years of age if it fits in a toilet paper roll) **Falls/rolling**—window guards and watch when on high surfaces **Infant walkers**—should not be used due to risk of falls down stairs and possible delay in motor skills
Late infancy (6 mo. to 2 yr.)	**Home safety**—walk at child's eye level to "get their view" (e.g., gates at top of stairs, cover sockets, hanging tablecloths, electrical cords, lock cabinets, store guns and ammunition separately, lower crib mattress, etc.) **Changing car seats**—at 1 year and 20 lb may face forward (back seat) **Ingestions**—ipecac in house, poison control center telephone number, lock away poisonous substances, cleaning equipment, family medicines **Water safety**—four-sided fences around pools, watch near toilets, buckets of water, bathtubs
Preschool (2–5 yr.)	**Traffic safety**—teach pedestrian safety, watch near streets **Playground safety**—check for energy-absorbing surfaces, observe on equipment higher than 3 feet **Pet awareness**—caution in approaching strange pets, especially when eating. Teach not to pull or tug on pets. **Fires**—avoid playing with matches, home escape plans **Caregiver**—discuss discipline skills; should know CPR **Dealing with strangers**

(continued)

Table 10.3.   *Continued.*

Development Age	Injury Topic—Specific Concerns
School age (5–12 yr.)	**Seatbelts**—after booster seat is too small **Bike safety**—always wear a helmet, know rules of the road **Sports protective gear**—such as mouth guards, helmets, and knee pads **Internet and TV safety**
Adolescence	**Alcohol and drug abuse** **Driving safety**—you and passenger should always wear a seat belt, defensive driving skills, follow the speed limit **Firearms**—guns should still be stored safely in house, if there at all, with ammunition separate, do not carry or use a weapon of any kind **Conflict resolution techniques**—negotiation and dealing with anger **Self-protection**—should never be emotionally, physically, or sexually abused in any way

car seats or unbelted passengers. Therefore specific counseling tips include the following:

1. *Buckle children 12 years of age and under in the back seat.*
2. *Use restraints appropriate for size and age.*
   a. ***Under 1 year and less than 20 pounds,*** use rear-facing car seats.
   b. ***For children 20 to 40 pounds and more than 1 year of age,*** use forward-facing car seats.
   c. ***With children 40 to 80 pounds (4 to 8 years),*** use booster seats.
   d. ***If the shoulder belt lies across the child's neck or the lap belt is across the abdomen,*** the child is not ready for seats belts.
3. *Make sure the car seat is properly buckled into the car and that the child is properly buckled into the car seat.*

B.   Injuries involving bicycles. Children 5 to 14 years of age have the highest injury rates on bicycles. Head injuries in the overall population account for one-third of injuries treated in emergencies departments, two-thirds of hospitalizations, and three-fourths of deaths related to bicycles. Helmets are very effective in preventing head injuries, decreasing risk of brain injuries by 88% according to one study. Specific counseling tips include the following:

1. *Follow the principle of "No helmet, no bike."*
2. *Set a good example.*

3. *Make sure helmets fit properly.*
4. *Measure the child's head for the parents and direct them to a reliable source to purchase the helmet.*
5. *Suggest helmet use for other sports in which participation makes one prone to head injury* (skate boarding, in-line skating, skiing, street hockey, horseback riding).

C. Injuries due to falls. Falls are a common reason that infants and children end up in the emergency department. Whether the fall is from a bed or out of a window, on the playground or in the house, certain precautions can be taken to prevent injuries:

1. *Don't leave infant unattended on sofa, bed, changing table.*
2. *Place a rug beneath the crib and changing table.*
3. *Check to see that crib rails are locked.*
4. *Move furniture away from windows.*
5. *Place safety gates on stairs.*
6. *Place window guards on windows on the second story and up.*
7. *Supervise indoor and playground activity.*
8. *Remind parents that trampolines are dangerous.*

D. Injuries from poisoning. More than 1 million children under the age of 6 years are unintentionally poisoned each year. Packaging regulations have greatly reduced the rates of poisoning deaths in children in this country. Despite that, poisonings continue at an astounding rate. Caretakers need to be counseled about locking up not only prescription medications and caustic cleaners but also items that might not be perceived as dangerous, such as vitamins (iron content can be toxic), mouthwash (high alcohol content), and acetaminophen. Storing chemicals in old food containers misleads the curious child and causes many poisonings. Counsel for parents includes the following:

1. *Don't overlook the danger over-the-counter medications and toiletries as potentially poisonous substances.*
2. *Don't store chemicals in food containers.*
3. *Flush expired medication.*
4. *Post the local Poison Control Center number near phone.*
5. *Keep a supply of Ipecac in the home.* (Instruct parents to call the local Poison Control Center before giving.)

E. Injuries from fires and scalding. Three-fourths of the deaths from fires are due to smoke inhalation. A 70% reduction in risk of death by fire occurs if a functioning smoke detector exists in the home. Tapwater scaldings account for 10% to 15% of burns in young children at high risk. A full-thickness burn will occur in less than 2 seconds with water from a water heater set at 140°F. By turning the temperature down to 120°F or lower, the time is extended to 10 minutes. Prevention of other scald burns is difficult, and continued education of caretakers is needed. Counseling tips include the following:

1. *Never drink hot drinks while holding a child.*
2. *Keep hot liquids away from the edge of a counter or table.*
3. *Avoid tablecloths.*
4. *Make the stove off-limits for children.*
5. *Cook on back burners with handles turned to the rear.*
6. *Set hot water heater below 120°F.*
7. *Test water before placing a child in the tub, and never leave a child in a bathtub unattended.*

  F.   Injuries from drowning. Among children 1 to 4 years of age, many drownings occur in swimming pools. The mortality from infant drowning (most commonly in bathtubs) has increased over the past 20 years. Many prevention strategies have been studied; the following have been found useful:

1. *Fence pools on all four sides with a height of 5 feet and a child-proof gate.*
2. *Keep rescue equipment and a phone at poolside.*
3. *Always supervise pool activity.*
4. *Never leave an infant or small child unattended in the tub.*
5. *Ensure that adult supervisors know how to swim.*

  G.   Injuries from firearms. Experts estimate that 40% of American homes have some type of firearm in the home. Firearms in a home increase the risk of suicide by a factor of 4.8 and the risk of homicide by a factor of 2.7. Most childhood unintentional shootings happen in or around the house. The American Academy of Pediatrics has developed a program to educate physicians about counseling families on the risks of firearms in the home. The effectiveness is not known. Strategies to be considered include counseling the parents to do the following:

1. *Store guns unloaded and in a locked case.*
2. *Store ammunition separately in a locked case.*
3. *Have trigger locks on guns.*
4. *Be aware of firearms in friends' houses.*
5. ***Have a gun-free home.***

VI. Conclusion
  As evident by the litany of statistics, one can see that injuries are a major cause of morbidity and mortality among the pediatric population. Any effort made to reduce these potential injuries will decrease the numbers of children harmed within the community in which one lives. Pediatricians can play a significant role by becoming involved with legislation, identifying children at increased risk for injury, implementing preventive strategies, and educating families about injuries at every well- or ill-child visit. The increased awareness of parents should increase their supervision and anticipation to prevent injury, ultimately reducing the morbidity and mortality of childhood injuries.

ADDITIONAL READING
American Academy of Pediatrics, Committee on Injury and Poison Prevention. *Injury prevention and control for children and youth,*

3rd ed. Elk Grove Village, IL: American Academy of Pediatrics; 1997.

Baker SP, O'Neil B, Ginsburg MJ, et al. *The injury fact book,* 2nd ed. New York: Oxford University Press; 1992.

Brenner RA, Smith GS, Overpeck MD. Divergent trends in childhood drowning rates, 1971 through 1988. *JAMA* 1994;271:1606–1608.

Centers for Disease Control. Child passenger restraint use and motor-vehicle related fatalities among children—United States, 1982–90. *MMWR* 1991;40:600–2.

DeHaven H. Mechanical analysis of survival in falls from heights of fifty to one hundred and fifty feet. *War Med* 1942; 2:586–596.

Division of Injury Control, Centers for Disease Control. Childhood injuries in the United States. *Am J Dis Child* 1990;144:627–652.

Eichelberger M. *Pediatric trauma: prevention, acute care, and rehabilitation.* St. Louis, MO: Mosby-Yearbook; 1993.

Feldman KW, Schaller RT, Feldman JA, McMillon M. Tap water scald burns in children. *Pediatrics* 1978;62:1–7.

Gordon JE. The epidemiology of accidents. *Am J Public Health* 1949;39:504–515.

Haddon W Jr. A logical framework for categorizing highway safety phenomena and activity. *J Trauma* 1972;12:193–207.

Hal MJ, Owings MF. Hospitalizations for injury and poisonings in the United States, 1991. Advance data from *Vital and Health Statistics,* National Center for Health Statistics 1994;252:1–12.

Haught K, Grossman D, Connell F. Parents' attitudes toward firearm injury prevention counseling in urban pediatric clinics. *Pediatrics* 1995;96:649–653.

Johnston C, Rivara FP, Soderberg R. Children in car crashes: analysis of data for injury and use of restraints. *Pediatrics* 1994;93:960–965.

Kahane CJ. *Fatality reduction by airbags: analyses of accident data through early 1996.* Washington, DC: National Highway Traffic Safety Administration; 1996. (Report no. DOT HS 808 470.)

Kellerman AL, Rivera FP, Somes G, et al. Suicide in the home in relation to gun ownership. *N Engl J Med* 1992;327:467–472.

National Center for Injury Prevention and Control. *Ten leading causes of injury death in the United States.* Atlanta: Centers for Disease Control and Prevention; 1996.

National Vital Statistics Reports, Vol 47, No. 19, June 30, 1999 (http://www.cdc.gov/nchs/data/nvs47_19.pdf).

Pearn JH, Wong RKY, Brown J III, Chung YC, Bart R Jr, Hammar S. Drowning and near-drowning involving children: a five-year total population study from the City and County of Honolulu. *Am J Public Health* 1979;69:450–454.

Rivara FP, Grossman DC, Cummings P. Injury prevention. *N Engl J Med* 1997;337:613–18.

Runyun CW, Bangdiwala SI, Linzer MA, Sacks JJ, Butts J. Risk factors for fatal residential fires. *N Engl J Med* 1992;327:859–863.

Thompson DC, Rivara FP, Thompson RS. Effectiveness of bicycle safety helmets in preventing head injuries: a case-control study. *JAMA* 1996;276:1968–1973.

Thompson RS, Rivara FP, Thompson DC. A case-control study of the effectiveness of bicycle helmets. *N Engl J Med* 1989;320:1361–1367.

Web Site

http://www.cdc.gov/ncipc/osp/data.htm (CDC National Center for Injury Prevention & Control)

11 ♣ Infant Dental Care

James F. Steiner

The American Academy of Pediatric Dentistry recommends a visit to the pediatric dentist when the first primary tooth erupts but at no later than 12 months of age. Before that first dental visit, oral health recommendations should be provided by the primary care physician. This chapter gives the health care provider the information necessary to recognize high-decay-risk behaviors, a description of oral physical examination findings, and anticipatory guidance recommendations to ensure optimal oral health.

I. History
The well-baby dental history should identify decay risk factors.

A. Ask about feeding practices—the more times per day children eat or drink, the greater the risk of caries.

Does the infant sleep with the nursing bottle or, if breast feeding, with the mother? If the child is eating table food, is the meal schedule regular, or is the child's eating and drinking unsupervised? Are multiple caretakers, such as child care centers or grandparents, involved in feeding?

B. Ask about oral hygiene routines. Daily brushing reduces caries risk. (*Who cleans the child's teeth? How are they cleaned? What is the frequency of cleaning? Is fluoride toothpaste used, and if so, how much?*)

C. Ask about fluoride availability. Dietary and topical fluoride reduces caries risk. (*Is the family's drinking water optimally fluoridated? If it is not, have fluoride supplements been prescribed?*)

D. Ask about nonnutritive sucking. (*Does the child suck a digit or a pacifier? What is the frequency and intensity of sucking? Is the pacifier worn on a cord around the neck? Before use, is the pacifier dipped in a sweetened liquid?*)

II. Oral Physical Examination
The physician should perform this part of the physical examination with the infant supine on the examination table. A bright light, a tongue blade, and gloves are needed.

A. Determine the number of teeth present. The mandibular primary incisors are the first primary teeth to erupt at approximately 6 months of age. The 20-tooth primary dentition is completed by 36 months of age. If no teeth have erupted by 12 months of age, refer the child to a pediatric dentist.

B. Look for plaque. Plaque is a soft, white material that collects on teeth along the gum line. *Streptococcus mutans* resides in plaque and converts dietary carbohydrates to acid. The acid demineralizes enamel, creating a chalky white line, which begins the decay process. Plaque should be cleaned from the teeth daily with a toothbrush to disrupt the caries process.

C. Remove plaque and look for demineralized enamel. If plaque is observed, it should be rubbed off with gauze, and the underlying enamel should be dried and inspected. De-

84

mineralized areas that appear chalky and whiter than the surrounding normal enamel are the initial clinical signs of dental caries. Daily tooth cleaning by the guardian is one way to stop the demineralization and prevent the formation of a cavity.

D. Examine for dental caries. If plaque is not removed regularly and the child's feeding practices are high risk, demineralization continues, developing caries. Caries is a light brown break in the enamel that will continue to enlarge slowly. When dental caries is suspected, refer the patient to a pediatric dentist.

III. Anticipatory Guidance

Providing oral health information for families during the first year of life can establish healthy oral hygiene routines. The physician should offer advice regarding the following:

A. Feeding practices. Bottle-fed children should be held when feeding and should not sleep with the bottle, which puts them at high risk for early-childhood caries (nursing caries) because of the presence of bacterial substrate in contact with the teeth for a prolonged period of time. The upper front teeth are the most severely affected; they can develop decay as early as 12 months of age in high-risk feeders. If the practice continues, decay eventually affects other newly erupted teeth as well.

Infants who sleep with their mothers and breast-feed unsupervised while their mothers sleep are likewise at high risk for early-childhood caries. The physician should advise caretakers at each well-baby visit that unsupervised sleeptime bottle- or breast-feeding is a high-risk behavior for dental decay. When weaning is introduced and table foods enter the diet, caretakers should be advised that children with unrestricted access to food and drink increase their risk for decay. The physician should recommend a feeding pattern of regular mealtimes and two snacks daily. Water should be the only liquid consumed between meals and snacks.

B. Oral hygiene. Cleaning the gum pads once daily using a clean, moist cloth or gauze without toothpaste should begin in early infancy. As teeth erupt, parents should change to an infant toothbrush and brush the teeth at least once daily to remove plaque. Brushes designed for infants and toddlers are available in pharmacies and supermarkets. At 24 months of age, a pea-sized amount of fluoride toothpaste can be placed on the toothbrush. Adults should supervise and assist with brushing until children develop the fine motor skills necessary to brush effectively, which usually coincides with the ability to tie shoes.

C. Fluoride. Water fluoridation reduces the incidence of dental caries 40% to 50%. If drinking water is not optimally fluoridated, the physician should prescribe fluoride supplements as indicated in Table 11.1. Supplements are available as liquid, chewable tablets, tablets, and vitamin/fluoride combinations in 0.25-, 0.50-, and 1.0-mg concentrations. Before

Table 11.1.   Recommended daily fluoride intake (mg/day) relative to the fluoride concentration in the local water supply

Patient Age	<0.3 ppm*	0.3–0.6 ppm*	>0.6 ppm*
6 months–3 years	0.25	0	0
3–6 years	0.50	0.25	0
6–16 years	1.00	0.50	0

*Fluoride concentration in drinking water in parts per million (ppm).

recommending fluoride supplements, the health care provider should determine the amount of fluoride in the patient's water supply. The local water department can be contacted for fluoride levels in the community water supply. If the family has well water, health departments and commercial laboratories can analyze well water for fluoride concentration. Fluoride toothpaste also prevents caries. Guardians should be advised to select a toothpaste that has the American Dental Association seal on the packaging. Fluoride products must be stored out of children's reach.

D.   Nonnutritive sucking. If an infant begins to suck a thumb or finger, caretakers should try to interest the infant in a pacifier, which is easier to discontinue. Pacifiers never should be hung on a cord around the baby's neck because of the risk of strangulation, nor should they be coated with honey or another sugary substance. The physician should encourage pacifier weaning at about 3 years of age. Thumb- or finger-sucking intervention should begin at 5 to 6 years of age. A very gentle technique to help children stop the sucking habit is described in the book *My Thumb and I*, which is listed in the "Additional Reading" section of this chapter.

E.   The first dental visit. Infants should be referred to the pediatric dentist when the first primary tooth erupts or at no later than 12 months of age. This establishes a dental home for the family. Dentoalveolar trauma is very common as the children begin to walk. Having a dental home will facilitate access to care if dentoalveolar trauma occurs.

ADDITIONAL READING

American Academy of Pediatric Dentistry. *Reference manual: pediatric dentistry special issue 1999–2000*; 21(5).

Hale KJ, Heller K. Fluorides: getting the benefits, avoiding the risks. *Contemp Pediatr* 2000;17:121–128.

Mayer CA. *My thumb and I: a proven approach to stop a thumb or finger sucking habit, for ages 6–10.* Glenview, IL: Chicago Spectrum Press; 1997.

Web Site

http://www.aapd.org (American Academy of Pediatric Dentistry)

12 ♣ Normal Speech and Language Development

Ann W. Kummer

The ability to communicate affects all activities of daily living, including the ability to learn and to develop social relationships. To answer questions from parents and to identify children at risk for a speech or language disorders, the primary care practitioner should be knowledgeable about the normal stages of communication development. Since a communication disorder can have a significant adverse effect on the developing child, early identification and intervention are important. In addition, early treatment often results in faster progress and a more favorable prognosis.

I. Definitions
   A. Speech (articulation). Speech, or *articulation,* can be defined as the physical production of individual sounds. It involves movement of the articulators (i.e., the lips, tongue, jaw, and velum) in coordination with respiration and phonation to form speech sounds, known as *phonemes.* These movements, and thus sounds, are produced in sequence to form spoken words.
   B. Language. Whereas speech is the physical component of verbal communication, *language* is the cognitive component. Language can be defined as the meaning or message conveyed between individuals. Although verbal language is the most common form of communication among humans, language can take other forms or modalities, such as the written form, signs, gestures, facial expressions, or even the taps of Morse Code. In assessing a child's language development, one must look at both receptive and expressive language.
      1. *Receptive language* is the child's ability to understand the language of others. The child typically demonstrates this understanding by appropriate responses to questions, requests, or commands.
      2. *Expressive language* refers to the child's ability to choose appropriate words to convey a message (semantics), to use the appropriate word forms (morphology), and to put the words together in an appropriate order in a sentence (syntax). Expressive language also includes the ability to use language in an appropriate way following the social rules of conversation (pragmatics). Both articulation and language skills begin to develop at birth. Although these skills develop concurrently, each component is discussed separately in this chapter for the sake of clarity. Table 12.1 summarizes the basic speech and language milestones of normal development.

II. Articulation Development
   A. Birth to 6 months
      1. *Articulation development* actually begins with the *birth cry.* With early cries, the infant must coordinate respi-

**Table 12.1.   Normal developmental milestones
for speech and language development**

2 Months
  Watches the speaker's face.
  Cries are differentiated by needs.
  Coos with vowel sounds.

4 to 6 Months
  Localizes to sound.
  Coos with intonation.
  Vocalizes in response to others.

6 to 9 Months
  Responds to name.
  Recognizes names of family members.
  Responds to simple commands accompanied by a gesture.
  Uses gesture for communication (pointing, reaching, waving
    for hi/bye).
  Imitates actions (as in Peek-a-Boo).
  Babbles using early developmental consonants (i.e., *b, m, w, d, n, g*).

10 to 12 Months
  Begins to point to some body parts following a command.
  Follows simple, one-part commands (i.e., "Get your shoe.").
  Gives objects to others upon verbal request.
  Jargons with different sound combinations.
  May begin to use first words.

12 to 18 Months
  Can identify many objects and pictures following a verbal
    command.
  Follows commands easily.
  Listens more to the meaning of conversations.
  Uses several single words.
  Communicates with a combination of words and gestures.

18 to 24 Months
  Understands concepts (adjectives, pronouns, plurals).
  Follows compound and complex commands.
  Uses two- to three-word combinations.
  Tries to tell about experiences.
  Begins to use more speech sounds, such as fricatives (*f, s, sh*).

2 to 3 Years
  Shows interest in explanations for "why" and "how" questions.
  Uses phrases and short sentences for communication.
  Begins to use more complex morphologic and syntactic forms.
  Speech is intelligible most of the time.

3 to 4 Years
  Uses long and structurally complex sentences.
  Tells stories and relates experiences from the past.
  Errors in syntax include regularization of irregular forms.
  Speech is intelligible to all listeners, although minor articulation
    errors are noted.

ration, phonation, and oral movements to produce a vocal sound.

2. *Purposeful sound making* begins at around 2 months of age, when the infant begins to coo. *Cooing* consists of sighs and various vowel sounds that the infant produces during "vocal play." Cooing is an important stage of articulation development because during this stage, the child learns to manipulate the oral mechanism to produce sounds in a purposeful manner. The child also learns to associate tactile/kinesthetic sensations with an acoustic result, thus developing an important oral/auditory feedback loop. Cooing becomes more intonated by 4 to 6 months of age as the child learns to produce contrasts in pitch and intensity.

B. Six to 12 months

1. *Babbling* begins at around 6 months and is characterized by the production of consonant sounds in a repetitive manner (e.g., ma ma ma, ba ba ba). Like cooing, babbling provides the child with an opportunity to practice sound production and to develop the oral/auditory feedback loop to produce sounds purposefully. During the babbling stage, the child learns to produce many of the early developmental phonemes, or speech consonants. When classified by place of production, these include the bilabial sounds (p, b, m), lingual/alveolar sounds (t, d, n), and velar sounds (k, g).

The babbling sounds are developed early because the place of production is easy to access and the manner of production is relatively easy. For some of the babbling sounds, the oral cavity is completely closed by either the tongue or the lips. Air pressure builds in the oral cavity and is released suddenly. Since the sudden release of air pressure is explosive in nature, these sounds are called *plosives*. Examples of plosives include /p/, /b/, /t/, /d/, /k/, and /g/. Other early sounds, called nasals, also require the oral cavity to be closed by the lips or the tongue. With these sounds only, the velum remains down during production, as in humming, resulting in nasal resonance. *Nasal sounds* include /m/, /n/, and /ng/.

2. *Early developmental sounds*, called *jargon*, are produced by the child at 9 to 10 months in a variety of combinations rather than in a repetitive manner. Since various intonational patterns are used with the sound combinations, the child may appear to be actually speaking, but in a foreign language. In fact, many parents report that their child is talking in sentences but just cannot be understood. Of course, jargon is merely sound practice and not meaningful speech.

C. Twelve months to 3 years. The next stage of articulation development involves the acquisition of sounds produced by forcing the air stream through a narrow opening, causing a high-frequency friction sound. These sounds, appropriately, are called *fricatives* and include /f/, /s/, /z/, and /sh/. Not only are these sounds more difficult to produce than the early developmental sounds, but they also require the assistance of teeth. Most of the fricative sounds develop between 12 months and 3 years of age. Once fricative phonemes are acquired, the child begins to produce affricate phonemes, such as /ch/ and /j/. *Affricate phonemes* combine a plosive sound with a fricative; for example, /ch/ is produced by combining /t/ plus /sh/, and /j/ is produced by combining /d/ and /zh/. Since the child needs to be able to produce both plosive and fricative sounds individually before these phonemes can be combined, affricates are developed after these other sounds; some children find producing them difficult.

D.   Three to 6 years. The last sounds to be developed are usually /l/, /r/, /th/, and occasionally /v/. These sounds require more fine motor control than early developmental phonemes; therefore many children have difficulty with one or more of these speech sounds until about the age of 6.

E.   Referral guidelines. During the first year of life, most of the early developmental sounds should be well established because they lay the groundwork for the development of the speech sounds. If the infant is not cooing by 4 months or babbling by 8 months, the physician should monitor the child's developmental progress closely and should consider a referral to a speech/language pathologist. Evidence of oral/motor dysfunction, such as difficulty with feeding or swallowing, should also prompt a referral. If the child is not producing a variety of sounds in different combinations by the age of 12 months, this may be reason for concern. By 3 years of age, the child should have acquired the use of enough speech sounds so that his or her speech is intelligible most of the time. If speech is very difficult to understand at this age, a referral should be considered. By age 6, the child should have essentially "perfect" speech, with no errors in articulation. If articulation errors persist after this age, a referral to a speech/language pathologist is indicated.

III.   Language Development

Because we cannot actually hear or see the process, the development of receptive language is inferred. More is known about the process that children go through in the development of expressive language, however, because it is more easily observed and documented.

A.   Newborns. At birth, the infant, aware of sounds in the environment, startles or cries in response to loud or sudden noises. Studies suggest that infants are aware of even the differences between similar speech sounds (e.g., p and b). Awareness and discrimination form the basis of later understanding. Expressive language development begins with early cries, which are reflexive and stimulated by physical or environmental conditions, such as hunger or pain. The infant soon learns, however, that these cries bring about a caregiver response, such as feeding or attention. As a result, the infant begins to use crying and various vocalizations to elicit a response. Within the first few months, most parents can distinguish their infant's cries of hunger, pain, and needing attention.

B. Two to 6 months. By approximately 2 months of age, the infant achieves and maintains eye contact with others as they speak. By 4 months, the infant begins to vocalize directly to others with cooing and learns to imitate and to take turns in sound production. In the first 6 months, the infant is taking in all that he or she hears in the environment and may be starting to understand some words and phrases. However, the infant does not demonstrate much understanding of language at this point.

Caregivers and other speakers in the environment unknowingly assist the infant in learning to listen to and to understand language by using a unique speaking style (sometimes called baby talk). This style of speech is characterized by the use of short utterances with very simple syntax. A small core vocabulary is used, and topics are limited to the here and now. The same utterance is often repeated, and verbal rituals or games, such as "so big" or "patty cake," are frequently used. The speaker will usually alter his or her tone of voice when speaking to an infant, tending to use a high pitch with great pitch variation and intonation. Facial expressions and gestures are exaggerated during speech to capture the infant's attention.

C. Six to 12 months. At 6 to 8 months of age, the infant begins to display an association of meaning to the sound combinations heard in speech. The child looks up in response to his or her name and responds to *no* and simple commands, such as "*Come here*." Gestures accompanied by vocalizations are used as a form of expressive language at this developmental stage.

By 7 to 8 months, most babies have begun to use a pointing or reaching gesture that may mean one of two things: "*I want that*" or "*Look at that*." This gestural form of communication proves very effective at this age and communicates all the child's needs at that time.

By 10 to 12 months of age, the child is usually able to point to body parts, common objects, and simple pictures following a request. The child demonstrates understanding by responding to many simple, one-part commands. The child also babbles and jargons to others and occasionally uses single words with gestures for communication.

D. Twelve to 18 months. After the first birthday, the child follows many simple commands and seems to understand much of what is said to him or her. Since comprehension precedes production, the child is able to understand far more than he or she is able to say.

First words begin to emerge at 9 to 18 months of age; most children use at least one or two words by their first birthday. Many first words sound much like babbling (e.g., *mama, dada, bye bye*). They become true words when these sound combinations are used in an appropriate and meaningful way.

The child's first words are typically holophrastic. In other words, **milk** may mean, *"I want the milk," "I don't want the milk,"* or *"I spilled the milk."* Most first words are substantive words, such as nouns or verbs. Some functional words, such as *all gone, no, more,* or *that,* also emerge as first words. A few social words are acquired early in development as well, such as *hi* or *bye bye.*

The development of vocabulary skills is a very complex process that involves much more than mere memorization of labels. For children to learn a simple word, such as *chair,* they must first develop a mental prototype of this word based on perceptual features, functional features, or both. For example, a chair has the perceptual features of four legs and a flat surface. These features also apply to a table or a sofa, however. A chair has the functional features of something to sit in, but this is also true of a sofa. The child needs to determine which perceptual and functional features most clearly define a word for understanding and appropriate use to occur. In the case of *chair,* the child needs to determine that this word refers to an object that has a seat and a back and that only one person can sit on at a time. Once this realization occurs, the child can use the word appropriately in novel situations.

Children often make mistakes while learning the meaning of words. They commonly overgeneralize a word category by including inappropriate things in the category. For example, the child may assume that all animals with a long nose, four legs, and a tail are dogs. As the child acquires a better understanding of the features of the word category, he or she may make the error of exclusion. For example, the child may assume a Chihuahua cannot be a dog because it is too small. The process of learning to code and categorize words appropriately is obviously very complex, yet it must take place for the development of much of the entire lexicon.

E. Eighteen to 24 months. At 18 to 24 months, the child understands more complex language, showing a comprehension of some concepts, such as adjectives, possessive pronouns, and plural forms. The child begins to follow many compound and complex commands and starts to combine words for short utterances. At first, words are combined without regard to syntactical order. Each word usually has a downward intonational contour, suggesting that the word represents a complete sentence. For example, the child may say *dish, broke,* and *Tommy* as three separate sentences. The child then learns to combine words in an appropriate syntactic order for two- and three-word utterances. When this occurs, the child may then say, *"Broke dish"* or *"Tommy broke dish."*

Although much is written about the two-word stage of language development, most children begin combining two, three, and even four words around the same time. By 2 years of age, the child should be combining at least two or three words together for short utterances.

F.   Two to 3 years. At 2 to 3 years, the child demonstrates an understanding of long and complex sentences and shows an interest in verbal explanations of why and how. The child understands most forms of syntax and follows everyday conversation easily. From this point on, receptive language continues to develop, primarily in the area of vocabulary and in understanding idioms or subtle meanings. At this stage, the child's expressive language consists of phrases and short sentences. The child uses different syntactical forms, such as pronouns, plurals, past tense, question forms, and negation. The child first learns the rules of syntax and then the exceptions to those rules. Therefore syntactic errors, such as the following, are very common in the normal developmental process: *"I talk gooder than you," "I runned outside," "I got stang by a bee," "I have two feets."* These errors actually show that the child has learned the rules and how to apply them; however, learning all the exceptions takes time. Therefore these errors of regularizing irregular syntactic forms may persist even past school age.

G.   Three to 6 years. By 3 years of age, the normally developing child communicates with long and structurally complex sentences and begins to develop the pragmatic skills that relate to the social rules of conversation. For instance, the child learns to initiate a conversation appropriately, usually by saying, *"Hi,"* followed by the listener's name. The child becomes aware that, in a conversation, the speaker needs to reference pronouns before using them. The speaker also needs to consider what the listener knows about the topic so that the conversation can be geared appropriately. The child learns that ending a conversation on the telephone without saying, *"Good-bye"* is not appropriate. At this stage, the child begins to understand that the meaning of what is said often has to be inferred. For example, *"Could you please pass the salt?"* is actually a command and does not require an affirmative answer, and the idiom *"Two heads are better than one"* is not meant to be interpreted literally. This pragmatic understanding takes years to develop, and errors in understanding and use of conversation are common in preschool and early school years.

H.   Referral guidelines. If the child does not use any single words by 16 to 18 months of age and cannot follow simple commands, a speech/language pathology assessment should be considered. If the child does not combine words for short utterances by the age of 2 or use complete sentences by the age of 3, an evaluation is indicated. Finally, if the child's sentence structures are noticeably defective or the child has difficulty communicating ideas effectively at age 4, a referral should be made for a language evaluation.

IV. Key Points
   A. Although speech and language development are very individual and minor variations occur in the rate and sequence of development, the health care provider should be knowledgeable about the stages of normal development and proactive in screening for communication difficulties.
   B. Whenever there is a suspicion that the child is not developing speech or language skills normally, the child should be referred to a speech/language pathologist for a professional evaluation.
   C. The primary care provider should always listen to parents' concerns because parents are usually good observers of their own children. If parents are worried about the child's speech and language development, a referral for evaluation is appropriate. Even if therapy is not recommended at that time, the speech/language pathologist can provide the parents with developmentally appropriate activities to stimulate speech and language acquisition in the home.
   D. Early intervention is very important and ultimately can affect the long-term prognosis for normal communication skills. Ideally, intervention should occur in the preschool years to take advantage of the brain's plasticity for developing speech and language skills. If the communication disorder persists into the school-age years, not only does the child have more difficulty acquiring language skills, but habit strength also makes the disorder more difficult to correct. An investment in early intervention can pay off in the future with regard to treatment and educational costs.

ADDITIONAL READING

Bloom L, Lahey M. *Language development and language disorders.* New York: John Wiley & Sons; 1978.

Coplan J. The Early Language Milestone Scale (ELM-2). Austin, TX: Pro-Ed; 1993.

Coplan J. Normal speech and language development: an overview. *Pediatr Rev* 1995;16:91.

Foster S. *The communicative competence of young children: a modular approach.* London: Longman; 1990.

Lindfors JW. *Children's language and learning.* Englewood Cliffs, NJ: Prentice-Hall; 1980.

Owens RE. *Language development: an introduction,* 4th ed. Needham Heights, MA: Allyn & Bacon; 1995.

Reed V. *An introduction to children with language disorders.* New York: Macmillan; 1986.

Skinner PH, Shelton RL. *Speech, language and hearing,* 2nd ed. New York: John Wiley & Sons; 1985.

Taylor, CM. An examination of the development of language in the normal child. *J Child Health Care* 1999;3:35–38.

Web Site

American Speech and Hearing Association Web Site. www.asha.org/publications.

13 ♣ Normal Motor and Cognitive Development

Nancy E. Lanphear

Developmental assessment of the young child is a key function of all physicians who provide primary care to infants and children. Development is a dynamic process that must be monitored throughout the child's growing years. Acquisition of normal motor milestones does not necessarily equate with normal cognition. Autistic children may have normal motor milestones, just as children with delayed motor milestones due to cerebral palsy may have normal cognition.

I. Normal Developmental Milestones

Developmental milestones are traditionally divided into five areas: gross motor, fine motor, cognitive, social adaptive, and language. The average ages and age ranges at which accomplishments in each of these areas occur in the normal infant are the basis of the Denver Developmental Screening Test-II (DDST-II). This is the most commonly, although not universally, utilized screen in pediatric well-child care. (The DDST-II, as shown in Appendix E, was updated and published in 1992 and contains the standard milestones in chronologic order.) The authors of the DDST-II suggest that it be administered in the standardized manner with specific tools. However, it is also useful as a reference for the primary care physician, since it shows the age range of acquisition of the developmental milestones. The primary care physician must remember that the Denver screens are most useful in identifying children who have global developmental delay or mental retardation and that it may not identify children with more subtle developmental issues. Because other areas of development are covered elsewhere in this book, this chapter will address primarily motor and cognitive development.

Pediatricians do not have the time in a typical office setting to administer the DDST-II personally, making this means of developmental screening impractical. One solution to this time constraint is to have ancillary office personnel trained in administration of the DDST-II administer the test routinely at selected visits or when the history and physical examination suggest the need for a quantitative tool. A more practical model would be the concept of "Developmental Surveillance." In this model, the pediatrician elicits developmental and behavioral milestones as part of routine well-child care and assesses for parental concerns about development, maintaining a high index of suspicion if concerns are reported. Parents are important guides to a child's development and have repeatedly been shown to report concerns accurately when delays are present. If delays are suspected based on the health care provider's history and physical examination, further assessment is planned at the time of the well-child check (e.g., referral to a pediatric developmentalist).

Early identification of a child with motor delay and/or delays in other areas is desirable so that an intervention program can be undertaken. Public laws that mandate an appropriate education in the least restrictive environment for all children with developmental problems have been in place since 1986. Children from birth to 3 years of age are entitled to free intervention services that may include an early childhood developmentalist, an occupational therapist, a physical therapist, and a speech therapist. The need is determined by assessment and family wishes. Every state has its own laws, which generally require local availability of resources and referral programs. The primary care physician must be aware of these resources to provide appropriate referrals as necessary.

II.   Cognitive Development

A number of methods can be used to determine cognitive development and intelligence. When testing these functions in children, the physician must recognize and accept that cognitive development and intelligence are affected by many factors besides genetics, many of which may not be readily apparent at the time of testing. These factors include environmental stimulation, cultural practices, motor function and development, and sensory function and development. As an infant and toddler, cognitive skills are assessed by observing a child's interaction with toys, obtaining language milestones, and observing problem-solving skills with standardized blocks, puzzles, and pegboards. Formal testing of cognitive skills is not typically performed by primary care physicians but is obtained by referral to an appropriate site, such as local or regional centers for developmental evaluation, psychologists, school systems, and some early-intervention systems.

Formal tests of cognitive development and intelligence include the following:

A.   **Bayley Scales of Infant Development** (0 to 2.5 years).
B.   **Gesell Developmental Schedule** (0 to 4 years).
C.   **Batelle Developmental Inventory Screening Test** (6 months to 8 years).
D.   **Stanford Binet IV** (2 years to adult).
E.   **Wechsler Preschool Primary Scale of Intelligence** (4 to 6 years).
F.   **Wechsler Intelligence Scale of Children** (5 to 15 years).

III.   Motor Development

During early childhood development, the primitive reflexes are replaced by voluntary motor control, which is under the control of higher cortical centers. Motor development in general proceeds in a cephalocaudad direction, characterized by the acquisition of oculomotor control at birth to 16 weeks, head and arm control (16 to 28 weeks), trunk and hand control (28 to 40 weeks), walking and running (second year), and mature motor control by

5 years. Observing symmetry of motor movements as well as the regular acquisition of developmental milestones is important. As infant sleep position has shifted from belly to back, children spend less time on their belly and may attain some of the prone milestones slightly later. Remind families to encourage babies to be on their bellies when awake. Motor development is a cumulative process, and higher-level skills are dependent on lower-level skills.

Significant delays in motor skills may indicate global developmental delay (mental retardation), primary motor delays (such as are seen in cerebral palsy), or environmental deprivation.

The following list outlines **typical fine and gross motor development**:

- **Two months**—with ventral suspension, head in same plane as body; lifts head on flexed forearms; hands open 75% of the time; active grasp of a toy.
- **Three to 4 months**—with ventral suspension, head held up beyond body plane; lifts head and chest off flat surface on extended forearms.
- **Four to 5 months**—slight head lag on pull to sit, rolls over prone to supine, crude reach and grasp, hands with midline play, toy to mouth, shakes rattle.
- **Six to 7 months**—bears full weight on legs if held standing, sits with support, begins to support self leaning on forearms.
- **Eight months**—independent sit; may assume quadruped position, good reach, developing palmar grasp patterns, bangs toy; takes two 1-inch cubes.
- **Nine to 11 months**—forward parachute, crawls, pincer grasp, pulls to stand, cruises, puts small toy in container but will not release.
- **Twelve to 14 months**—pivots in sitting, attains independent walking (average 12 months, range 9 to 15 months), releases toys into container, may show preference for one hand.
- **Fifteen to 18 months**—creeps up stairs, stoops and recovers, begins stiff run, walks with pull toy, turns pages of a book, scribbles in imitation and then spontaneously.
- **Twenty-four months**—walks up and down stairs, rarely falls, kicks large ball, tower of 6 cubes, turns door knob, overhand throw.
- **Three years**—pedals a tricycle, stands on one foot for a second, jumps from bottom of step, unbuttons, zips and unzips, tower of nine to 10 cubes.
- **Four years**—stands one foot for 5 seconds, hops on one foot, buttons clothes, pours from pitcher.
- **Four and a half years**—heel-to-toe maneuver, catches a bouncing ball.
- **Five to 7 years**—skips, ties shoelaces, copies or writes first name, rides a two-wheeler.

IV.   Primitive Reflexes in the Infant

Normal motor development depends on an intact peripheral and central nervous system, normal muscle tone, the presence and later integration of primitive reflexes, and the development of postural and righting reflexes. Persistence of primitive reflexes can interfere with normal motor development.

In addition to the routine developmental milestones suggested by the DDST-II or on the list of milestones, the neurologic examination of the infant should include an evaluation of several primitive reflexes that, although normal in the first 3 or 4 months of life, should disappear at certain ages. Persistence should alert the physician to neurodevelopmental abnormalities, such as cerebral palsy. At the same time, certain postural reflexes develop as neurodevelopmental maturation occurs. These primitive and postural reflexes are described in the following paragraphs.

   A.   Moro reflex (Fig. 13.1). The infant is cradled in a semi-reclined position of about 45 degrees; the head is supported with the examiner's hand. Keeping the hand and forearm under the head and trunk, the examiner drops the infant's body downward and back. The sudden loss of support should produce a good Moro response without letting the baby's head fall back unsupported. The young infant responds (positive Moro) by extending the arms from the body and quickly opening the hands and fingers. This movement is good for early detection of asymmetry in the upper extremities. The response should disappear at approximately 4 months of age.
   B.   Asymmetric tonic neck reflex (Fig. 13.2). The infant is placed in a prone position (on the back). Keeping the neck in line with the body and stabilizing the trunk with one hand, the head is gently turned to one side and held for about 10 seconds, watching the child's arms. With a positive response, (e.g., head turned to the left), the infant responds by flexing the right elbow and straightening the left arm. The asymmetric tonic neck reflex is normally present in infants 1 to 4 months old.
   C.   Pull to sit (Fig. 13.3).
      1.   *Under 4 months:* The head lags behind the body.
      2.   *Four to 5 months:* The infant keeps the head in line with the body.
      3.   *More than 5 months:* The head leads the body.
   D.   Body lying prone (Fig. 13.4).
      1.   *Birth to 2 months:* Head in line with the body.
      2.   *Two to 4 months:* Head elevated to about 45 degrees.
      3.   *Six months:* Head elevated to 90 degrees.
   E.   Sitting posture. With the child in the sitting position, the observer notes the curvature of the back. Normal responses are the following:
      1.   *Less than 4 months:* Completely rounded back.
      2.   *Four months:* Extension or straightening of back to the level of the third lumbar segment.

(*text continues on page 103*)

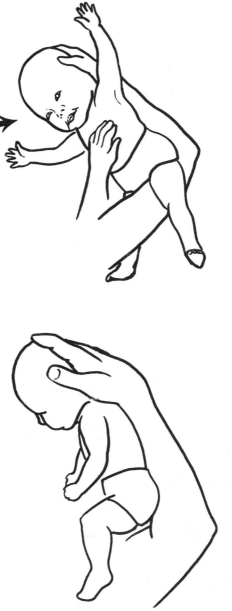

Figure 13.1. Moro reflex.

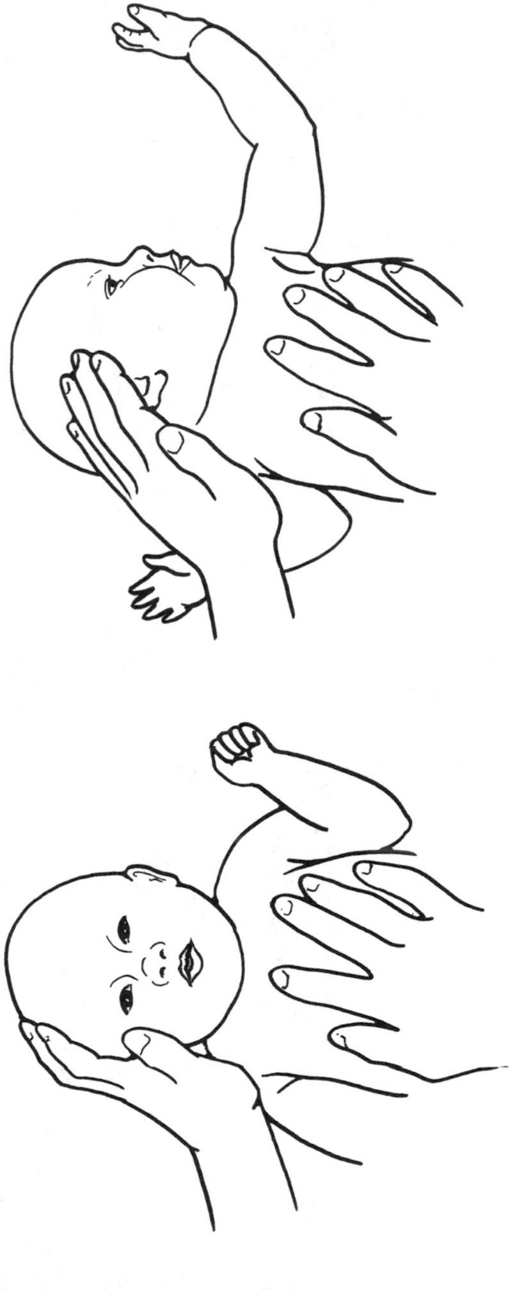

Figure 13.2.   Asymmetric tonic neck reflex.

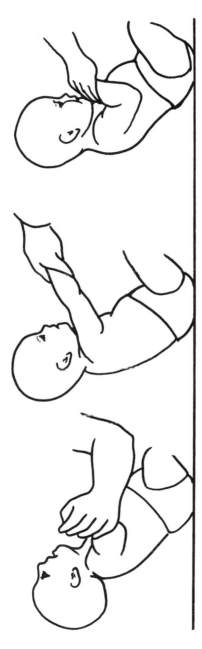

Figure 13.3. Pull to sit.

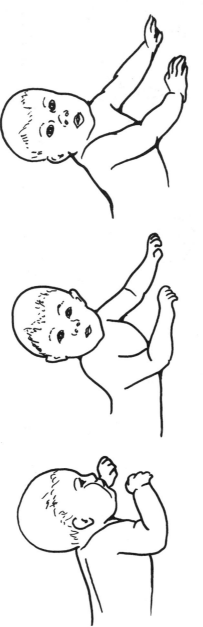

Figure 13.4. Body lying prone.

3. *Six months:* Extension or straightening upper and lower back, and propping forward with hands.

4. *Seven months:* Extension or straightening upper or lower back, and propping forward with hands.

5. *Eight months:* Sitting erect with no difficulty.

F. All fours (Fig. 13.5)—refers to child's ability to assume the all-fours position.

1. *Three and a half months:* Infant props on forearms/hands (Fig. 13.5A).

2. *Five months:* Infant supports self on hands (Fig. 13.5B).

3. *Seven to 9 months:* Infant on hands and knees (Fig. 13.5C).

4. *Ten to 12 months:* Child in plantigrade position on hands and feet (Fig. 13.5D).

G. Head in space. The infant is held in vertical suspension and tilted slowly, first sideways each way, then forward and backward. For an infant with poor head control or a premature newborn, be careful to prevent hyperextension of the neck when tilting the child backward.

When tilted, the infant should try to adjust the head so that it remains upright regardless of the body position, with the eyes and mouth horizontal and the nose vertical. This reaction normally begins to appear at about 1.5 months of age and is complete by 4 months.

H. Downward parachute (Fig. 13.6). The test for the downward parachute response should be attempted only after the child has demonstrated head control. The child is lifted vertically some distance from the examination table. Once the legs are somewhat flexed, the child is rapidly lowered 2 to 3 feet to simulate the feeling of falling. If no response is elicited by lowering to the tabletop, lower the child to the floor. The normal infant at about 4 months of age reacts by straightening and spreading the legs and turning feet outward.

I. Standing ability. To test the infant's ability to stand, hold the child upright above the examining table. Note whether the child can support the body's weight well. Normal development of this ability is as follows:

1. *Five months:* Able to support own weight; legs are semiflexed.

2. *Eight months:* Able to stand with support, with trunk slightly forward and hips flexed.

3. *Ten months:* Able to stand erect with support.

4. *Twelve months:* Able to stand independently.

Primitive supporting reactions are tested by holding at least part of the infant's weight. An infant younger than 2.5 months immediately stiffens the legs in extension ("positive supporting"). If the child is between 2.5 and 5 months of age, the legs may collapse as the infant is lowered toward the table ("astasia").

(*text continues on page 106*)

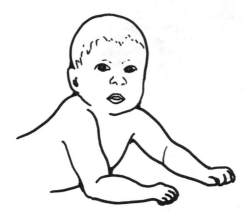

A.

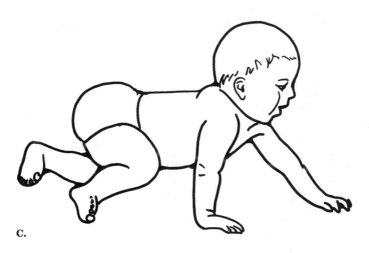

C.

Figure 13.5.   All fours. Figures are lettered A through D according to their chronological order in normal development.

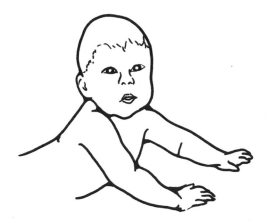

B.

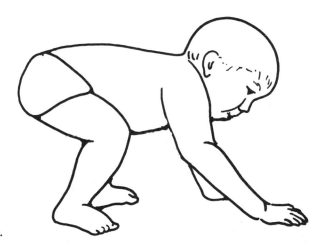

D.

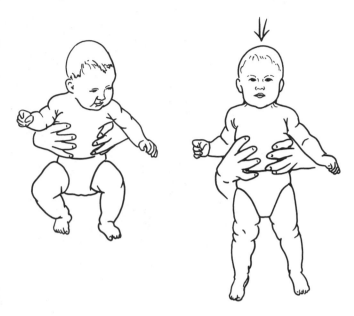

Figure 13.6.   Downward parachute.

J.   Sideways parachute (Fig. 13.7). After the age of 6 months, a normal infant attempts self-protection from falling by extending the arm and open hand.

K.   Forward parachute (Fig. 13.8). Like the other parachute reactions, this should not be tested until the child has demonstrated head control. The infant is held firmly at mid-trunk level, with back to the examiner. The child is suspended vertically above the table, then tilted forward suddenly. A normal infant reacts by straightening arms in front of the body and extending the fingers. This reaction may be seen in infants as young as 7 months. Asymmetry in the upper extremities can be detected in this maneuver.

L.   Backward parachute (Fig. 13.9). Again holding the child in the sitting position, the infant is gently tipped backward. Usually a child 9 months of age or older reacts to the sudden imbalance by either extending both hands behind the body or by rotating to one side to catch the body with the hand. This should not be tested in a child who does not have good head control to avoid rapid flexing and extension of the neck.

(*text continues on page 110*)

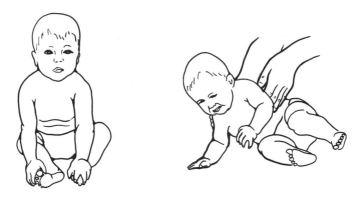

Figure 13.7.   Sideways parachute.

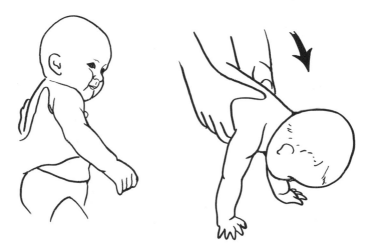

Figure 13.8.   Forward parachute.

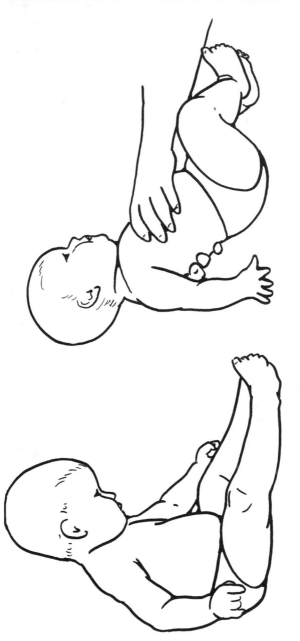

B.

A.

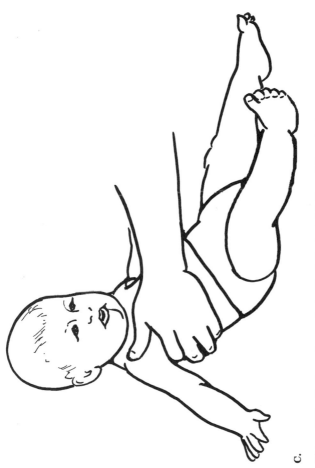

C.

Figure 13.9. Backward parachute. The lettering of A, B, and C on the figures indicates the order of progression in the parachute test.

ADDITIONAL READING

Bayley N. *Manual for the Bayley Scales of Infant Development.* San Antonio: Psychological Corporation; 1969.

Frankenberg WK, Dodds J, Archer P, et al. The Denver II: a major revision and restandardization of the Denver Developmental Screening test. *Pediatrics* 1992;89:91–97.

Frankenberg WK, Thornton SM, Cohrs ME. *Pediatric developmental diagnosis.* New York: Thieme-Stratton; 1981.

Gesell A, Amatruda CS. *Developmental diagnosis.* New York: Harper & Row; 1967.

Thorndike RL, Hagen EP, Sattler JM. *The Stanford-Binet Intelligence Scale: guide for administering and scoring,* 4th ed. Chicago: Riverside; 1986.

Wechsler D. *The Wechsler Pre-school and Primary Scale of Intelligence (WPPSI).* New York: Psychological Corporation; 1967.

Wechsler D. *Wechsler Intelligence Scale for Children—Revised Manual (WICS-R).* New York: Psychological Corporation; 1974.

Web Site

http://snapper.utmb.edu/pedi/MedicalEducation/H&D/ (Health and Development Curriculum)

14 ♣ Preparticipation Sports Physical

Raymond C. Baker

The primary purpose of the preparticipation sports physical (PSP) is to perform a focused health assessment to uncover physical conditions that might negatively influence the young athlete's ability to compete safely and effectively and to ensure that such competition is appropriate to the athlete's age and body habitus. More specifically, the physician can identify conditions that predispose the athlete to injury or sudden death as related to the type of sports under consideration. Secondary objectives of the sports physical are (a) to provide the primary care physician the opportunity to have input into the athlete's choice of sports activities, (b) to identify contagious diseases and suggest appropriate precautions necessary to prevent spread to other athletes during competition, and (c) to perform a more comprehensive health maintenance supervision visit for adolescents with a history of noncompliance with routine health care.

The PSP should precede sports participation by 6 to 8 weeks, when possible, to allow time to evaluate any abnormalities that might be uncovered by the examination. Although the primary care provider's office is ideal for the PSP, especially when part of a comprehensive health maintenance visit, effective sports physicals can be performed on groups of athletes with several physicians manning stations focused on individual components of the examination, such as review of history (perhaps from a questionnaire completed by the athlete); vital signs and growth parameters; visual acuity; head, ears, eyes, nose, and throat examination; cardiorespiratory and genital (males) examination; neuromusculoskeletal examination; and finally review of the findings, fitness determination, and written documentation (often a legal requirement). The method is often less costly to the athlete and parent (local physicians may volunteer their services in the spirit of community) and may offer a better opportunity to identify specific abnormalities when specialized physicians take part.

HISTORY

The medical history is the most important part of the PSP and uncovers up to three-fourths of conditions that might affect participation in sporting activities. A questionnaire may be used in the interest of time, but the physician still needs to review the findings with the athlete to clarify and to expand responses before proceeding. The important elements of the PSP medical history follow:

I. **Assessment of General Health**
   A. **Illnesses requiring hospitalization.**
   B. **Surgery,** especially when resulting in loss of a paired organ.

C. Chronic illness requiring ongoing medical care, physician visits, and/or chronic medications (e.g., seizure disorder, diabetes, asthma).

D. Allergic conditions, especially asthma and insect reactions.

E. Heat related illness.

F. Menstrual history.

G. Medications, supplements, or vitamins, especially used for the purpose of weight loss or improved athletic performance.

H. Immunization history, especially most recent tetanus booster.

I. Drug or alcohol use.

J. Recent gains or losses of weight or body image distortion.

II.   **Orthopedic/Injury History**

A. Significant extremity injury, especially a fracture or sports-related injury necessitating missing more than three consecutive days of usual activities or practice.

B. Head trauma with concussion, because of increased risk of "second impact syndrome."

C. Chronic lower back pain, when suggestive of spondylolysis/spondylolisthesis.

D. Accident prone, both at home and in sports—parents are a better source of this information.

III.   **Cardiopulmonary History**

Several conditions have been associated with sudden death in athletes—hypertrophic cardiomyopathy, congenital coronary artery anomalies, aortic rupture with Marfan syndrome, myocarditis, dilated cardiomyopathy, dysrhythmias, aortic stenosis, and premature atherosclerosis. Asthma is likewise an important diagnosis to uncover, if not previously recognized, in order to begin appropriate treatment to maximize the athlete's performance. The history should include questions focused on the following conditions:

A. Syncope or dizziness during or after exercise— associated with hypertrophic cardiomyopathy and congenital coronary artery anomalies.

B. Chest pain during or after exercise—same associations as A.

C. Fatigue that occurs more easily than that of peers during exercise.

D. Abnormalities of the heart (racing, "skipped a beat," "flopping around in my chest")—associated with congenital coronary artery anomalies.

E. Heart murmur or hypertension on previous examinations—associated with aortic stenosis.

F. Family history of death from heart problems before age 50—associated with hypertrophic cardiomyopathy, Marfan syndrome, premature atherosclerosis.

IV. Targeted Review of Systems
  A. Glasses/contacts required or has difficulty seeing blackboard.
  B. Dental appliances or braces.
  C. Skin rashes—might suggest contagion (folliculitis, impetigo, herpes simplex, molluscum contagiosum, verrucae, tinea, pediculosis, scabies).
  D. Numbness or tingling in extremities—might suggest previous spinal cord injury.
  E. Recurrent headaches.
V. Physical Examination
    The physical examination for the PSP should focus on those areas that are likely to determine fitness for athletic participation: growth parameters, blood pressure, heart and respiratory rate, and cardiovascular and musculoskeletal systems. In addition, the examination should assess muscular development and physical maturity (inferred from Tanner's stages of sexual maturity) to allow the physician to help determine the risk for contact/collision sports.
  A. Growth parameters—height, weight, and weight for height.
  B. Blood pressure (measured with appropriate-sized cuff in the right arm with the athlete seated), **heart, and respiratory rate.**
  C. Eyes—visual acuity; anisocoria (usually physiologic), which should be documented should head injury occur during sports participation.
  D. Lungs—auscult at rest and after brief period of exercise (e.g., jumping jacks) for evidence of bronchospasm.
  E. Heart—rhythm, including normal sinus arrhythmia, and murmurs.
  F. Abdomen—organomegaly increases risk of traumatic rupture.
  G. Genitalia (males)—Tanner stage of sexual maturity correlates with muscular growth and maturity, an important factor in determining eligibility for contact/collision sports. Examination for inguinal hernia, varicocele, and testicular mass.
  H. Skin—impetigo, folliculitis, tinea corporis, molluscum contagiosum, herpes simplex infection, and scabies.
  I. Musculoskeletal system (Table 14.1)
VI. Sports Participation Eligibility
    Following the history and physical examination of the athlete, the physician is usually ready to complete the appropriate documentation indicating eligibility for sports participation. The vast majority (98%) of sports physicals result in a clean bill of health and eligibility for sports participation. However, some abnormalities uncovered during the course of the history and physical examination will require further evaluation, treatment, and possible referral before eligibility can be sanctioned. The physician should discuss these issues with the athlete and the

Table 14.1.   Assessment of musculoskeletal system

Test/Instructions	Purpose of Test and Abnormalities of Importance
Stand, facing examiner	Acromioclavicular and sternoclavicular enlargement (sprain); asymmetric hips (leg length discrepancy or scoliosis); swelling of knee, ankle (sprain); asymmetry of thigh muscle bulk suggesting previous knee injury
Extension, flexion, lateral rotation, lateral bending of neck	Decrease suggests cervical injury or congenital deformity
Shrug shoulders	Trapezius strength
Arms abducted to 90 degrees resisting examiner's downward pressure	Deltoid strength
Hands clasped behind head in position of shoulder abduction and external rotation	Decreased range of motion (ROM)/pain suggests prior shoulder injury (rotator cuff, sub/dislocation, acromioclavicular sprain)
Hands clasped behind the lower back in position of shoulder adduction and internal rotation	Decreased ROM/pain suggests prior shoulder injury (rotator cuff, sub/dislocation, acromioclavicular sprain)
Flexion/extension of elbows	Decreased ROM suggests previous injury
Pronation/supination of forearms with upper arms adducted, elbows flexed to 90 degrees	Decreased ROM suggests previous injury
Spread fingers; make fist	Decreased ROM suggests previous injury
Stand on heels, toes	Muscle strength of anterior/posterior (calf) muscles, ankle sprain
Stand with back to examiner	Shoulder/tip of scapula asymmetry/pelvic tilt suggest scoliosis or leg length discrepancy; asymmetry of calf muscle bulk suggestive of previous knee/ankle injury
Stand and bend backward from waist	Decrease/pain suggests spondylolysis or spondylolisthesis
Bend forward at waist, legs straight, and touch toes	Decreased with hamstring tightness; kyphoscoliosis if posterior ribs on one side
Duck walk three or four steps with buttocks on heels	Inability to completely flex and support weight suggests previous knee/ankle injury

athlete's parents so that the expectations are clear. The following abnormalities require further evaluation and treatment before the athlete can be cleared for participation in sports activities:

A. Growth parameters and history suggestive of an eating disorder.

B. Hypertension—moderate to severe.

C. Cardiac abnormality—murmurs (other than recognizable functional murmurs), arrhythmias (other than sinus arrhythmias).

D. Bronchospasm (wheeze)—untreated reactive airways disease can significantly influence athletic performance and stamina.

E. Decreased visual acuity—uncorrected.

F. Organomegaly on abdominal examination.

G. Skin—impetigo, folliculitis, tinea corporis, molluscum contagiosum, herpes simplex infection, and scabies unless affected areas can be completely covered during the sporting activity (contact sports only).

H. Symptomatic inguinal hernia, testicular mass, varicocele.

I. Postconcussion syndrome—history of recent concussion with symptoms of postconcussion syndrome (cognitive/memory impairment, irritability, headache, depression, anxiety, fatigue, dizziness).

J. Orthopedic injury/condition—sprains, strains, subluxation/dislocation, muscle contusion, overuse injury, fracture, scoliosis.

The final determination of eligibility for sports participation depends on many variables. Although the history and physical examination are important and may be the deciding factors, other factors also influence the determination of eligibility: athlete's age, musculoskeletal maturity, type of sport, and intensity of the sporting activity (degree of competition). A complete discussion of these many factors is beyond the scope of this chapter. Furthermore, the physician performing the PSP may or may not have the interest or expertise to make these determinations with the limited information presented here. The reader is referred to and encouraged to consult *Preparticipation physical examination,* 2nd ed., written by the American Academy of Family Physicians, the American Academy of Pediatrics, the American Medical Society for Sports Medicine, the American Orthopaedic Society for Sports Medicine, and the American Osteopathic Academy of Sports Medicine.

ADDITIONAL READING

American Academy of Family Physicians, the American Academy of Pediatrics, the American Medical Society for Sports Medicine, the American Orthopaedic Society for Sports Medicine, and the American Osteopathic Academy of Sports Medicine. *Preparticipation physical evaluation,* 2nd ed. New York: McGraw-Hill; 1997.

Andrews JS. Making the most of the sports physical. *Contemp Pediatr* 1997;14:183–205.

Callahan LR. The evolution of the female athlete: progress and problems. *Pediatr Ann* 2000;29:149–153.

Cavanaugh RM, Miller ML, Henneberger PK. The preparticipation athletic examination of adolescents: a missed opportunity? *Curr Probl Pediatr* 1997;27:109–120.

Corrado D, Basso C, Schiavon M, et al. Screening for hypertrophic cardiomyopathy in young athletes. *N Engl J Med* 1998;339:364–369.

Glover DW, Maron BJ. Profile of preparticipation cardiovascular screening for high school athletes. *JAMA* 1998;279:1817–1819.

Gomez JE, Lantry BR, Saathoff KNS. Current use of adequate preparticipation history forms for heart disease screening of high school athletes. *Arch Pediatr Adolesc Med* 1999;153:723–726.

Harris S. The preparticipation examination. In: Reider B. *Sports medicine: the school-age athlete,* 2nd ed. Philadelphia: WB Saunders; 1996:95–114.

Krowchuk DP. The preparticipation athletic examination: a closer look. *Pediatr Ann* 1997;26:37–49.

Maron BJ, Shirani J, Poliac LC, et al. Sudden death in young competitive athletes: clinical, demographic, and pathologic profiles. *JAMA* 1996;276:199–204.

Maron BJ, Thompson PD, Puffer JC, et al. Cardiovascular preparticipation screening of competitive athletes: a statement for health professionals from the sudden death committee (clinical cardiology) and congenital cardiac defects committee (cardiovascular disease in the young), American Heart Association Circulation. *Circulation* 1996;94:850–856.

Patel DR, Gordon RC. Contagious diseases in athletes. *Contemp Pediatr* 1999;16:139–164.

Web Site

http://www.physsportsmed.com/ppe_ad.htm
http://www.physsportsmed.com/children.htm

15 ♣ Adolescent Health Maintenance Supervision— Overview

Thomas S. Webb

INTRODUCTION

The adolescent visit is an underutilized yet extremely valuable opportunity to have a significant impact on the health and well-being of the developing teen. Although well-child checks are frequent during infancy and early childhood, many families taper the number of routine physicals during the school-aged years. Most medical interventions are for illness only. This is especially unfortunate for the adolescent, who is experiencing radical physical and emotional changes. Both parents and teens are struggling with issues of maturity, independence, responsibility, and communication. The provider can guide both parents and teens through the physical and developmental changes of adolescence, screen for potential risk-taking behaviors, and influence lifestyle and health decisions during these formative years.

Adolescence is typically defined as falling between the ages of 12 and 21. It is divided into three periods, early (12 to 14), middle (15 to 17), and late (18 to 21) adolescence. Changes occur in physical (puberty), cognitive, and psychosocial (adolescence) development at different times and independent rates during each of the three periods. Therefore reviewing the physical changes of puberty independently of the cognitive and psychosocial development of adolescence is necessary.

I. Puberty

The physical changes of puberty include alterations in body mass composition, a significant increase in skeletal growth velocity, the development of secondary sex characteristics, the "switching on" of the reproductive organs, and an increase in energy requirements and nutrient utilization.

II. Body Mass Composition

Puberty affects males and females very differently in body mass composition. Females decrease in lean body mass from about 80% to 75% total body weight. Adipose mass increases from an average of 15% to 27%. Conversely, males increase in lean body mass, from 80% to 90% and decrease adipose mass from 14% to 11%. For both sexes bone mass increases (males more than females), and epiphyseal plates mature.

III. Growth Spurt

An increase in skeletal growth velocity, the "growth spurt," generally starts during early adolescence and peaks in the later years of early adolescence or in the early part of middle adolescence. Females enter their growth spurt usually 1.5 to 2 years before males. In both sexes, the growth spurt lasts 2 to 3 years, averages 2.5 to 6 inches per year, and accounts for up to 25% of final adult height. Nutrition, sleep habits, and the general state of health can have a significant impact on the genetic potential of the growth spurt.

IV. Sexual Maturity (Tanner) Staging

The development of secondary sex characteristics usually occurs "silently." Because breast enlargement, penile enlargement, testicular development, and pubic hair development are usually embarrassing to both parent and teen, questions and concerns are often not addressed unless prompted by the health care provider. The usual but not universal progression of puberty is outlined in Appendix D.

V. Menarche/Spermarche

The development of the reproductive organs occurs frighteningly early in adolescence. Spermatogenesis begins during Tanner stage II at an average age of 13.5, usually before the growth spurt or significant pubic hair development. Menarche usually starts after the female growth spurt and during Tanner stage III, which often corresponds to age 13 to 14 also. However, menarche and ovulation are not synonymous, and many of the first year's menstrual cycles are anovulatory, which can result in irregular menstrual cycles and random fertility. Nutritional status and body fat composition have a significant impact on menarche and the menstrual cycle.

VI. Nutritional Requirements

After birth, the accelerated growth during puberty is second only to that in infancy. Total nutrient needs during this age are higher than at any other time in life. Optimal nutrition is necessary for achieving full genetic potential in linear growth, lean body mass, and sexual maturation. Skeletal growth requires adequate nutrients for bone mineralization, especially calcium and vitamin D. Tissue synthesis and increased red cell production require iron, nitrogen, zinc, and vitamin B-12. The other B vitamins—thiamine, niacin, and riboflavin—are needed to support the high energy demands of puberty. Fortunately, a balanced Western diet including milk, high-quality animal protein, grains, fruits, and vegetables usually suffices. Vegans, "crash" dieters, and low-income adolescents are at greater risk for malnutrition, however. In addition, teens with chronic medical problems, especially those with chronic infection, inflammation, malabsorption, or neuromuscular problems, are at significantly increased risk for nutritional deficiencies.

Although pubertal growth depends on the availability of increased calories, most adolescent nutritional needs are applied to the basal metabolic rate, a function of the lean body mass, and activity level. Only 5% to 6% of total intake is utilized for growth. Therefore excessive caloric intake or insufficient activity places the adolescent at risk for obesity.

VII. Cognitive

Adolescent cognitive processes develop independently of the physical changes of puberty. The teenager passes from concrete, egocentric thinking in early adolescence to more formal, "decentered" thought processes that allow the mature adolescent to grasp abstract ideas, consider several alternatives, and plan for the future. Awareness of this cognitive progression is important to the health care provider for several reasons. Concrete questions should be posed to the early teen, whereas more open-ended questions may be used with a late adolescent. The greatest risk-taking behaviors usually occur when physical maturity precedes cognitive development. Most important, delays or interruptions of cognitive development can have significant effects on education, employment, and independent living success.

VIII. Psychosocial

Psychosocial development can be characterized by the four I's. During adolescence the teenager focuses on body *image,* initially compared with peers, then with societal norms. Early adolescent identity focuses on normalcy compared with others, which develops into a sense of *individuality.* Throughout adolescence, the teenager strives for increasing *independence* from family. Finally, the adolescent attempts to form adult (and sexual) *interpersonal* relationships.

IX. Legal Issues

Providing care to adolescents often raises legal concerns, especially in areas of consent, confidentiality, and payment for care. The exact laws and statutes are state specific, but the concepts are similar.

A. Consent. Providing medical care to patients requires informed consent. In young children, this implies parental consent; however, consent for medical treatment of adolescents becomes complicated. At some point, the decision of the patient overrides the wishes of the parent. Generally, states recognize the age of 18 (or 19 in some states) as the age of majority, when a teenager can make independent, legally binding decisions. Before this age, the teenager is considered a minor and the responsibility of the parent.

There are exceptions to this age limit, also state specific, which can include the following:

1. *Mature minors.* Usually a minimum of 14 years old, these adolescents can provide informed consent for medical care if they can demonstrate an understanding of the risks and benefits of receiving care, the treatment is necessary according to conservative medical opinion, and good reason exists to avoid parent consent.

2. *Legally emancipated minors.* These adolescents have undergone formal court proceedings to declare independence from their parents. Typical reasons for emancipation include marriage, military service, or living separately and financially independently from parents.

3. *Medically emancipated minors.* These teenagers are not formally emancipated but are deemed capable of seeking medical care independently. Typical adolescents in this category are those who are pregnant, parents, runaways, homeless, or high school graduates.

4.   *Specific medical services.* State statutes may permit minors to receive medical care without parental consent for emergencies, sexually transmitted diseases, pregnancy-related care, contraception, abortion, substance abuse, and/or mental health services.

B.   Confidentiality. Legal issues surrounding confidentiality also vary by state. In general, an adolescent who can provide informed consent should receive the same confidentiality as an adult patient. Most states support confidentiality for minors seeking treatment for sexually transmitted diseases, pregnancy-related care, substance abuse, and mental health. There are some states that require parental notification for certain procedures (i.e., abortion); however, the teenager must have the option to seek a judicial bypass. Confidentiality can be breached for any patient who may be harmful to himself or others.

X.   Payment

Health care providers must contemplate payment issues with minor patients seeking confidential or independent medical care. Insurance billing may breach patient confidentiality if the parent receives the claim. Financially independent minors often have poor or no insurance, which may adversely affect compliance and continuity unless costs and payments are discussed proactively. Health care providers can financially help their patients and themselves by familiarizing themselves with any federal- or state-funded programs that can assist the adolescent patient.

XI.   Relationship

The method for conducting the adolescent visit depends on whether the patient and family have an established relationship with the provider. If a previous relationship exists, the provider can use the family's existing trust to introduce this next stage as a natural progression in the health care experience. If the family is new to the provider, outlining distinctly for the adolescent and parent the format and flow of the visit, the issues of consent and confidentiality, and the goals of the visit is important.

XII.   The Adolescent Visit

A.   History. An extended visit is necessary to perform complete interviews with both parent and adolescent and a comprehensive physical examination. Some primary care physicians use a preprinted questionnaire (see Appendix I) that the patient or patient and parent can complete in the waiting area before the visit. This may act as a springboard for discussion with the adolescent during the interview. Developmental stage, cognitive ability, and confidentiality must be carefully considered for this to be useful.

The interview should begin with both parent and patient in the room. If this is the first visit, the physician should introduce himself to the adolescent first and then the parent. The family should understand that the visit begins with both parent and patient. The adolescent is then seen alone for a confidential interview, followed by the physical examination with or without the parent, depending on the adolescent's preference. The parent will feel more comfortable knowing the private interview is part of the developmental process in which the adolescent begins an individual relationship with the health care provider. Reassure the parent that any indication of potential harm to the child or others will be relayed and that open communication with the parent will be encouraged.

The interview process should be performed with the patient clothed. The provider should observe the interaction between parent and child. Is it positive, obtrusive, or antagonistic? Does the child answer the health provider's questions or turn toward the parent for responses? Basic past medical history, family history, social history, medications, and review of systems can be asked of both the patient and parent during this time. Parental questions and health concerns can be addressed together also. If the parent becomes vague or appears uncomfortable, ask the adolescent to leave the room so the parent can speak freely. (Hearing and vision examinations could be done at this time.)

Once the parents have provided historical information and their questions have been addressed, the adolescent should be interviewed alone. This provides the opportunity to explain or reinforce confidentiality, to develop trust, and to encourage open communication with the parent. Nonjudgmental screening for high-risk behaviors and frank discussion and education regarding sexuality, substance use, and safety should occur.

Begin the interview with general questions about school, friends, and hobbies. Assess the patient's cognitive and psychosocial development using developmentally appropriate questions. When broaching sensitive topics, repeat your assurances and limitations of confidentiality. Don't make assumptions about the teen's sexual orientation, level of experience, or knowledge. Open-ended, gender-neutral, explicit questions produce better answers. A teen who is performing oral sex may not consider himself or herself "sexually active"; thus an opportunity to screen for sexually transmitted infections could be inadvertently missed. A similar approach is useful when discussing drug use, body image, and dieting issues and when screening for physical and sexual abuse.

One recommended approach includes first asking about the behaviors of the adolescent's peer group (*"Do you know anyone who smokes/drinks/uses marijuana/dates/kisses/ has oral sex/male–female sex/etc.?" "Do any of your friends do this?" "Have you ever. . .?" "Do you have any questions about. . .?"*). Adolescents are often closely aligned in behaviors with their peer group; therefore even if they deny these behaviors, the prudent approach is to perform appropriate screening, education, and risk reduction interventions. Remaining neutral and allowing the teen the opportunity to ask questions on these subjects facilitates the exchange of valuable information for the health care provider and patient.

Important topics to review include the following:
1. *Adequate sleep and aerobic exercise.*
2. *Nutrition*—iron intake, calcium and vitamin D intake, balanced diet.
3. *Eating disorders*—body image, dieting, purging.
4. *Tobacco use*, including smokeless tobacco.
5. *Alcohol use.*
6. *Prescription, over-the-counter, and recreational substance use* (including huffing, steroids, pep pills).
7. *Nutritional supplements, "organic" products.*
8. *Sexual activity/behaviors*—abstinence, birth control, infection control, specific behaviors, sexual identity.
9. *Depression, suicidal ideation or attempts.*
10. *Abuse*—emotional, physical, sexual.
11. *School problems, attendance.*
12. *Stealing, violence, weapons use or possession, gang activity, legal trouble, incarceration.*
13. *Homelessness, institutionalization*—past or present.
14. *Work/career plans*—current and future.

B. Physical examination. Although yearly check-ups are the most desirable, a minimum of three comprehensive physical examinations should occur, one at each of the three stages of adolescence. The teen should make the decision about whether the parent stays in the room. The health provider should step out while the patient disrobes; appropriate covering should be available. Important components of the comprehensive examination are the following:
1. *Blood pressure.*
2. *Growth parameters* (height, weight, weight for height) *and body mass index.*
3. *Vision screen*—myopia can develop or worsen in puberty.
4. *Tanner staging.*
5. *Scoliosis screening and musculoskeletal development.*
6. *Skin*, especially acne.
7. *Evidence of iron deficiency.*
8. *Pelvic examination*, if sexually active or over age 17.

C. Laboratory screening that is recommended at each visit includes the following:
1. *Complete blood count* (CBC), looking for iron deficiency anemia.
2. *Total cholesterol in adolescents with a family history of coronary artery disease or hypercholesterolemia or if the family history is unknown.*
3. *Urinalysis for leukocyte esterase* (LE) *in males believed to be sexually active.* A positive LE is sensitive for an asymptomatic chlamydial infection and warrants treatment.
4. *HIV serology in high-risk patients*, which includes the following:
   a. **More than one sexual partner in the last 6 months.**

   b. *Previous history of a sexually transmitted infection.*
   c. *Intravenous drug use.*
   d. *Sex with an intravenous-drug-using partner.*
   e. *Previous history of sex for drugs.*
   f. *Male/male sex.*
   g. *Living in a high-HIV-prevalence area.*
  5. *Pap smear in females believed to be sexually active or more than 17 years of age regardless of sexual history and for males participating in anal intercourse.*
  6. *Tuberculosis testing with purified protein derivative* (PPD) *if high risk*, which includes the following:
   a. *Low socioeconomic status.*
   b. *Residence in areas with high prevalence of tuberculosis.*
   c. *Exposure to tuberculosis.*
   d. *Immigrant status.*
   e. *Homelessness.*
   f. *History of incarceration.*
   g. *Employment or volunteer work in health care setting.*

D. **Immunizations.** The immunization record should be examined to ensure that basic immunizations have been given. Special attention should be given to the following:
  1. *Catch-up immunizations* for the adolescent who failed to receive immunizations previously.
  2. *Hepatitis B vaccine*, if not given previously.
  3. *Varicella vaccine* (if history is negative/unknown for disease and previous immunization; varicella serology may verify the former).
  4. *Measles, mumps, rubella (MMR) booster*, if not given previously.
  5. *Tetanus-diptheria, adult strength (Td) booster*, recommended at the early adolescent visit if more than 5 years have passed since the previous booster (at 4 to 6 years). Subsequently, Td boosters are recommended every 10 years.

XIII. Concluding the Adolescent Visit
  After the history and physical examination are completed, the primary care provider should sit down with the adolescent (usually alone; occasionally with both adolescent and parent, depending on the findings, recommendations, and circumstances) and discuss the findings of the examination and laboratory testing (if results are available; if not, make arrangements to contact the adolescent with the results) and provide anticipatory guidance in areas suggested by the history and physical examination. This discussion should be unhurried and informal, allowing the adolescent the opportunity to ask questions and to respond to suggestions. Many physicians provide adolescents and parents written information, which expands and supplements issues raised during the visit. Finally, follow-up should be arranged, and information should be given to the adolescent and parents regarding how and when to contact the office for appointments, information, or referrals.

ADDITIONAL READING

American Academy of Pediatrics Committee on Psychosocial Aspects of Child and Family Health. *Guidelines for health supervision III,* 3rd ed. Elk Grove Village, IL: American Academy of Pediatrics; 1997.

American Academy of Pediatrics. *Recommendations for preventative pediatric health care (RE9535).* Elk Grove Village, IL: American Academy of Pediatrics; 2000.

Committee on Psychosocial Aspects of Child and Family Health, American Academy of Pediatrics. *Guidelines for health supervision III,* 3rd ed. Elk Grove Village, IL: American Academy of Pediatrics; 1997.

Fox CE, III. *Put prevention into practice: clinician's handbook of preventive services,* 2nd ed. Washington, DC: U.S. Department of Health and Human Services; 1998.

Green M, Palfrey JS, eds. *Bright futures: guidelines for health supervision of infants, children, and adolescents,* 2nd ed. Arlington, VA: National Center for Education in Maternal and Child Health; 2000.

McAnarney ER, Kreipe RE, Orr DP, Comerci GD. *Textbook of adolescent medicine.* Orlando, FL: Harcourt Brace Jovanovich; 1992.

Neinstein LS. *Adolescent health care: a practical guide,* 3rd ed. Baltimore: Williams & Wilkins; 1996.

Pickering LK, ed. *2000 red book: report of the Committee on Infectious Diseases,* 25th ed. Elk Grove Village, IL: American Academy of Pediatrics, 2000.

U.S. Preventative Services Task Force. *Guide to clinical preventive services: report of the U.S. Preventative Services Task Force,* 2nd ed. Washington, DC: U.S. Department of Health and Human Services; 1995.

For Parents and Caregivers

Greydanus DE, ed. *Caring for your adolescent: ages 12 to 21.* Elk Grove Village, IL: American Academy of Pediatrics; 1991.

Web Sites

http://www.brightfutures.org/http://www.aap.org

http://www.ama-assn.org/adolhlth/adolhlth.htm (AMA Adolescent Health On-Line—includes Guidelines for Adolescent Preventative Services [GAPS])

II

Well-Child Visits by Age and Developmental Stage

16 ♣ Well-Child Visits: Prenatal

Raymond C. Baker

The prenatal visit of expectant parents with the primary care physician is the first step toward forging a strong bond between physician and family. Among primary care providers, a considerable variation in the types of prenatal visits that may be offered to prospective parents ranges from brief get-acquainted visits to extended visits during which a medical history, parental counseling, and office tours may take place. Some providers offer group prenatal visits where several families meet with the physician. This has the advantage of economy of time and adds an element of group sharing that many families find appealing.

The prenatal visit should accomplish several objectives from both the parents' and the physician's perspectives. For the **parents**, the prenatal visit offers the opportunity to evaluate the practice itself, based on information, such as call and fee schedules, insurance issues, hours, emergency coverage, the opportunity to see the same physician at each visit, and links with other physicians and facilities (referral patterns, admitting hospital). Most important, parents have the opportunity to evaluate the "personality" of the office and to see if it meets their needs—sociable versus businesslike, formal versus informal, child friendly versus clean and neat. Some families find convenient appointment times more important than continuity and timeliness more important than stickers and lollipops. Since many more families have two working parents, efficiency sometimes has to be a consideration when selecting a practice.

For the **physician**, the prenatal visit is a time to obtain medical information *from* the family that will influence the care of the infant and to provide information *to* the family.

I.   **Medical Information**
   A.   **Pregnancy**—illnesses, medications, smoking, alcohol, recreational drugs, previous pregnancy outcomes.
   B.   **Family history**—health of family members, familial diseases.
   C.   **Social history**—planned versus unplanned pregnancy, marital status, educational background, home environment, work, support systems.
   D.   **Delivery hospital and obstetrician.**
   E.   **Plans to breast-feed, circumcise.**
II.   **Information to Discuss with the Family**
   A.   **Nutrition**—breast versus bottle, maternal nutrition.
   B.   **Circumcision**—pros and cons.
   C.   **Preparations for the baby**—crib, clothing, supplies, car seat, finances, sibling preparation, books or other reading materials about infant care and parenting (see later).
   D.   **Safety issues**—car seats, smoke/carbon monoxide detectors, fire extinguisher, water heater temperature (120°F).
   E.   **Psychosocial issues**—parenting, babysitting, impact of an infant on the family, impact on siblings, going back to work.

   F.   Office and physician issues—appointment schedules
   for well-child care, emergency care, hours, after-hours availability, fees, insurance, telephone triage, method for notifying
   the physician of the birth.
 III. Closure
   A.   Entertain questions from the family.
   **B.   Provide written materials from the office and sug-
   gest commercially available reading materials.**
   **C.   Provide a business card with office telephone
   number, after-hours emergency number, and office
   address.**

ADDITIONAL READING

American Academy of Pediatrics Committee on Psychosocial Aspects
   of Child and Family Health. *Guidelines for health supervision III,*
   3rd ed. Elk Grove Village, IL: American Academy of Pediatrics;
   1997.
Green M, Palfrey JS, eds. *Bright futures: guidelines for health supervision of infants, children, and adolescents,* 2nd ed. Arlington, VA:
   National Center for Education in Maternal and Child Health;
   2000.

Books for Parents

Brazelton TB. *Touchpoints: your child's emotional and behavioral
   development.* Reading, MA: Addison-Wesley; 1992.
Markel H. *The practical pediatrician: the A to Z guide to your child's
   health, behavior, and safety.* New York: WH Freeman; 1996.
Schmitt BD. *Your child's health,* rev. ed. New York: Bantam Books;
   1991.
Shelov SP, Hannemann RE, eds. *Your baby's first year,* reprint ed.
   New York: Bantam Books; 1998.
Shelov SP, Hannemann RE, DeAngelis CD. eds. *Caring for your baby
   and young child: birth to age 5,* rev. ed. New York: Bantam Doubleday Dell; 1998.

17 ♣ Well-Child Visits: Newborn

Raymond C. Baker

The newborn visit in the hospital should be performed within the first 24 hours after birth, usually in the morning following birth. With early discharges the rule now, only one examination and contact with the infant and parents is possible before discharge, so this contact must be complete and must anticipate the parents' needs. The physician should review the maternal, birth, and nursery records before the examination to help direct the discussion with the parents and the examination of the infant. Important points in the perinatal history to note are the following:

I. Perinatal History
 A. Previous pregnancies and complications
 B. Maternal health during pregnancy and prenatal care, including serologic screening (hepatitis B, syphilis, HIV, rubella) and screening cultures for infection (gonorrhea, *Chlamydia,* group B streptococcus).
 C. Length of gestation, complications of delivery, Apgar scores, and birth weight.
 D. Resuscitation efforts/requirements in the delivery room.
 E. Screening tests performed.
  1. *Newborn metabolic screening tests,* as required by state law.
  2. *Blood type of mother and infant.*
  3. *Hearing screening* (evoked otoacoustic emissions or auditory brainstem response).
  4. *Blood glucose.*
 F. Nursery course (feeding, elimination, growth parameters, nursing observations of infant with parents).
 The examination ideally is performed in the presence of the parents so the physician can reassure parents during the examination and explain abnormalities on the examination. This is a good time to anticipate and answer questions the parents have about the infant and infant care, such as common skin conditions (dryness, facial rashes, erythema toxicum, transient pustular melanosis, mottling, and acrocyanosis), birth marks, conjunctival hemorrhages, gynecomastia, molding of the skull and cephalohematoma, normal infant movements (startle response, jitteriness, and chin quivering), cord care, circumcision care, bathing, feeding and weight gain, and elimination. The examination itself should be thorough with an emphasis on detecting congenital abnormalities and abnormalities related to the birth process itself.

II. Physical Examination
 A. Weight, length, and head circumference plotted on standard growth charts.
 B. Assessment of gestational age.
 C. Skin—jaundice, pigmented lesions, hemangiomata, Mongoloid spots, erythema toxicum, transient pustular melanosis,

xerosis, evidence of birth trauma (bruising, forceps marks, petechiae).

D. Head—fontanels, head shape.

E. Head, ears, eyes, nose, and throat—red reflex, nasal patency, external auditory canal and tympanic membranes, palate.

F. Cardiorespiratory—heart murmur, breath sounds.

G. Gastrointestinal/genitourinary—abdominal masses, kidney enlargement, cord, genitalia (vaginal discharge, circumcision, testes in scrotum), anal placement and patency.

H. Neuromusculoskeletal—clavicles for fracture, extremity anomalies, hips, symmetric movement of extremities, symmetric Moro reflex, suck reflex.

At the end of the examination, the physician should sit down with the parents and discuss the results of the physical examination, any screening tests that have been performed, and the infant's overall health. This usually leads to questions from parents that the physician, in answering, can use to lead into providing both general advice about the new baby and anticipatory guidance.

III. Anticipatory Guidance

A. Feeding and nutrition (breast or formula, formula preparation, feeding, burping).

B. Sleep habits of newborns and sleep position (back or side) **and crib safety.**

C. Skin and diaper care and bathing (e.g., recommend the kitchen sink, which is easier on the back than a tub, daily bathing not necessary, sparing use of mild soap).

D. Circumcision and cord care.

E. Vaginal discharge and bleeding.

F. Visitors and visiting.

G. Proper clothing for ambient temperatures.

H. Sibling reactions to the newborn.

I. Sneezing and hiccups.

J. Safety precautions. Avoidance of direct sun exposure, crib safety, pacifiers, water heater temperature, smoke and carbon monoxide detectors, fire extinguisher, car seats, cigarette smoking (*all* smoking must be done outside the home/apartment), precautions against being left alone on changing table or bed and with siblings, pets, and young children.

IV. Closure

At the end of the visit, the health care provider should identify problems and suggest a management plan, arrange for the first office visit, and explain to parents what to do in case of an emergency and how to contact the practice for problems. Many physicians also provide families with written materials to support and supplement the discussion about infant care.

Finally, the health care provider should review the infant's nursing orders and write any additional orders that might be indicated as a result of the history, physical examination, and discussion with the infant's parents. Specifically, the first hepatitis B vaccine should be given before discharge from the hospital.

ADDITIONAL READING

American Academy of Pediatrics Committee on Psychosocial Aspects of Child and Family Health. *Guidelines for health supervision III,* 3rd ed. Elk Grove Village, IL: American Academy of Pediatrics; 1997.

Green M, Palfrey JS, eds. *Bright futures: guidelines for health supervision of infants, children, and adolescents,* 2nd ed. Arlington, VA: National Center for Education in Maternal and Child Health; 2000.

Books for Parents

Brazelton TB. *Touchpoints: your child's emotional and behavioral development.* Reading, MA: Addison-Wesley; 1992.

Markel H. *The practical pediatrician: the A to Z guide to your child's health, behavior, and safety.* New York: WH Freeman; 1996.

Schmitt BD. *Your child's health,* rev. ed. New York: Bantam Books; 1991.

Shelov SP, Hannemann RE, eds. *Your baby's first year,* reprint ed. New York: Bantam Books; 1998.

Shelov SP, Hannemann RE, DeAngelis CD. eds. *Caring for your baby and young child: birth to age 5,* rev. ed. New York: Bantam Doubleday Dell; 1998.

18 ♣ Well-Child Visits—Early Postnatal: 1 to 2 Weeks

Raymond C. Baker

Because early discharge has become the standard of care in most areas of the country, many birth hospitals have shared with the primary care provider the responsibility for early follow-up with postdischarge nurse visits to the home some time during the first week of life. The home health nurse visits the homes of newborn infants within the first 1 or 2 days of discharge, evaluates feeding and nutrition, and assesses for problems, such as jaundice, that formerly would have been noticed while the infant was still hospitalized. The nurse may also obtain blood for newborn screening (for phenylketonuria, hypothyroidism, galactosemia, hemoglobinopathy, and others, depending on state law) if this was not done in the hospital. Problems identified at the home visit are then reported to the primary care physician of record. Breast-fed infants, particularly with first-time breast-feeding mothers, require close attention to prevent dehydration and jaundice exacerbation that may occur before milk letdown.

Most primary care physicians have also reacted to the policy of early discharge by instituting an early postnatal visit, usually within 1 to 2 weeks of birth—earlier for breast-feeding infants. The objectives of the early postnatal visits are (a) to evaluate nutrition and the establishment of weight gain, (b) to monitor breast feeding to avoid problems with dehydration and jaundice, (c) to reevaluate for congenital abnormalities and problems related to birth, (d) to check newborn metabolic screen results, and (e) to answer questions and provide anticipatory guidance to parents. Specific historical information that is important at the visit includes the following.

I. **History**
   A. **Nutrition.** Frequency, duration, quantity, retention in bottle-fed infants; frequency, duration, evidence of adequate intake (satiety, adequate urine output, sounds of swallowing, milk leakage from breasts), and nipple symptoms in mother in breast-fed infants.
   B. **Stool and urine output.**
   C. **Sleep habits of infant.**
   D. **Crying patterns.**
   E. **Infant development.** Fixes and follows parent's face, lifts head slightly when prone, blinks to light, and startles with sound.
   F. **Maternal sleep, nutrition (especially for breast-fed infants), mood, coping with child care.**
   G. **Cigarette smoke exposure.**
II. **Physical Examination**
   The physical examination should include all growth parameters plotted on appropriate growth charts. The examination should emphasize documentation of weight gain and reevaluation

for congenital abnormalities with specific attention to the following:

A. Skin—jaundice, diaper dermatitis.

B. Head—head shape, fontanels.

C. Eyes—red reflex.

D. Mouth—oral thrush, intact palate.

E. Nose—patent.

F. Heart and lungs—murmur, breath sounds symmetric.

G. Abdomen—masses or organomegaly.

H. Neuromusculoskeletal—Developmental dysplasia of hips, symmetric movements, suck reflex.

III. Anticipatory Guidance

Following the examination, the physician should sit down with the parents and discuss the results of the examination and ask for questions that have arisen about the baby. At the time of delivery and the newborn visit, parents often do not ask too many questions at a time when Mom is tired and Dad is overwhelmed with feelings of joy and responsibility. However, after they have had a week or two of complete responsibility for the baby's care, many questions arise as a result of the many minicrises at home involved with taking care of a new baby. This aspect of the early postnatal visit is probably the most important. In answering questions, the physician should address other issues that are pertinent to the infant's physical and developmental age.

A. Nutrition. In bottle-fed infants, review mixing formula, warming formula (avoid microwave), feeding schedule (especially for premature infants, who require a regular feeding schedule), and avoidance of bottle propping. In breast-fed infants, review maternal nutrition, including adequate fluids and rest, and common problems in breast feeding (frequency of feeds, stool consistency, concerns about milk sufficiency, and sore nipples). Discuss occasional bottle feeds (with expressed breast milk or formula), anticipating the babysitter or father feeding infant. Anticipate the possible need for vitamin D, iron, and fluoride supplementation.

B. Elimination. Review variation in stools and change in stool pattern, especially in breast-fed infants (transition from several liquid stools per day to infrequent stools by 1 to 2 months).

C. Sleep. Review sleep patterns and suggest that the mother nap while the infant does (if she takes responsibility for all night-time activities) or the father sharing with night duty. Review sleep position.

D. Behavior and parenting. Crying, up to 3 hours per day, peaking at 4 to 8 weeks, especially in the evening, is normal in young infants. Babies cry for several reasons, not just hunger. Review consoling techniques. Remind parents that feeding and sleeping schedule will become regular at 1 to 2 months of age. Encourage personal time for parents. Discuss sibling interactions with infant and the need for individual

attention to siblings. Encourage visual and language stimulation of infant. Observe for evidence of postpartum depression.
E.   Safety. Remind parents about car seats, water heater set to 120°F. Smoke/carbon monoxide detectors, bathing safety, and smoking. Avoid leaving the infant unattended on bed or changing table and with siblings. Discuss harmful effects of shaking infant. Keep home free of cigarette smoke (and discuss smoking cessation programs).
F.   Anticipated development by 2-month visit.
   1.   *Has moderate head control in upright position.*
   2.   *Holds head up in prone position.*
   3.   *Smiles and coos responsively.*
   4.   *Recognizes and interacts with primary caregivers.*
   5.   *Holds briefly object put in hand.*
IV.   Closure
   Ask for questions or concerns. Provide written materials to supplement and support infant care. Recommend health-related items to keep in the home—acetaminophen or ibuprofen, thermometer, saline nose drops. Review with parents how and when to call for problems. Arrange the next well-child visit for 2 months of age unless a problem is identified that requires earlier follow-up.

ADDITIONAL READING

American Academy of Pediatrics Committee on Psychosocial Aspects of Child and Family Health. *Guidelines for health supervision,* 3rd ed. Elk Grove Village, IL: American Academy of Pediatrics; 1997.

Green M, Palfrey JS, eds. *Bright futures: guidelines for health supervision of infants, children, and adolescents,* 2nd ed. Arlington, VA: National Center for Education in Maternal and Child Health; 2000.

Books for Parents

Brazelton TB. *Touchpoints: your child's emotional and behavioral development.* Reading, MA: Addison-Wesley; 1992.

Markel H. *The practical pediatrician: the A to Z guide to your child's health, behavior, and safety.* New York: WH Freeman; 1996.

Schmitt BD. *Your child's health,* rev. ed. New York: Bantam Books; 1991.

Shelov SP, Hannemann RE, eds. *Your baby's first year,* reprint ed. New York: Bantam Books; 1998.

Shelov SP, Hannemann RE, DeAngelis CD. eds. *Caring for your baby and young child: birth to age 5,* rev. ed. New York: Bantam Doubleday Dell; 1998.

19 ♣ Well-Child Visits—Infancy: 2, 4, 6, and 9 Months

Raymond C. Baker

The first year of life is a time of rapid growth in both size and development. The birth weight triples, and the infant changes from a dependent, passive organism into an interactive, mobile bundle of energy with curiosity, personality, and presence. Well-child care during this time lays the foundation for lifelong preventive medicine and effective parenting to optimize the genetic potential of the infant. Because neurocognitive and motor development is rapid during this time and many preventive measures need implementation, well-child care visits are closely spaced and timed to coincide with this developmental progression. Traditionally, visits are suggested at 2, 4, 6, and 9 months of age, corresponding to the recommended immunization schedule.

TWO-MONTH VISIT

I. History

By 2 months of age, infants have developed the beginnings of interactive personalities, responding to parents with smiles and cooing and eliciting parental responses. Feeding and sleeping patterns are fairly well established, which brings some degree of consistency to the home. At the same time, 2-month-old infants are still demanding care, attention, and entertainment. This is a good age to explore with the parents sibling reactions to the new baby and parents' responses to these reactions (which may not be entirely positive).

The visit should begin with several open-ended questions from the physician to prompt parents to think about the first 2 months with their new baby and their management of their new roles as parents. *How is your baby doing? How are you handling your new roles as mother and father? Do you have any concerns for or issues with your baby you would like us to talk about? Has your baby had any illnesses since I saw you last?* As parents talk, the physician should observe the interaction of parents and infant, response to the baby, and parents' interactions with each other (consider postpartum depression).

After addressing parental concerns, the physician can ask more focused questions about feeding, sleep and crying behavior, elimination, and development. Normal development in a 2-month-old might include the following:

A. **Major motor**—holds the head and upper chest up in the prone position.

B. **Fine motor**—briefly holds a rattle (reflexively).

C. **Language**—responds to new sounds by becoming quiet and looking toward the focus, coos in response to verbal stimulation.

D. **Social**—tracks and follows objects visually, especially parents' movements; smiles socially.

II.   Physical Examination

Doing a complete physical examination in front of the parents at every visit and making positive comments as the examination progresses is important. The ongoing conversation has the added effect of stimulating and distracting the infant so that crying is less likely to occur. As at any age, the physician should progress from observational, noninvasive maneuvers to more invasive, from using the hands to instruments, and from comfortable to less comfortable maneuvers. Several important physical examination features are especially important at this visit:

A.   Growth parameters plotted on standard growth curves.

B.   Red reflex and strabismus.

C.   Torticollis, developmental hip dysplasia, and metatarsus adductus.

D.   Cardiac murmurs.

E.   Abdominal masses/organomegaly.

F.   Neurologic abnormalities (symmetry, strength, tone).

G.   Overall evidence of good care (cleanliness, skin condition, clothing).

H.   Developmental assessment to document historical information.

III.   Screening Procedures

No screening laboratory procedures are usually needed at the 2-month visit in healthy, term infants. Hematocrit and/or hemoglobin should be considered in infants with low birth weight or premature delivery, history of hemolytic disease, blood loss, or use of formulas with low-iron.

IV.   Routine Immunizations (DTaP #1, IPV #1, HIB #1, SPN #1, HBV #2)

Routine immunizations at the 2-month visit include the first combined diphtheria/tetanus/pertussis vaccine (DTaP), inactivated poliomyelitis vaccine (IPV), and conjugated *Haemophilus influenzae* type b vaccine (HIB), and the second hepatitis B virus (HBV) vaccine (assuming the first HBV vaccine was given in the hospital). A heptavalent, conjugated pneumococcal vaccine (Prevnar-SPN) has recently been approved by the FDA and is recommended as a routine immunization. The first dose is given at the 2-month visit.

V.   Anticipatory Guidance

After the physical examination, the physician should sit down with the parents and discuss the results of the examination and address topics in anticipatory guidance as follows:

A.   Nutrition. Encourage breast feeding and discuss breast pumping (working mothers) or formula supplementation while the mother is unavailable; feeding intervals of 3 to 4 hours, longer at night; and supplementation (vitamin D for exclusively breast-fed infants with darkly pigmented skin and limited sunlight exposure, iron for premature or anemic infants). Discuss the avoidance of honey and the introduction of solids at 4 to 6 months.

   B. Elimination. Four to six wet diapers per day are normal; constipation determined by consistency, not frequency; breast-fed infants may stool only once every 2 to 3 days, formula-fed infants usually stool at least once per day.
   C. Sleep. Sixteen hours or more per day of sleep is normal; consistency is important. Infant should be put in the crib while still awake and should not be given a bottle in bed. Avoid bottle propping.
   D. Behavior and parenting. Discuss spending time with infant—playing, cuddling, talking; attention to siblings while infant is asleep and engaging siblings in care of infant; establish a bedtime routine; and need for babysitter, to allow parents a break from the infant and time to themselves. Address family planning; discuss babysitting/day care selection.
   E. Development. By next visit expect increased vocalization, smiling, head control, reaching, rolling.
   F. Safety. Car seat safety (rear facing, back seat), sleep position, smoke detectors, sun exposure, water heater thermostat at 120°F. Avoid cigarette smoke in house/apartment; avoid leaving the infant unattended (high places or with siblings/pet); avoid drinking hot liquids while holding infant.
VI. Closure
   Ask parents for any last questions or concerns. Set next well-child appointment. Review with parents procedures for contacting office. Give parents written educational materials.

FOUR-MONTH VISIT
   I. History
   By 4 months of age, infants have become friendly and responsive, with increasing interest in their environment and the people in their environment. Using smiles, they seek interactions with people and respond with coos, squeals, and laughs. Most infants are sleeping through the night. Crying behaviors have decreased as a result of the infant's ability to self-stimulate (hands to face, hands to midline), increased interest in and stimulation by the environment, and cognitive ability to interact more with people. The 4-month-old is beginning to manipulate the environment by rolling, pivoting, and enjoying the touch and feel of surrounding toys and blankets.
   The visit should begin with open-ended questions to encourage dialogue (e.g., *"How is your baby doing?" "How has your baby changed since our last visit?" "Do you have any questions or concerns you would like us to talk about?"*). As the discussion unfolds, the physician should observe maternal/paternal/infant interactions and should look for evidence of appropriate nurturing behaviors.
   After addressing any concerns or questions the parents raise, the physician should progress to more focused questions to explore feeding, sleep and crying behavior, elimination, and

development. Normal development in a 4-month-old might include the following:

    A.   Major motor—rolls, good head control, raises body with arms in prone position.

    B.   Fine motor—reaches and grasps objects, brings hands to midline and plays with hands, beginning to release voluntarily.

    C.   Language—coos in response to parents, blows bubbles, indicates needs with differential cry.

    D.   Social—smiles readily to respond and to initiate interaction, laughs and squeals, differentiates family members.

II.   Physical Examination

    The physician, making positive comments as the examination progresses, should perform a complete examination in front of the parents. Continued dialogue with the parents during the examination may bring up issues they had forgotten previously and gives the physician the opportunity to address some of the points of anticipatory guidance. The 4-month-old infant is usually cooperative and interactive during the examination, allowing the physician to role-model appropriate interactive behaviors, such as responsive mimicry of the infant's vocalization and language stimulation. Important features of the physical examination are the following:

    A.   Growth parameters plotted on standard growth curves.

    B.   Red reflex and ability to track the examiner's head.

    C.   Cardiac murmur.

    D.   Abdominal masses/organomegaly.

    E.   Examination for developmental dysplasia of hips (asymmetric gluteal folds, leg length discrepancy, hip range of motion), **metatarsus adductus.**

    F.   Neurologic examination.

    G.   Developmental assessment to document historical information.

III.   Screening Procedures

    No screening procedures are routine at the 4-month visit. Hemoglobin and/or hematocrit may be considered in the preterm infant or the infant at increased risk of anemia (e.g., use of formulas with low iron).

IV.   Routine Immunizations (DTaP #2, IPV #2, HIB #2, SPN #2)

V.   Anticipatory Guidance

    A.   Nutrition. Encourage breast feeding with vitamin D and iron supplementation as indicated; give formula-fed infants no more than 32 ounces per day, usually in four to five bottles; avoid honey; introduce solids at 4 to 6 months beginning with iron-fortified cereal, spacing new solids at 3- to 4-day intervals; emphasize continued importance of breast milk or formula in infant's diet; avoid bottles in crib and bottle propping.

B. Elimination. Infant should pass stools easily; grunting and face turning red are normal (as long as stools remain soft); stool pattern may change with introduction of solids.

C. Sleep. Most infants sleep through the night by 4 months of age with two to three naps for a total of up to 16 hours of sleep per day; encourage establishing a pattern of daytime feeding, nighttime sleeping, and consistency.

D. Behavior and parenting. Encourage playing with the infant and language stimulation; discuss babysitting/day care selection, bedtime routine, including putting the infant to bed awake to encourage self soothing and ability to go to sleep (may use transitional object, such as blankie, toy), sibling rivalry and the importance of "special time" with siblings while infant is asleep or partner is taking care of the infant; encourage both parents to share care for the infant; age-appropriate toys.

E. Development. By next visit, expect increased vocalization and babbling, reaching, grasping, and transferring; infant may begin sitting by 6 months of age.

F. Injury/illness prevention. Use car seats; avoid leaving infant unattended on high places; avoid hot liquids while holding infant; provide only age-appropriate toys (without small detachable objects, sharp edges); avoid cigarette smoke in the home (and discuss smoking cessation programs with parents); discuss sun safety and pet safety. Discuss respiratory illnesses and home management of common self-limiting illnesses, calling the office, hygiene measures to prevent spread, and risks of antibiotic overuse.

VI. Closure

Ask for any last questions or concerns. Set next well-child appointment. Review with parents procedures for contacting office. Give parents written educational materials.

SIX-MONTH VISIT

I. History

The 6-month-old infant is a truly delightful creature! At this age, infants are anxious to interact with caregivers and often initiate interactions by smiling, vocalizing, and laughing. They love face-to-face reciprocal play and respond readily to adoring parents. Because they are still immobile and are not yet irresistibly drawn to explore their environment as they will be when they begin to crawl, they are happy participants in interactive games with parents and siblings. At the same time, they may begin to show distinct preferences and attachments to their primary care providers and may resist strangers, including the physician. However, they are usually fairly easily won over by a gentle and nonthreatening approach so that the visit to the doctor is a pleasant one. That will change!

The visit should begin with open-ended questions to encourage dialogue ("*How is your baby doing?*" "*What new things have you noticed since our last visit?*" "*Do you have any questions or concerns you would like us to talk about?" "Has your baby had any illnesses since our last visit?"*). As the discussion unfolds, the physician should observe maternal/paternal/infant interactions and look for evidence of appropriate nurturing behaviors.

After addressing parental concerns, the physician should ask more focused questions about the infant, including feeding (solid food introduction, preferences, supplements, behaviors), sleep (especially night waking or night feeding, naps), elimination, behavior (personality/temperament, reaction to strangers), family (child care for working parents, exposure to cigarette smoke), and development. Normal development in a 6-month-old might include the following:

   A.   **Major motor**—rolls both ways, sits with support.
   B.   **Fine motor**—grasps and transfers rattle, plays with hands, raking grasp at small objects.
   C.   **Language**—turns head toward voice/sound, babbles reciprocally, imitates sounds, makes sounds at play.
   D.   **Social**—initiates social interaction, may react when parent moves away or toy/object is removed, may resist strangers (early stranger anxiety).
II.   **Physical Examination**
   The physician should perform a complete examination in front of the parents, making positive comments as the examination progresses. Continued dialogue with the parents during the examination may bring up issues they have forgotten previously and diverts the infant's attention from the parent, allaying anxiety the infant may have with the physician. The caregiver should remain visible to the infant during the examination; this will become increasingly important in older infants, when stranger anxiety has become fully developed. Important features of the physical examination follow.
   A.   **Growth parameters plotted on standard growth curves.**
   B.   **Red reflex and strabismus.**
   C.   **Tooth eruption** (should stimulate a brief discussion of teething in general).
   D.   **Developmental hip dysplasia and tibial torsion.**
   E.   **Muscle tone and symmetry of movement.**
   F.   **Cleanliness, evidence of neglect, abuse.**
   G.   **Developmental assessment to document historical information.**
III.   **Screening Procedures**
   No screening procedures are routine at the 6-month visit. Hemoglobin and/or hematocrit may be considered in the preterm infant or the infant at increased risk of anemia (e.g., use of formulas with low iron).
IV.   **Routine Immunizations (DTaP #3, IPV #3, HIB #3, SPN #3, HBV #3)**
   The third HBV vaccine must be at least 4 months from the first dose and 2 months from the second dose, and the infant must be at least 6 months of age. Therefore some physicians delay the

third dose of HBV to a later visit. The PRP-OMB conjugate HIB vaccine (PedvaxHIB and ComVax) does not require a third dose in the primary series. The third (booster) dose of IPV can be given any time from 6 months to 18 months of age.

The availability of combination vaccines may affect the timing of immunizations in order to keep the numbers of injections to a minimum. For example, the use of ComVax (HBV plus conjugate HIB) may decrease the number of injections required at some of the visits (2 and 6 months). In the future, other combination vaccines that further reduce the number of injections needed at each visit will likely become available. Some parents are reluctant for their infants to receive too many injections at a single visit because of concerns about pain and unfounded concerns about side effects of the vaccines. The health care provider should specifically address these concerns when immunizations are discussed.

V. Anticipatory Guidance

A. Nutrition. Breast or formula feeding should be continued; solids should be given two to three times per day, beginning with iron-fortified cereal and introducing a new food every 3 or 4 days as tolerated; parents should not be putting the bottle into the crib with the infant (propped or held), to reduce risk of nursing caries; until after 12 months of age, parents should not be feeding the infant honey; parents should supplement vitamin D and flouride (if local water supply has less than 0.3 ppm flouride) for exclusively breast-fed infants; begin giving infant a sipper cup.

B. Sleep. Infant should be sleeping through the night supplemented by two naps per day and should be put to bed while still awake; if infant wakens at night, he or she should be comforted with words and patting (in the crib) but not fed or picked up; encourage bedtime routine.

C. Hygiene and health habits. If any teeth have erupted, advise parents to clean daily with soft brush or wash cloth wrapped around a finger (no toothpaste).

D. Sexuality. Infants commonly explore their genitalia during diaper changes.

E. Behavior and parenting. Encourage language stimulation and social games, such as peek-a-boo, pat-a-cake, and so-big; allow infant to explore environment but do set limits using distraction; at bedtime or stressful times (parents leaving infant with sitter), provide infant with transitional object, such as a favorite toy or blankie.

F. Development. By next visit expect infant to crawl, get to sitting position, perhaps cruise; begin finger feeding, two-syllable utterances (*mama, baba, dada*), pincer grasp.

G. Injury prevention. Child-proof the home: put plastic plugs in electrical outlets; eliminate dangling electrical cords; keep sharp objects out of reach; keep plastic wrappers, bags, and balloons out of reach; keep medications and poisonous household products locked in cabinets out of reach; suggest syrup of ipecac and provide the number of local poison information center; keep gates at stairs; avoid possible exposure to hot liquids, surfaces, and appliances (iron, curling iron); and lower water heater temperature. Be careful of exposure to the sun; advise against walkers, especially with stairs and excessive use; give information about car seats; provide information about pet safety; avoid leaving infant unattended on high surfaces, with siblings, or with pets.

VI.   Closure

Ask for any last questions or concerns. Set next well-child appointment. Review with parents procedures for contacting office. Give parents written educational materials.

NINE-MONTH VISIT

I.   History

By 9 months of age, infants have achieved mobility! This opens a whole new world to them and to parents. At this age, infants have an insatiable curiosity about their environment and will put exploration of that environment above everything else, including feeding, cuddling, and sleeping. The infant who loved to sit in Mom's lap, play pat-a-cake, and make faces now wants to wriggle off her lap and see the world. The mouth becomes an important sensory organ, and tasting objects achieves similar importance to seeing, feeling, and manipulating them. These daring activities require constant surveillance by parents and limitation of setting. Because the infant has gained object permanence, many actions previously ignored now produce anxiety and protest, such as parents leaving the room or waking in the night and not seeing parents. All these activities change the parents also as they see emerging independence and loss of "our little baby."

The visit should begin with open-ended questions to encourage dialogue (*"How is your baby doing?" "How are you coping with your baby now that he / she can get around?" "What other things have changed since our last visit?" "Has your baby had any illnesses since the last visit?" "Do you have any questions or concerns you would like us to talk about?"*). As the discussion unfolds, the physician should observe the parents' attitudes toward the infant, their relationship with each other, and methods of coping with their baby's antics.

After addressing parental concerns, the physician should ask more focused questions about the infant, including feeding (self-feeding, preferences, supplements, taking from cup), sleep (especially night waking and naps), elimination, behavior (personality/temperament, reaction to strangers, reaction to limit setting, method for making wants known), family (coping with the infant's exploratory behaviors, changes in the family constellation), and development. Normal development in a 9-month-old might include the following:

A.   Major motor—sits well, gets into sitting position, may cruise.

B. **Fine motor**—developing pincer grasp and ability to manipulate small objects, feeding self.

C. **Language**—responds to name and verbal cues, such as *"wave bye-bye,"* understands a few words, such as *"no"* (of course, understanding and responding appropriately are two different things!), imitates speech.

D. **Social**—enjoys social games; evidences stranger anxiety.

II. **Physical Examination**

Although variable, many 9-month-old infants have fully developed stranger anxiety, which may affect the physical examination and cause some resistance by the infant. The physician should keep the infant in the mother's lap most of the time and begin friendly overtures to the infant (smiling, touching the hands, feet, tickling) during the interview. The introduction of examining instruments should be slow, allowing the infant to explore them first. The physical examination itself should progress from the least invasive aspects, such as inspection/observation and palpation, to more invasive maneuvers, such as the use of the stethoscope, otoscope, and tongue blade. Although much of the physical examination can be performed with the infant in the mother's lap, the physician should not compromise the examination because of the infant's anxiety. Important features of the examination at this age are the following:

A. **Growth parameters plotted on standard growth curves.**

B. **Red reflex and strabismus.**

C. **Tooth eruption.**

D. **Cardiac murmurs.**

E. **Abdominal examination for masses or organomegaly, testes position.**

F. **Hips for developmental dysplasia and lower extremities for tibial torsion.**

G. **Neurologic examination, muscle tone, grasp, symmetry.**

H. **Cleanliness, evidence of neglect, abuse.**

I. **Developmental assessment to document historical information.**

III. **Screening Procedures**

A. **Complete blood count (CBC) at the 9-, 12-, or 15-month visit** (ideally includes mean corpuscular volume [MCV], red cell distribution width [RDW]).

B. **Blood lead if at increased risk** (depends on local prevalence of lead toxicity and other risk factors, such as sibling with lead toxicity, older housing, recent renovations in the home) at 9- or 12-month visit.

C. **Tuberculin testing if risk factors present** (low socioeconomic status [SES], exposure history, increased prevalence locally, immigrant status).

IV. **Immunizations**

No immunizations are recommended at this visit if previous immunizations given at appropriate intervals.

V.   Anticipatory Guidance

A.   Nutrition. Breast feeding or formula feeding should continue; practice with sipper cup; establish routine mealtimes of three or four per day with solids, including soft table foods and pureed foods; offer finger foods, such as toast, bread, biscuits, cereals; wean from bottle to cup by 12 to 15 months; continue vitamin D and fluoride supplements if local water supply has less than 0.3 ppm fluoride if breast-fed.

B.   Elimination. Stools may vary with changes in diet.

C.   Hygiene and health habits. Advise parents to clean teeth daily with soft brush or wash cloth wrapped around a finger (no toothpaste). Avoid bottle in bed to prevent dental caries.

D.   Sleep. Infant should continue two naps per day; put to bed while still awake—may go through a phase of night waking (manage by keeping transitional object in crib with infant, comfort with words and patting in the crib, but avoid feeding or picking up); encourage bedtime routine.

E.   Sexuality. Genital exploration is normal.

F.   Behavior and parenting. Discuss separation anxiety and age-appropriate discipline for actions that are now resulting from the infant's new-found mobility and exploration drive (distraction and diversion; environmental engineering; no hand slapping or other physical deterrents). Promote language stimulation by parents. Discuss sibling rivalry, which may intensify now that the infant has mobility and can "get into sibling's stuff."

G.   Development. By next visit expect infant to pull to stand, cruise, and perhaps take independent steps, to develop pincer grasp, to desire to pick up small objects, to feed self both bottle and finger foods, to have vocabulary of three words, including *mama* and *dada*.

H.   Injury prevention. Review child-proofing the home (gates, window screen safety devices, poisons, medications, cabinet locks, small objects that can be put in mouth, electrical sockets and cords); recommend syrup of ipecac and poison information number; use car seats; discuss domestic violence exposure; advise against walkers.

VI.   Closure

Ask for any last questions or concerns. Set next well-child appointment. Review with parents procedures for contacting office. Give parents written educational materials.

ADDITIONAL READING

American Academy of Pediatrics Committee on Psychosocial Aspects of Child and Family Health. *Guidelines for health supervision,* 3rd ed. Elk Grove Village, IL: American Academy of Pediatrics; 1997.

Green M, Palfrey JS, eds. *Bright futures: guidelines for health supervision of infants, children, and adolescents,* 2nd ed. Arlington, VA: National Center for Education in Maternal and Child Health; 2000.

Books for Parents

Brazelton TB. *Touchpoints: your child's emotional and behavioral development.* Reading, MA: Addison-Wesley; 1992.

Markel H. *The practical pediatrician: the A to Z guide to your child's health, behavior, and safety.* New York: WH Freeman; 1996.

Schmitt BD. *Your child's health,* rev. ed. New York: Bantam Books; 1991.

Shelov SP, Hannemann RE, eds. *Your baby's first year,* reprint ed. New York: Bantam Books; 1998.

Shelov SP, Hannemann RE, DeAngelis CD. eds. *Caring for your baby and young child: birth to age 5,* rev. ed. New York: Bantam Doubleday Dell; 1998.

20 ♣ Well-Child Visits—Toddler: 12, 15, and 18 Months

Raymond C. Baker

The second year of life, the toddler age, is an age of exploration and developing independence. Toddlers learn to walk, which drastically widens their range of territory and play activities. The toddler's overestimation of his/her ability often leads to falls, tears, parental comfort, and fresh starts. Toddlers learn the rudiments of speech and how that speech allows access to a new world of interaction. A useful and provocative word, *no*, enters the vocabulary, and the toddler quickly learns the power of speech and the reactions it can elicit. At the same time that the toddler's geographic range increases, so does the need for limit setting; and, with that, the first real element of conflict comes between toddler and parent. How parents set those limits—consistency, firmness, methods, and choices—and temper them with love and tolerance lays the groundwork for the parent/child relationship that will endure through childhood. For parents the toddler years are a time of intensity, pride, and gratification but require humor and patience to enjoy them and foster nurturing and growth.

From the primary care provider's perspective, the physical examination during the toddler years can be the most difficult to perform. The toddler has well-developed stranger anxiety and seeks the protection of the parent during the examination, often clinging to the parent and attempting to ward off overtures from the physician. Even the most patient of physicians does not especially look forward to an afternoon in the office when scanning the appointment book and noting a predominance of 15-month-olds for well-child-care visits! The best approach to the toddler visit is for the physician to concentrate on the history and anticipatory guidance and to make the examination itself brief and focused. A good sense of humor and an armamentarium of colorful distractions help.

TWELVE-MONTH VISIT

I. History

The 12-month-old has achieved a new perspective on the world. Instead of crawling around the room with all the good stuff out of reach, the 1-year-old is cruising, perhaps walking independently, which brings a whole new world within his grasp. This new mobility increases the range of activity and brings a level of self-confidence that marks the beginnings of independence from doting parents. Experimental steps bring falls. Fingers touching forbidden objects on the coffee table bring a new kind of look on parents' faces and a disagreeable word, *no-no*, probably coupled with being picked up (with less gentleness than a cuddle) and put down elsewhere. This newfound autonomy is especially evident during mealtime, when food seems to have become less a means of nourishment and more an art form and play activity.

The visit should begin with some open-ended questions to parents to encourage dialogue (*"How are you and the baby doing?"* *"What new things is the baby doing now?"* *"Has the baby had any illnesses since our last visit?"* *"Do you have any concerns or questions for me?"*). As the interview unfolds, the physician should make overtures to the child by smiling, offering toys, and gently touching the infant's hand or foot to help allay fears and establish some sense of rapport. Some toddlers can be won over; many will resist and cling even more tightly to the caregiver.

After exploring the parents' questions and concerns, the physician should ask more focused questions about nutrition and mealtime behaviors (self-feeding, use of cup, use of spoon), sleep (night waking, naps), elimination, behavior (play activities, interactions with siblings and baby sitter, temperament, exploration of attitudes about discipline—how parents were disciplined, how they plan to discipline, what they do when the infant touches things that are forbidden), family (changes in family constellation, moves, new jobs, children entering school), and development. Normal development in a 12-month-old might include the following:

    A. Motor—sits without support, crawls, pulls to stand, cruises, may walk independently, uses pincer grasp to pick up small objects.

    B. Language—points with index finger, uses vocabulary of *mama* and *dada* plus one other word, imitates speech.

    C. Social—plays social games, feeds self, drinks from cup, looks for hidden objects, bangs blocks together.

II. Physical Examination

    Because most 1-year-olds have significant stranger anxiety and may resist the examination, the physician should keep the infant in the mother's lap for most of the examination. After making friendly overtures to the infant during the interview, the physician should begin the examination slowly (after washing hands and warming them with warm water). The introduction of examining instruments should be slow, allowing the infant to explore them first. The physical examination itself should progress from the least invasive aspects, such as inspection/observation, to more invasive maneuvers, such as palpation, leaving the use of the otoophthalmoscope and tongue blade until the end of the examination. Although much of the physical examination can be performed with the infant in the mother's lap, the physician should not compromise the examination because of the infant's anxiety. Important features of the examination at this age are the following:

    A. Growth parameters plotted on standard growth curves.

    B. Red reflex and strabismus.

    C. Tooth eruption and nursing caries.

    D. Hip and extremity examination (for hip dysplasia, tibial torsion).

    E. Abdominal examination for masses and organomegaly, testicular descent.

F.   **Cleanliness, evidence of abuse or neglect.**
G.   **Developmental assessment to document historical information.**

III.   **Screening Procedures**

A.   **Complete blood count (CBC)** (ideally includes mean
corpuscular volume [MCV], red cell distribution width [RDW])
if not done at 9-month visit. May be deferred to the 15-month
visit if infant is on iron-fortified formula.

B.   **Blood lead if at increased risk** (depends on local prevalence of lead toxicity and other risk factors, such as a sibling
with lead toxicity, older housing, recent renovations in the
home) if not done at 9-month visit.

C.   **Tuberculin testing if risk factors present** (low socioeconomic status [SES], exposure history, increased prevalence
locally, immigrant status) if not done at 9-month visit.

IV.   **Immunizations**

If the toddler is beyond the first birthday at the 12-month
visit, varicella vaccine (VAR), combined measles/mumps/rubella
vaccine (MMR), booster doses of HIB and DTaP (if at least
6 months from the third in the primary series), and the booster
dose of conjugate pneumococcal vaccine (SPN) may be given. The
booster dose of IPV can also be given at this age if not given previously. The recommendations for administering varicella vaccine
are 12 to 18 months of age; MMR, 12 to 15 months; HIB, 12 to 15
months; SPN, 12 to 15 months; and DTaP, 15 to 18 months. Decisions regarding the timing of the administration of these vaccines
depend on several factors, including parental concerns, cost, compliance with well-child visits, availability of combination vaccines,
and, of course, vaccine-related issues (allergic and other reactions).

Possible immunizations include **DTaP booster, HIB
booster, VAR, MMR, SPN booster, IPV booster**.

V.   **Anticipatory Guidance**

A.   **Nutrition.** Diet should consist predominantly of table
food eaten three times a day with the family plus two or three
snacks (avoid nuts, hard candy, popcorn, grapes, hard raw
fruits/vegetables that require chewing and might be aspirated); wean from bottle/breast to cup and vitamin D cow's
milk (limit to 24 ounces per day) and other liquids (avoid liquids with high sugar content); continue fluoride supplementation if fluoride content of drinking water is less than 0.3
ppm; encourage self-feeding; anticipate typical mealtime
behaviors of messiness with self-feeding and pickiness.

B.   **Elimination.** Toilet training should usually be delayed
until 2 years of age.

C.   **Hygiene and health habits.** Clean teeth with soft
brush or damp cloth; avoid putting bottle in crib with infant
(to prevent nursing caries).

D.   **Sleep.** Encourage bedtime ritual to help transition;
allow at least one nap per day; cover nighttime waking management.

E.   **Behavior and parenting.** Discuss limit setting using
distraction and *no-no* or stern statement ("no hitting") with

distraction. Emphasize positive reinforcement for good behaviors (cuddling, praise, positive comments) and ignoring negative behaviors. Encourage language stimulation and looking at picture books. Avoid physical discipline. Avoid television, especially as a babysitter.

F. Socialization and family. Encourage one-on-one time with toddler and siblings and play among toddler and siblings; share limit-setting behavior with other family members for consistency.

G. Development. By next visit, expect the child to begin using a spoon (with considerable spillage!), self-feeding consistently (all table food), walking independently, using several single words, communicating with gestures, employing jargon speech, understanding and following simple commands, liking to look at picture books with parent, and playing games with parent.

H. Safety. Child-proof the home; discuss sun safety and sunscreen use; use gates on stairs; correctly use car seats; supervise closely outdoor play, guns, and smoke alarms; emphasize water/tub safety; avoid domestic violence; practice pet safety; and keep syrup of ipecac and the telephone number of local poison information center on hand.

VI. Closure
Ask for any last-minute questions or concerns. Set next well-child appointment time. Give parents written educational materials.

FIFTEEN-MONTH VISIT
I. History
By 15 months of age, toddlers have achieved locomotion in the upright position and delight in practicing that new feat *all day long!* They are bundles of energy, walking about constantly and exploring the new world opened up to them, touching, poking, prodding, tasting, and, when possible, carrying or dragging their finds to new locations. (Is it any wonder the house of a 15-month-old is always a mess?) The downside of this behavior is that toddlers have to be watched every minute they are awake and that limits must be set on their insatiable curiosity to prevent injury to themselves and chaos for parents.

The visit should begin with open-ended questions to parents to encourage dialogue and acknowledge the challenges of the toddler (*"How are you and the baby doing?"* *"What new things is your toddler doing since we met last?"* *"Is he keeping you busy?"* *"Have there been any illnesses since we last met?"*).

After discussing the parents' questions and concerns, the physician should move on to more focused questions about nutrition (diet, preferences, changes in appetite, pica behaviors), elimination, sleep (nighttime waking, naps, difficulty going to sleep), family changes and reactions to the toddler, behavior (new activities, reaction to limit setting and parents' handling of the toddler's misbehaviors, toddler's communication, temperament), and development. Normal development in a 15-month-old might include the following:

    A.   Motor—self-feeding with fingers/spoon, scribbling with crayon, independent walking.

    B.   Language—five to 15 single words, jargon speech, comprehension of single commands, ability to point to one or two body parts when asked, gestures.

    C.   Social—Exchanges toys, tests limits, enjoys games with parents/siblings, communicates likes and dislikes, understands and demonstrates function of objects (e.g., telephone).

II.   Physical Examination

    Most primary care providers agree that the 15-month visit is the most difficult from the perspective of cooperation by the toddler. Stranger anxiety and separation issues peak at this age. Therefore experienced physicians perform the physical examination quickly and in the parent's lap as much as possible and use distraction techniques (brightly colored toys and mobiles, continual dialogue with parents and toddler). Even then, some toddlers react with tears and resistance. The provider's reaction must reflect calmness, consistency, humor, firmness, and affection while still setting limits. This is a crucial opportunity to role-model these characteristics that a parent needs to deal with a rambunctious toddler. Important features of the examination at this age are the following:

    A.   Growth parameters plotted on standard growth curves.

    B.   Observe interactions with parents; watch for reactions to limit setting and parental reactions to the toddler's behaviors (which may serve as a springboard for discussions of behavior management).

    C.   Tooth eruption, caries.

    D.   Skin examination for congenital lesions (hemangiomas, cafe au lait spots, and skin tags/pits).

    E.   Location of bruises and other skin trauma that might suggest inadequate supervision or abuse. Bruising in certain locations (knees, shins, forehead), however, is not uncommon at this age because of the reckless abandon with which many toddlers careen around their environment.

    F.   Developmental assessment to document historical information.

III.   Screening Procedures

    CBC (ideally includes MCV, RDW) if the toddler is at increased risk for iron deficiency (intake of more than 24 ounces per day of cow's milk, receipt of cow's milk before 12 months of age, dietary history of inadequate iron intake). Many health care providers prefer to perform the CBC on the 15-month visit since the incidence of iron deficiency is likely to be higher as a result of the introduction of cow's milk at 12 months of age.

IV.   Immunizations

    If not given at the 12-month visit, administer MMR, VAR, booster HIB, booster SPN, and booster DTaP; administer the booster IPV if not given at 6, 9, or 12 months.

V. Anticipatory Guidance

A. Nutrition. Discuss picky eating in the toddler age group, messy eating, eating with fingers and with spoon (with considerable spillage!), eating three meals per day with the family, weaning from a bottle, the limitation of cow's milk to 24 ounces per day, and avoidance of small hard foods that might be aspirated.

B. Elimination. Toilet training should be delayed in most instances until 24 months, but parents should observe child's interest in toileting and behaviors around urination and defecation that might be helpful when the time comes.

C. Hygiene and health habits. Brushing teeth with soft brush (no toothpaste) or damp cloth; avoid nursing caries.

D. Sleep. Establish a bedtime ritual; keep a transitional object in the crib; lower the mattress in the crib if toddler displays any climbing activity. Maintain the afternoon nap.

E. Socialization and family. Encourage imitative play (e.g., dusting, dolls, ball) and representational play activities (e.g., combing hair, spoon-feeding doll). Encourage language stimulation through books.

F. Behavior and parenting. Discuss temper tantrums, limit setting, feeding, positive reinforcement for good behaviors (and ignoring most less acceptable behaviors). Avoid television, especially as a babysitter. Discuss time-out technique with parents and recommend it as the primary limit-setting and disciplinary means for the 2-year-old. Supplementary written instructions on the time-out technique are helpful to emphasize its importance in child rearing.

G. Development. By next visit, expect walking up stairs, climbing activities, use of spoon and fork, scribbling with crayons, use of 10 to 20 words (may make two-word phrases), and pretend play activities.

H. Safety. Discuss car safety, stair safety, crib safety (may need to lower mattress if child is a climber), dangers of small objects that can be detached and put in mouth (especially as part of toys), water/sun safety, water heater temperature, gun safety, and exposure to domestic violence.

VI. Closure

Ask for any last-minute questions. Set next well-child appointment. Give parents written educational materials.

EIGHTEEN-MONTH VISIT

I. History

The 18-month-old toddler is a paradoxical blend of curiosity, defiance, charm, and cuddle. Having mastered walking and other major motor skills, the toddler is now working on socialization and communication skills. The toddler continues striving for independence while at the same time needing the love and comfort of a parent to turn to for cuddling after a fall. Quiet play with an older sibling can quickly escalate into a major throw-me-down-on-the-floor-and-kick-and-scream tantrum over who gets to push the toy baby carriage. The toddler's word *no* may mean "No" or it may mean "Johnny just took my toy, and I won't eat my lunch until you make him give it back for me." This is a time when parents need patience, humor, diplomacy, and sometimes clairvoyance. Parents' management of this age is often a test of these skills tempered with pride at their toddlers' achievements during this period of rapid development.

The visit should begin with open-ended questions to encourage parents to voice their frustrations with their toddler and raise areas of problems for discussion. For example, the physician might begin by saying, *"How are you doing with your baby? Many parents find this a difficult age. Are you having any particular problems right now? Has Mary had any illnesses since our last visit?"* During the discussion the physician should watch the toddler/parent interaction and parents' reactions to the toddler's behavior. The stress of the office visit sometimes brings out the best or the worst in children (and their parents), but both provide fodder for discussion. Because this is a common age for abuse, the physician should be observant of any behaviors that might suggest a need for preventive counseling.

After discussing the parents' concerns and questions, the physician should ask more focused questions about nutrition and mealtime behaviors (diet, snacks, milk intake, family meals, decreased appetite), elimination (interest in potty training), sleep and bedtime behaviors (nighttime ritual, naps, problems going to sleep), family (siblings, changes in family structure, toddler's interactions with siblings), behavior (temperament, tantrums, handling of defiant behaviors), and development. Normal development in an 18-month-old might include the following:

    A. Major motor—walking, running, climbing stairs.

    B. Fine motor—scribbles with crayon, uses spoon and fork, stacks three or four blocks, throws a ball.

    C. Language—uses 10 to 20 words, may have two-word phrases, points to body parts on command, understands commands.

    D. Social—enjoys playing with siblings, parents, and other children. Enjoys reading and naming pictures, making animal sounds, and pretending as part of play.

II. Physical Examination

The examination of an 18-month-old may be similar to the previous visit, with tears and resistance to the physician, or the toddler may allow some parts of the examination to proceed easily with the use of distraction techniques. The prudent course of action is to do as much of the examination as possible on mother's lap. Important features of the physical examination at this age are the following:

    A. Growth parameters plotted on standard growth curves. Sharing this information with parents, especially if they have concerns about diet, may be helpful as it can demonstrate normal growth and the slow-down in growth during the second year.

   B. Eyes for strabismus.
   C. Tooth eruption and caries.
   D. Gait and extremities for developmental rotational deformities.
   E. Abdominal examination for masses or organomegaly.
   F. Evidence of abuse or neglect.
   G. Developmental assessment to document historical information.

  III. Screening Procedures
       Lead screen for children at increased risk at this visit or 2-year visit. May also consider CBC if child is at increased risk for iron deficiency.

  IV. Immunizations
       If not given at the 12- or 15-month visit, administer MMR, VAR, booster HIB, booster SPN, and booster DTaP; consider booster IPV if not given at 6, 9, or 12 months.

   V. Anticipatory Guidance
   A. Nutrition. Encourage three meals a day with the family plus healthy snacks; avoid arguments over eating, but limit the amount of time given for it; limit cow's milk intake to 24 ounces per day; allow self-feeding with spoon and cup; limit the amount of sugar and sodium in diet.
   B. Elimination. Discuss toilet-training preparation (watching for behavioral signs of urination/defecation, continence; interest as evidenced by watching siblings and interest in the potty chair); encourage waiting until 24 months, but suggest purchase of potty chair—allowing toddler to sit on it (clothed) may help the child's comfort level and prepare him for the "real thing."
   C. Hygiene and health habits. Ensure daily teeth care and regular bathing.
   D. Sleep. Discuss bedtime ritual, naps, night waking, and resistance to falling asleep.
   E. Sexuality. Genital manipulation/touching is common. Masturbation may be a self-comforting behavior with stress. Encourage correct terms for genitalia when appropriate.
   F. Socialization and family. Encourage including the toddler in family activities and recreation; suggest that parents manage disputes among siblings without taking sides; allow older siblings the right to have their own things (i.e., off-limits to the toddler).
   G. Behavior and parenting. Discuss temper tantrums and management; remind parents that toddlers are selfish and seldom share; initiate discussion of behavior management and discipline; avoid television, especially as a babysitter.

H. Development. By the next visit, expect the child to run, jump, walk up and down stairs, throw a ball overhand; use a fork and spoon, climb; child should have 50-word vocabulary and short phrases; child should help brush teeth and assist in dressing self.

I. Safety. Discuss car, water, and sun safety; window safety; guns; and exposure to domestic violence.

VI. Closure

Ask for any last-minute questions. Set next appointment time. Give parents written educational materials.

ADDITIONAL READING

American Academy of Pediatrics Committee on Psychosocial Aspects of Child and Family Health. *Guidelines for health supervision,* 3rd ed. Elk Grove Village, IL: American Academy of Pediatrics; 1997.

Green M, Palfrey JS, eds. *Bright futures: guidelines for health supervision of infants, children, and adolescents,* 2nd ed. Arlington, VA: National Center for Education in Maternal and Child Health; 2000.

Books for Parents

Brazelton TB. *Touchpoints: your child's emotional and behavioral development.* Reading, MA: Addison-Wesley; 1992.

Markel H. *The practical pediatrician: the A to Z guide to your child's health, behavior, and safety.* New York: WH Freeman; 1996.

Schmitt BD. *Your child's health,* rev. ed. New York: Bantam Books; 1991.

Shelov SP, Hannemann RE, eds. *Your baby's first year*, reprint ed. New York: Bantam Books; 1998.

21 ♣ Well-Child Visits— Early Childhood: 2 to 3 Years

Raymond C. Baker

The early childhood years, ages 2 and 3, are a time of extraordinary development. The child achieves major accomplishments in fine motor skills, social skills, cognitive skills, and language skills. The dependency of infancy gives way to developing independence and the "I can do it myself" age. This emerging independence is a source of great pride to the child. At the same time, it is a time of spills, falls, bumps, and scrapes as the child overestimates his abilities. For parents, early childhood offers a mixture of intense pleasure and pride as the child becomes much more interactive because of exponential advances in cognition and language. Limit setting remains essential to balance the child's emerging independence, and use of the time-out means of behavior management replaces distraction and redirection.

TWO-YEAR VISIT
I. History
The 2-year-old has mastered the art of getting around and now concentrates on communication and social skills. The toddler speaks in two- and three-word phrases and has a considerably larger receptive language. Although enjoying the company of other children, the child is selfish with toys and tends to play alongside other children rather than with them. Curiosity still drives the toddler to get into things that are forbidden, leading to continued conflict with parents and the need for limit setting. The need for independence and autonomy leads to the toddler imitating parents, thus preparing the way to the "I can do it myself" phase that will begin in the next year.

The visit should begin with open-ended questions that will encourage dialogue with parents ("*How are things going?*" "*What new things is Johnny doing?*" "*What do you enjoy about this age?*" "*Are there some difficult things about this age?*"). A review of the behaviors indicated by the parent on the Preschool Children's Behavior Checklist (Appendix G) during this part of the history serves as a good trigger to discuss normal age-appropriate behaviors and behavior management techniques. Part of this discussion may occur later as part of anticipatory guidance. As the interview progresses, the physician should watch the activity of the toddler and reactions of the parent to it. The child's reaction to the physician's overtures will probably portend the level of ease of the examination. A 2-year-old can go either way—clinging to parents and crying at the approach of the physician or remaining interactive and playful.

After addressing the parents' questions and concerns, the physician can ask more focused questions about feeding and mealtime behaviors, sleep, elimination, and toilet training (begun? child's willingness to sit on the potty? any successes?), family life and interactions with siblings and playmates, behavior (use or limit setting, time-outs, positive reinforcement), and development. Normal development by age 2 might include the following:

A.   Major motor—walks and runs well, goes up and down stairs, throws ball overhand, jumps in place.

B.   Fine motor—uses spoon and fork, is able to open doors, stacks 5 to 6 blocks, kicks a ball, brushes teeth (but requires supervision and help), dresses with help.

C.   Language—has a 50-word (and more) vocabulary, uses two- and three-word phrases; follows two-step commands; uses pronouns.

D.   Social—imitates adults, plays parallel.

II.   Physical Examination

This visit is probably the last well-child visit where the physician can expect some degree of resistance from the child during the examination. Although the child may have overcome, because of improved cognition and reasoning, much of the stranger anxiety that caused the resistance previously, some positive or negative associations between the doctor and the office setting may have developed. For example, the 2-year-old may make a connection between a painful procedure (the last immunization or finger stick) and the office setting, especially if he sees (or hears) other tearful youngsters in the office. Some 2-year-olds, however, engage with the physician and find the physical examination experience yet another lark in their unending quest for new and fun activities.

Several important physical examination features are important at this age:

A.   Growth parameters plotted on standard growth curves.

B.   Strabismus, vision and hearing (informal, subjective assessment).

C.   Dental caries.

D.   Abdominal examination for masses or organomegaly.

E.   Extremities for rotational deformities, genu valgum.

F.   Cleanliness, evidence of abuse or neglect.

G.   Developmental assessment to document historical information

III.   Screening Procedures

Conduct lead and tuberculin testing if the child is at increased risk.

IV.   Immunizations

No immunizations are routine at 2 years of age for all children. For children living in certain states with an increased incidence of hepatitis A (Arizona, Alaska, California, Idaho, New Mexico, Nevada, Oklahoma, South Dakota, Utah, Washington), hepatitis A vaccine is recommended routinely (in 2 doses, 6–12 months apart, beginning at 2 years of age). The child's immunization record should be reviewed at every well-child visit to check for completeness and to catch-up immunizations as indicated.

V. Anticipatory Guidance

A. Nutrition. Discuss diet, which includes low-fat milk, limited fat and processed sugar, and fruit and vegetable snacks; discuss food preferences and pickiness; recommend vitamin/mineral supplements only if diet is inadequate. Child should drink exclusively from a cup or glass.

B. Elimination. Discuss potty training readiness and technique; allow the child to watch parents/siblings using the toilet to encourage him/her to want to imitate. When possible, potty chair purchase should be an "event" that allows the child to take ownership (e.g., putting the child's name on it).

C. Hygiene and health habits. Emphasize tooth brushing and bathing; recommend first dental appointment at age 2 or 3.

D. Sleep. Discuss important of bedtime ritual and nap.

E. Sexuality. Discuss child's curiosity about genitalia, and encourage use of correct anatomic terms.

F. Socialization and family. Discuss shared family meals and consistency of limit setting with all family members; discuss family outings that include the 2-year-old (with appropriately limited time and activity).

G. Behavior and parenting. Discuss time-out technique and preference over physical discipline; discuss limit setting and offering choices; limit television to no more than 1 hour per day, preferably with the parent (avoid the temptation to use the television as a babysitter).

H. Development. By the next visit (3 years), expect walking up stairs using alternating feet, peddling a tricycle, interest in crayons, self-dressing, playing using pretend activities, and knowing name/sex; speech—50% to 75% should be intelligible by nonfamily members—with short sentences with appropriate syntax, understanding of prepositions, and many "why" questions.

I. Safety. Discuss car seats, water/sun safety (including sunscreen), street safety (supervision), playground safety, pet safety, syrup of ipecac and local poison information center telephone number, stove safety (handles of pots on stove turned inward), guns, smoke detectors, and exposure to violence (domestic, television).

VI. Closure

Ask for any last-minute questions. Advise about timing of next well-child appointment time. Give parents written educational materials.

THREE-YEAR VISIT

I. History

The 3-year-old has become a truly interactive youngster with the ability to communicate understandably with family members and others (when he or she wants to!). The child remains egocentric and resists sharing. The 3-year-old can participate more easily with family outings, such as trips to the store or park, without all the accoutrements a baby needs, although he or she may want to take along a favorite transitional object. Though still requiring limits (and testing them regularly), increased language abilities allow the child to respond well to choices. The 3-year-old child's appearance and actions significantly change, clearly showing that he or she has left infancy and toddlerhood to take a place in the family constellation as a full-fledged participant.

Although the primary care provider always interacts with the young patient with words, actions, and gestures, regardless of age, as part of the interview and physical examination, the 3-year visit is the first visit in which the physician can expect some meaningful communication from the child. A portion of the interview should be devoted to questions directed to the child, perhaps with parental supplementation and interpretation. This give and take with the child is important for language assessment and to develop a relationship with the child to aid in cooperation. Questions might include the following: *"What are your favorite foods?" "Do you use the potty?" "Do you have a pet?" "What is your favorite toy?"*

The physician should begin the interview with the parents with open-ended questions to encourage dialogue (*"How are things going at home?" "What new things can Elizabeth do now that she's 3?" "Has she had any illnesses since our last visit?" "Do you have any special concerns or questions today?"*). A review of the behaviors indicated by the parent on the Preschool Children's Behavior Checklist (Appendix G) during this part of the history serves as a good trigger to discuss normal age-appropriate behaviors and behavior management techniques. Part of this discussion may be addressed later as part of anticipatory guidance. During the interview, the physician should watch the child to see how she reacts to the parent's responses. Does she listen and participate in the discussion, or does she ignore the conversation and occupy herself with play activities?

After addressing the parent's concerns, the physician should ask more focused questions about nutrition (appetite, food preferences, variety of diet, supplements, milk intake), elimination (potty training, accidents, and the parent's reaction to accidents), sleep (bedtime ritual, naps, night-time fears), family (change of job/home, siblings, alcohol/drug/tobacco use, exposure to violence), behavior (temperament, discipline management, limit setting), and development. Normal development by age 3 might include the following:

    A.   Major motor—pedals tricycle, jumps in place, walks up and down stairs alternating feet.

    B.   Fine motor—uses eating utensils, scribbles and copies circle with crayon, dresses with supervision, stacks eight to 10 blocks, dresses and undresses with supervision.

    C.   Language—speaks in short sentences with 50% to 75% intelligible to nonfamily members, understands prepositions, asks "Why?" and "What's that?"

    D.   Social—engages in pretend play, plays interactively, listens to short stories, knows name and sex.

II. Physical Examination

Most 3-year-olds will cooperate for most of the physical examination if it is done slowly and if the physician provides careful explanations at each step. Three-year-olds are fearful of pain and may remember previous visits and injections (especially if an older sibling has primed them for the visit). Therefore offering reassuring explanations are helpful, such as *"I'm going to look in your ear with a light; I'll be very careful and it won't hurt."* Many 3-year-olds will sit on the examining table, especially if the parent stands next to them. Important aspects of the physical examination are the following:

A. Growth parameters plotted on standard growth curves.

B. Blood pressure.

C. Vision and hearing.

D. Speech and language evaluation (articulation, syntax, fluency).

E. Gait and rotational deformities, genu valgum.

F. Hip range of motion.

G. Cleanliness, evidence of abuse or neglect.

H. Developmental assessment to document historical information.

III. Screening Procedures

No screening procedures except blood pressure are usually necessary at this visit, unless the child is at increased risk (tuberculosis, lead). If the family history is positive for elevated cholesterol, consider a cholesterol level. This can be delayed if the child does not tolerate venipuncture well according to parental history.

IV. Immunizations

No immunizations are routine at 3 years of age (except the booster hepatitis A vaccine in children in selected high-incidence states—see earlier). However, the child's immunization record should be reviewed at every well-child visit to check for completeness and to catch-up immunizations as indicated.

V. Anticipatory Guidance

A. Nutrition. Discuss balanced diet and limited junk foods; vitamin/mineral supplementation is usually unnecessary; foods should not be used as rewards; encourage mealtimes as times for family conversation, giving each child the opportunity to talk.

B. Elimination. Discuss toilet training with family, including resistance, problems, and expectations.

C. Hygiene and health habits. Encourage tooth brushing under supervision with small amount of fluoridated toothpaste; discuss fluoride supplementation, if needed, and bathing.

D. Sleep. Discuss bedtime ritual; address nighttime fear management if fear is present (e.g., fear of monsters under the bed might necessitate parent and child doing a monster hunt before bedtime).

E. Sexuality. Genital exploration is normal; encourage use of correct terms for genitalia; introduce the concept of

"private areas of the body." Be prepared to answer questions at this age level about where babies come from and the differences between boys and girls.
   F.   School. Discuss the selection of preschool; anticipate separation anxiety at preschool.
   G.   Socialization and family. Encourage family play activities, sibling play activities with the child, family outings, limiting television to 1 hour, exposure to violence (domestic or television); if the mother is pregnant, discuss sibling rivalry and management.
   H.   Behavior and parenting. Discuss the importance of choices, firm limits, consistency, and the time-out technique. If parents have chosen spanking as a form of discipline, encourage other methods, but at same time discuss appropriate spanking technique.
   I.   Development. By next visit expect hopping/balancing on one foot, going up and down stairs alternating feet, drawing a person with three to six body parts, use of scissors, beginning recognition of alphabet/numbers, extensive vocabulary that is virtually 100% intelligible, the abilities to play simple board games and to dress and undress, and toilet training.
   J.   Safety. Discuss car seats, water/sun safety, street safety, keeping medications out of reach, guns, exposure to violence, limiting television to 1 hour per day, preferably with parent(s). The situation may necessitate the discussion of a new baby in the house.
  VI.   Closure
   Ask for any last-minute questions. Set next well-child appointment time. Give parents written educational materials.

ADDITIONAL READING

American Academy of Pediatrics Committee on Psychosocial Aspects of Child and Family Health. *Guidelines for health supervision of infants,* 3rd ed. Elk Grove Village, IL: American Academy of Pediatrics; 1997.

Green M, Palfrey JS, eds. *Bright futures: guidelines for health supervision of infants, children, and adolescents,* 2nd ed. Arlington, VA: National Center for Education in Maternal and Child Health; 2000.

Books for Parents

Brazelton TB. *Touchpoints: your child's emotional and behavioral development.* Reading, MA: Addison-Wesley; 1992.

Markel H. *The practical pediatrician: the A to Z guide to your child's health, behavior, and safety.* New York: WH Freeman; 1996.

Schmitt BD. *Your child's health,* rev. ed. New York: Bantam Books; 1991.

Shelov SP, Hannemann RE, DeAngelis CD, eds. *Caring for your baby and young child: birth to age 5, revised ed.* New York: Bantam Doubleday Dell; 1998.

22 ♣ Well-Child Visits—
Preschool Age: 4 to 5 Years

Raymond C. Baker

The preschool ages of 4 and 5 years mark the child's entry into a world of ordered social interaction and structure as the child begins preschool and kindergarten. All the cognitive and physical skills the child has attained by this age have led to this first world away from parents and family. The school experience allows, indeed requires, a degree of independence that has previously been practiced daily with ever larger excursions from the family embrace. School is simultaneously frightening, exhilarating, and sobering as the child begins a journey of *formal* education with books and concepts and *informal* education in relationships and social interaction. The reaction to the first day of preschool, as any preschool teacher can relate, varies from tears at separation from parents to a triumphant exploration of the classroom, with the child giddy at the prospect of new friends and new activities. Parents' reactions often reflect those of their youngster, including both tears and pride. With the emerging independence also comes increasing responsibility for behavior and self, including such chores as picking up toys and depositing dirty clothes in a clothes hamper and such personal tasks as teeth brushing, dressing, and bathing. The need for supervision with many of these activities continues but with fewer interventions as cognitive and fine motor abilities mature.

A trip to the physician is a very memorable experience for preschool children, one they will talk about and play act for weeks to come. Primary care providers must always be aware of the impact of their actions, words, and attitudes when interacting with impressionable young children. To a busy physician, picking up the next chart may sometimes feel like the visit is "just another well-child check-up" among many. To the child, however, it is a major event. The health care provider must enter each examining room with a caring and friendly demeanor and interact with the youngster as though that child was the most important child in the world.

FOUR-YEAR VISIT

I. History

The 4-year-old has well-developed communication skills and the irrepressible need to display them. With these language skills and an insatiable curiosity about the world and its inhabitants, the 4-year-old constantly questions the workings of everything with *why, who, what, when,* and *where* questions. He becomes an expert in testing limits set by parents and siblings, with little real understanding of the frustration that testing causes. At the same time, he is learning to understand emotions of sadness, anger, fear, and guilt in himself and his family members. He has acquired the skill of making friends and engaging in play activities, including make-believe. The 4-year-old has achieved bowel and bladder control (although he or she may still have nocturnal enuresis) and has developed a sense of privacy and modesty—at least some of the time. The same youngster who may prance around naked at one time of the day may later demand privacy when using the potty chair.

The interview should include questions directed to the child. This gives the child ownership of the visit, increases rapport with the child, and allows the physician to evaluate speech and language. Parents usually listen with pride at their child's conversation and may add or supplement the information. The interchange between parent and child are important clues to how nurturing or critical the parent/child relationship is. Questions might include the following: *"How old are you?"* *"Do you go to preschool?"* *"What do you like best about school?"* *"What do you like to do with your parents?"*

The physician should begin the interview with the parents with open-ended questions to encourage dialogue (e.g., *"How are things going at home?"* *"How is Johnny doing in school?"* *"Has he had any illnesses since our last visit?"* *"Do you have any special concerns or questions today?"*). A review of the behaviors indicated by the parent on the Preschool Children's Behavior Checklist (Appendix G) during this part of the history serves as a good trigger to discuss normal age-appropriate behaviors and behavior management techniques. Part of this discussion may be addressed later as part of anticipatory guidance. During the interview the physician should watch the child to see the reactions to the parent's responses. Does the preschooler listen and join in the conversation, sit quietly, or play with toys in the examination room?

After addressing the parent's concerns, the physician should ask more focused questions about nutrition (eating habits, mealtime behavior, diet), elimination (accidents and parents' reaction to them, nocturnal enuresis), sleep (bedtime ritual, sleep disturbances—nightmares or night terrors), family (change of job/home, siblings, alcohol/drug/tobacco use, exposure to violence), behavior (discipline management, limit setting, interaction with children in preschool), and development. Normal development by age 4 might include the following:

A.   Major motor—pedals tricycle, hops on one foot, walks up and down stairs alternating feet.

B.   Fine motor—draws circle and cross, draws a person with 3 to 6 body parts, cuts with scissors, dresses and undresses with minimal supervision, brushes teeth.

C.   Language—speaks in full sentences fully intelligible to nonfamily members, asks questions, talks about daily activities, uses tenses, may stutter; counts, may know alphabet, shows interest in learning letters and numbers.

D.   Social—plays using pretend activities, shows ability to take turns and share, plays simple board games (Candyland, Hi-Ho Cherry-O).

II.   Physical Examination

The physical examination at this age is usually met with interest (and a lot of questions!) and mild anxiety, which can usually be allayed by careful explanations of each step. The child will usually sit on the examining table during the examination as long as the parent is within sight, and the examination can proceed from head to foot. The physician should talk to the child as the examination progresses to answer questions and explain the parts of the examination. Important features of the physical examination are the following:

   A. Growth parameters plotted on standard growth curves.
   B. Blood pressure.
   C. Strabismus and visual acuity.
   D. Ear examination for chronic changes, hearing.
   E. Mouth for dental caries and dental hygiene.
   F. Abdominal examination for masses or organo-megaly.
   G. Gait, spine, extremities for rotational deformities.
   H. Cleanliness and evidence of abuse or neglect.
  III. Screening Procedures
       Perform lead and tuberculin testing if child is at increased risk. Cholesterol if at child is at increased risk and can tolerate venipuncture without undue fear and resistance (may be postponed to the 5-year visit). Blood pressure screening and vision and hearing screening are also appropriate at this visit.
  IV. Immunizations
       Immunizations should include **IPV, DTaP, and MMR** at this visit or the 5-year visit.
   V. Anticipatory Guidance
   A. Nutrition. Discuss balanced diet; serve small portions with an opportunity to ask for more; offer variety but respect limited food preferences; discuss mealtime as family time, with each child having the opportunity to talk; limit refined sugar and salt intake; provide healthy snacks between meals (fruits, raw vegetables).
   B. Elimination. Discuss normal nighttime urinary continence while praising daytime control; anticipate regression with new sibling or other life changes.
   C. Hygiene and health habits. Encourage tooth brushing with small amount of fluoridated toothpaste with supervision and help (general rule: a child is able to brush teeth without help when able to tie shoes), annual dental checkups, and regular bathing.
   D. Sleep. Stress the importance of the bedtime ritual; acknowledge that nighttime fears ("monsters under the bed"), nightmares, and sleep terrors are common at this age (explain difference and management).
   E. Sexuality. Sexual curiosity about genitalia and masturbation is normal as it shows curiosity about boy/girl differences. Use correct anatomic terms; answer questions about sex at age-appropriate level ("Where do babies come from?"). Children may attempt to touch genitalia of parent, which should lead to discussion of private areas of body; brief episodes

of sexual play among children are common, which should also stimulate discussion of private areas of body.

F.   School. Encourage preschool if not already enrolled; stress importance of parent/teacher contact.

G.   Socialization and family. Emphasize the importance for the child to have opportunity for peer play (school, neighbors, church activities); pretend play is common.

H.   Behavior and parenting. Review behavior management; stress the use of time out as an important technique at this age; child can understand limited consequences of rule breaking (applied consistently and when appropriate to the rule broken); praise for good behavior is much more effective than negative reinforcement for bad behaviors.

I.   Development. By next visit anticipate hopping, skipping, balancing on one foot, shoe tying, mature pencil grasp and use of pencil to draw squares, circles, triangles, print some letters (in name); child will be able to relate stories using full sentences, use appropriate tenses and pronouns, count, and name colors.

J.   Safety. Discuss car seats and water/sun safety; anticipate bicycle helmets; discuss stranger precautions, including telling parent if approached or touched inappropriately, pet safety, the importance of a fire plan in home, 911 instructions, guns, and exposure to violence; limit television to 1 hour per day.

VI.   Closure

Ask for any last-minute questions. Advise about next well-child appointment time. Give parents written educational materials.

FIVE-YEAR VISIT

I.   History

By 5 years of age, most children have entered a school setting and experienced the structure needed to listen, respond to the teacher, and attend to learning tasks. While this may come easily for some children, it may challenge others, depending on innate temperament and experiences at home. Perhaps the greatest learning task of this age is learning how to sit quietly and attend to the teacher without being distracted by others in the class. From the primary care provider's perspective, the 5-year-old should be an active participant in the history and physical examination. The physician should speak directly to the child while asking age-appropriate questions. This helps develop a special rapport between child and physician and fosters the concept of independence that is developing in the child. Questions for the child might include the following: *"How are you today?" "Do you have any questions for me about your body or your health today?" "How are you doing in school?" "What is your teacher's name?" "What do you like best about school?" "Do you ride the school bus?" "Who is your best friend at school?" "What is your address?"*

As the child answers, the physician can look to parents for supplemental information or questions that arise. The physician should likewise ask the parents several open-ended questions to encourage dialogue. A review of the behaviors indicated by the parent on the Preschool Children's Behavior Checklist (Appendix G) during this part of the history serves as a good trigger for discussing normal age-appropriate behaviors and behavior management techniques. After discussing issues raised by the parents and the checklist, the physician should ask the child and parent more focused questions about the following areas:

A. **Nutrition.** Diet and appetite; snacks, mealtime behavior.

B. **Elimination.** Fecal soiling, enuresis.

C. **Sleep.** Bedtime, sleep disturbances.

D. **School.** Social skills, school avoidance behaviors, and results of parent/teacher conferences.

E. **Family.** Family activities/outings, recent stresses (move, job change, divorce), sibling interactions, child's interaction with new baby, television habits, smoking/alcohol/drug exposure.

F. **Behavior.** Self-dressing, shoe tying, bicycle riding, letter/number recognition, counting, ability to sit still during storytelling and meals.

G. **Development.** Normal development at 5 years of age might include the following:

1. *Motor*—balance on one foot, hop/skip.

2. *Fine motor*—tie shoes; show mature pencil grasp and pencil use and ability to draw some numbers and letters (especially name).

3. *Language*—relates a story using full sentences, correct tenses, and pronouns; counts at least to 10 and knows colors.

4. *Social*—dresses and undresses without supervision (except to pick out matching clothes!); sits quietly in class and listens to teacher without being distracted by classmates.

II. **Physical Examination**

The 5-year-old cooperates well with the physical examination and does not feel afraid, except perhaps for injections. However, the child should be able to distinguish between the examination itself (and not be afraid) and the injection by the nurse, which may cause some anxiety. Most 5-year-olds tolerate injections fairly well, sometimes even bragging "*I like shots!*" The physician can use the examination to maintain a running conversation with the child, to supplement the history, and to assess the child's language development. This interaction also helps to form a bond with the physician. Important features of the physical examination are the following:

A. **Growth parameters and blood pressure.**

B. **Vision and hearing screening, check for strabismus.**

C. **Dentition, including caries, oral hygiene, dental injuries, malocclusion, tooth eruption and shedding.**

D. **Cleanliness and evidence of abuse or neglect.**

III.   Screening Procedures
Vision and hearing screening, blood pressure screening. Risk assessment for tuberculosis, lead, hyperlipidemia, and screening tests as appropriate.

IV.   Immunizations
If not given at the 4-year visit, administer **DTaP, IPV, and MMR**.

V.   Anticipatory Guidance
  A.   Nutrition. Discuss healthy diet; limit junk foods, candy, processed sugar, sodium, and soda; encourage at least one meal per day with the whole family; emphasize healthy snacks.

  B.   Elimination. Episodic nocturnal enuresis still common enough that major intervention is unnecessary; if present, parent can eliminate fluids within the hour before bedtime and encourage the child to help change sheets on wet mornings. Discuss etiology of nocturnal enuresis, and emphasize that it is not deliberate.

  C.   Hygiene and health habits. Discuss with child and parent regular teeth brushing twice a day with supervision and the importance of regular exercise; limit television/computer games to 1 hour per day; prohibit television in child's room.

  D.   Sleep. Discuss adequate sleep needs and regular bedtime (8:00 to 8:30 P.M. on school nights).

  E.   Sexuality. Encourage parents to answer questions about sexuality frankly and at age- and interest-appropriate level. Suggest using a picture book on sexuality. Encourage parents to discuss inappropriate touching with the child.

  F.   School. Encourage parent/teacher meetings; encourage/praise child's schoolwork. The refrigerator is a good place to display child's work.

  G.   Socialization and family. Encourage family outings, meals, and sharing school stories.

  H.   Behavior and parenting. Encourage chores for the child (picking up toys, dirty clothes in hamper, taking dirty dishes to sink after meals), playing with peers, praise of the child, and reading with and without parents.

  I.   Safety. Review car, water, sun, street, and bicycle safety and the use of smoke detectors and the importance of a fire plan; discuss guns and exposure to domestic and/or television/movie violence.

VI.   Closure
Ask for any last-minute questions. Advise about next well-child appointment time. Give parents written educational materials.

ADDITIONAL READING

American Academy of Pediatrics Committee on Psychosocial Aspects of Child and Family Health. *Guidelines for health supervision of infants,* 3rd ed. Elk Grove Village, IL: American Academy of Pediatrics; 1997.

Green M, Palfrey JS, eds. *Bright futures: guidelines for health supervision of infants, children, and adolescents,* 2nd ed. Arlington, VA: National Center for Education in Maternal and Child Health; 2000.

Books for Parents

Brazelton TB. *Touchpoints: your child's emotional and behavioral development.* Reading, MA: Addison-Wesley; 1992.

Markel H. *The practical pediatrician: the A to Z guide to your child's health, behavior, and safety.* New York: WH Freeman; 1996.

Schmitt BD. *Your child's health*, rev. ed. New York: Bantam Books; 1991.

Shelov SP, Hannemann RE, DeAngelis CD. eds. *Caring for your baby and young child: birth to age 5,* rev. ed. New York: Bantam Doubleday Dell; 1998.

23 ♣ Well-Child Visits—Elementary School Age: 6 to 11 Years

Raymond C. Baker

By the time of entry into the formal education of elementary school, the child has matured cognitively, physically, and socially with an emerging sense of self in the family, the classroom, and the world. The child has learned to function independently of parents in the classroom and with friends. This independence coincides with a growing sense of what is right morally and spiritually. Even though developing independence is a critical stage of the school-aged child, family values remain a major force in the child's life, molding and shaping self-image and a sense of self-worth. The value parents put on education and other life activities is reflected in how much value the child puts into learning and other aspects of his life. Unfortunately, other forces that may be less concerned with the child's best interests are also at work during these critical years—television, movies, cigarette and alcohol advertising, and even exposure to drug use—all of which suggest a glamor of certain lifestyles far from what parents want for their child. The child looks to parents and other family members to put these external forces into proper perspective relative to the family's value system.

The child's developing autonomy extends to health care as the child assumes greater responsibility for health and hygiene measures and for his relationship with the health care provider. The provider can form a therapeutic alliance with the child and can interact directly with him on health care issues, albeit with continued parental supervision and sanction. Health supervision visits are well suited to open discussions between health care provider and the school-aged child about health care, school, and other age-related behaviors. As the child gets older (10 years), the provider may find spending time alone with the child for these discussions appropriate, anticipating the time when, as a teenager, most of the visit involves the provider and the patient without the parent in the room.

SIX-YEAR VISIT

I. History

By 6 years of age, most children have begun elementary school in either kindergarten or first grade. Most of the anxiety about separation from parents and functioning independently in the school setting has been resolved by this age, and the child is able to enjoy school and the new social interactions it brings. First graders, proud of their accomplishments in school and on the playground, bask in praise from parents and teachers. The 6-year-old is learning about safety rules, such as street safety, but needs consistent reminders, role modeling, and limit setting. Friends have become increasingly important and may influence the 6-year-old's behavior, making consistent enforcement of family and house rules important.

In the pediatric office setting, the first grader is anxious to please and cooperates with the history and physical examination, now that most fears about injections are put in proper perspective. The physician can address many questions directly to the child and expect totally frank answers.

The interview should be directed primarily to the child with supplementation from the parent and begins with open-ended questions to allow the parent or child to bring up questions or concerns (*"How are you getting along in school?"* *"Who is your favorite teacher?"* *"Do you have something special you would like to ask me about today?"* *"Are you worried about anything?"*). A review of the behaviors indicated by the parent on the Pediatric Symptom Checklist for School-Age Children (Appendix H) during this part of the history serves as a good trigger to explore normal age-appropriate issues and behaviors. Part or all of this discussion may be addressed later as part of anticipatory guidance. The interview should then focus on several important areas:

    A. **Nutrition.** Balanced diet, junk foods, appetite.
    B. **Elimination.** Enuresis or fecal soiling, regularity.
    C. **Sleep.** Bedtime, dreams, nighttime fears.
    D. **School.** Performance, parent/teacher conferences, socialization with classmates.
    E. **Family.** Family outings, house rules, discipline.
    F. **Behavior and development.** Bicycle riding, tying shoes, sports participation, learning letters and numbers, anger management, and conflict resolution.

  II. **Physical Examination**
    Important features of the examination are the following:
    A. **Growth parameters, blood pressure.**
    B. **Vision testing, hearing testing** (unless tested and normal at last visit or at school).
    C. **Speech and language evaluation by physician—** articulation, fluency, syntax, ability to count to 20 and recite the alphabet.
    D. **Coordination and strength.**
  III. **Screening Procedures**
    No screening procedures are usually indicated at this age unless the patient is at high risk for tuberculosis or hyperlipidemia.
  IV. **Immunizations**
    No immunizations are needed at this visit.
  V. **Anticipatory Guidance**
    A. **Nutrition.** Advise a well-balanced diet, avoiding junk foods and excessive candy. Recommend family meals at least once per day, including time to talk about the day's activities. Avoid using food/candy as rewards. Encourage regular exercise.
    B. **Elimination.** If nocturnal enuresis persists, discuss management.

   C.   Hygiene and health habits. Encourage twice-daily teeth brushing and regular bathing.
   D.   Sleep. Advise adequate sleep with bedtime between 8:00 and 9:00 P.M.
   E.   Sexuality. Advise answering questions about sexuality frankly and at an age-appropriate level. Encourage age-appropriate books on sexuality.
   F.   School. Encourage parent/teacher conferences and praise for child's schoolwork. If school performance is a problem, advise parents of the school's legal obligation to evaluate the child for learning disabilities/problems and also of ways to initiate the process.
   G.   Socialization and family. Encourage reading, family outings, family discussions about house rules, and chores.
   H.   Behavior and parenting. Discuss behavior management, house rules, and consequences for breaking house rules (avoiding physical discipline); discuss conflict resolution and anger management and showing affection; limit television/computer games to 1 hour per day; avoid television in the child's room.
   I.   Safety. Review the use of a bicycle helmet and car/street/water/sun safety; prohibit smoking in the house; discuss guns and exposure to violence; discuss inappropriate touching.
VI.   Closure
   Ask for any last-minute questions. Advise about next well-child appointment time. Give parents written educational materials.

SEVEN- TO 9-YEAR VISITS
   I.   History
   Children from 7 through 9 years of age have achieved greater responsibility in their own day-to-day activities, including areas, such as personal hygiene and household chores (e.g., keeping their rooms tidy, feeding pets, setting the table, and making their beds). While clearly viewed as "chores," these activities at the same time give the child a sense of accomplishment and competency. Schoolwork during the second through fourth grades is becoming more complex, with book reports, school projects, and other homework, which adds to the sense of responsibility. As peers become more important, often including best friends, the child begins to see parents as just like everyone else's parents, rather than the all-knowing icons of previous years (a major difficulty for some parents!).
   The physician should address most questions directly to the child, who should be able to provide most of the pertinent history with supplementation from the parent. The interview should begin with open-ended questions to encourage the child and parents to bring up areas of concern or questions (*"How are things going at home?" "How about school—do you enjoy it?" "What are your favorite subjects in school?" "How is homework going?"*). A review of the behaviors indicated by the parent on the Pediatric

Symptom Checklist for School-Age Children (Appendix H) during this part of the history serves as a good trigger to explore normal age-appropriate issues and behaviors. Part or all of this discussion may be addressed later as part of anticipatory guidance.

The physician can then ask the child more focused questions in several areas. Each area of questioning may have related questions addressed to the parent, with the physician looking for areas of concern or those that raise questions:

  A. Nutrition. Diet, including snacks, concerns about weight, junk food.

  B. Elimination. Enuresis, fecal soiling, frequent urination.

  C. Sleep. Bedtime, sleep disturbances, sleepovers.

  D. School. Parent/teacher conference results, grade cards, likes and dislikes, homework.

  E. Hygiene. Bathing, brushing teeth.

  F. Behavior. House rules and consequences (television, homework), hobbies, competitive sports, reading, television/computer games, anger management.

  G. Health and safety. Bicycle helmet, sports safety.

 II. Physical Examination

    Important features of the examination are the following:

  A. Growth parameters and blood pressure.

  B. Speech—free of articulation errors, fluent.

  C. Visual acuity, hearing screening—if child, parent, or teacher has any concerns.

  D. Observation of age-appropriate attentiveness, social abilities, relationship with parents.

  E. Early signs of puberty (underarm odor/sweat, growth spurt, secondary sex characteristics).

  F. Scoliosis.

  G. Coordination, muscle strength and tone in children participating in sports activities.

 III. Screening Procedures

  A. A screening urinalysis. Perform once during the early school-aged years.

  B. Tuberculin testing if at high risk.

  C. Cholesterol determination if at high risk and not done previously.

  D. Vision and hearing screening.

  E. Blood pressure screening.

 IV. Immunizations

    No immunizations are recommended at this age, unless catch-up immunizations are needed.

 V. Anticipatory Guidance

  A. Nutrition. Emphasize balanced diet, regular exercise, and limited junk foods.

  B. Hygiene and health habits. Discuss teeth brushing twice a day, regular dental visits, regular bathing, and tobacco, alcohol and drug use.

  C. Sleep. Cover bedtime and sleep requirements (9 to 10 hours per night).

D.   Sexuality. Answer questions about sexuality frankly and at an age-appropriate level; discuss school sex education with child; encourage mother to prepare daughters for onset of menses.

E.   School. Discuss homework, encouragement, and praise for successes.

F.   Socialization and family, relationships. Encourage reading, hobbies, family outings, and chores; discuss overnights and personal/private space for child.

G.   Behavior and parenting. Discuss house rules, consequences for breaking house rules, television/computer game limits, anger management, and conflict resolution.

H.   Safety. Emphasize car/water/sun safety; discuss interaction with strangers (telephone, stranger at the door when alone in house), guns, exposure to violence, fire safety, and smoke detectors.

VI.   Closure

Ask for any last-minute questions. Advise about next well-child appointment time. Give parents written educational materials.

TEN- TO 11-YEAR VISITS

I.   History

The preadolescent, 10 to 11 years of age, stands on the brink of the tumultuous teenage years, which will bring dramatic changes in physical and psychological make-up. These two preadolescent years often set the stage for these subsequent changes. Some children at this age, girls more than boys, are already entering adolescence physically. Independence from parents grows as the child shows greater reliance on peers for style, attitudes, and values. This developing independence and allegiance to peers, often misunderstood and resisted by parents, brings them into conflict with the child. The primary care provider is in a good position to help parents understand this growing autonomy as a desirable trait, which can be fostered and channeled into positive behavior. Parents should be encouraged to give the child more responsibility and choices, such as chores done on the child's own timetable, an allowance, and freedom to pick out clothing, which will very likely be greatly influenced by peers (and don't expect the clean-cut, tailored look!).

Preadolescents continue to need parental approval and praise in order to enhance and to maintain their self-esteem and self-confidence. School performance, extracurricular activities, and sports are all areas that parents can use to find areas in which their child excels. Because risk-taking behaviors, physical and otherwise, might be seen in this age group due to peer pressures, both parents and the health care provider must address these behaviors in a positive, nonconfrontational manner.

Much of the health supervision visit interview can be directed to the child, perhaps even with the parent out of the room, depending on the child's wishes and the circumstances.

Questions should cover a wide variety of issues, including nutrition and diet, school performance and homework, risk-taking behaviors or exposure to these behaviors in peers (smoking, alcohol use, drug use, physical recklessness), hobbies, anger management, and sexuality (such as sex education at school, sexual abuse, early sexual exploratory behaviors [depending on the stage of pubertal development], discussions the child has had with parents, and any questions the child might have). A review of the behaviors indicated by the parent on the Pediatric Symptom Checklist for School-Age Children (Appendix H) during this part of the history serves as a good trigger to explore normal age-appropriate issues and behaviors. Part or all of this discussion may be addressed later as part of anticipatory guidance.

II. Physical Examination
The physical examination should be comprehensive, with appropriate draping to respect the child's modesty. The health care provider may want to ask the child if he or she wants the parent in the room when the genitalia are examined. Even at this age, and certainly at subsequent ages, if the parent is not present, a third person (nurse or nursing assistant, same gender as patient preferably) should be present. Important features of the examination at this age are the following:

   A. Growth parameters plotted on standard growth curves with close attention to children below the 5th percentile or above the 95th percentile on weight for height graph or body mass index.

   B. Scoliosis examination (and check for leg length discrepancy) **with orthopedic referral as needed.**

   C. Sexual maturity rating.

   D. Dental caries/injuries/malocclusion/hygiene.

III. Screening Procedures
No screening procedures are usually necessary at this visit, unless at increased risk for tuberculosis or hyperlipidemia. Perform routine blood pressure, vision, and hearing screens.

IV. Immunizations
None are usually indicated at this visit. However, if the child has missed the HBV immunization series, it should be given now before onset of puberty and sexual activity.

V. Anticipatory Guidance

   A. Nutrition. Discuss a balanced diet with snacks, especially in the context of over- or underweight children, avoidance of junk foods, and participating in regular exercise.

   B. Hygiene and health habits/high-risk behaviors. Encourage regular (twice-daily) tooth brushing, flossing, and dental check-ups; avoid cigarettes/drugs/alcohol; discuss sports training and injuries; limit television/computer games to 1 hour per day with no television in child's room.

   C. Sleep. Encourage a regular bedtime, with 9 to 10 hours of sleep per night.

   D. Sexuality. For pubertal adolescents, encourage sexual abstinence.

  E. School. Discuss homework issues and house rules regarding homework; encourage reading.
  F. Socialization and family, relationships. Encourage parents to get to know the child's friends, especially if overnights are planned; encourage family outings and meals together; discuss appropriate supervision of child with friends.
  G. Behavior and parenting. Emphasize house rules and the consequences for breaking them; encourage parents to spend individual time with the child; discuss chores and allowance; encourage parents to prepare child for menarche/nocturnal emissions/sexual feelings; suggest appropriate books to cover sexuality.
  H. Safety. Discuss participation in competitive sports with appropriate training and supervision, car/sun/water safety, bicycle helmets, padding for roller blading/skateboarding, guns in the home, alcohol in the home, and exposure to violence.
VI. Closure
  Ask for any last-minute questions. Advise about next well-child appointment time. Give parents written educational materials.

ADDITIONAL READING

American Academy of Pediatrics Committee on Psychosocial Aspects of Child and Family Health. *Guidelines for health supervision of infants,* 3rd ed. Elk Grove Village, IL: American Academy of Pediatrics; 1997.

Green M, Palfrey JS, eds. *Bright futures: guidelines for health supervision of infants, children, and adolescents,* 2nd ed. Arlington, VA: National Center for Education in Maternal and Child Health; 2000.

Books for Parents

Kutner L. *Your school-age child: from kindergarten through sixth grade.* New York: Avon Books; 1997.

Nathanson LW. *The portable pediatrician's guide to kids: your child's physical and behavioral development from ages 5 to 12.* New York: Harper Perennial; 1996.

Schmitt BD. *Your child's health*, rev. ed. New York: Bantam Books; 1991.

Schor EL, ed. *Caring for your school-age child: ages 5 to 12.* New York: Bantam Books; 1995.

24 ♣ Health Maintenance Visits— Early Adolescence: 12 to 14 Years

Thomas S. Webb

Early adolescence is characterized by rapid changes in physical characteristics. These pubertal changes coexist with the adolescent's heightened concern with appearance, normalcy, and desire for peer acceptance. The adolescent is preoccupied with body image, development of secondary sex characteristics, menstruation, nocturnal emissions, and concerns surrounding masturbation and sexual feelings.

During this period, the adolescent strives for greater independence from parental control. The teen becomes less interested in family activities, challenges parental input and authority, and focuses on same-sex friendships. Cognitively, the early teen remains in Piaget's concrete operational thought stage, with little insight and limited abstract reasoning skills. Foresight and judgment are poor, and decisions are viewed as absolutely right or wrong.

THE EARLY ADOLESCENT VISIT

An extended visit is necessary to perform complete interviews with both parent and adolescent and a comprehensive physical exam. The interview should begin with both parent and patient in the room together. If this is the first visit, the physician should introduce himself to the adolescent first and then to the parent. The adolescent is then seen alone for a confidential interview, followed by the physical exam with or without the parent present, depending on the adolescent's preference. The parent will feel more comfortable knowing the private interview is part of the developmental process in which the adolescent begins an individual relationship with the health care provider. Reassure the parent that any indication of potential harm to the child or others will be relayed and that open communication with the parent will be encouraged.

I. **History**

The interview process should be performed with the patient remaining clothed. The provider should observe the interaction between parents and child. Is it positive, cooperative, or antagonistic? Does the teenager answer the health provider's questions or turn to the parents for responses? Basic past medical history, family history, social history, medications, and review of systems can be asked of both patient and parents during this time. Parental questions and health concerns can be addressed with both together. If the parents become vague or seem uncomfortable with the adolescent in the room because of the information they want to discuss, the adolescent can be asked to step out of the room so the parents can speak freely. The hearing and vision examinations could be performed during this time.

Following the joint interview, the physician should ask the parents to leave and should interview the adolescent alone. The confidential interview begins with general questions about school, friends, and hobbies. Assess the patient's cognitive and psychosocial development using developmentally appropriate questions. Repeat your assurances and limitations of confidentiality. When possible, conduct the interview with open ended, non-judgmental questions. Some clinicians have the adolescent complete a preprinted questionnaire (such as the Adolescent Previsit Questionnaire in Appendix I) that can be reviewed as part of this discussion.

A. **Questions for the parent:**
1. How is your teenager doing in general? At home? At school?
2. How is everyone getting along?
3. Are there any changes or new stressors in the family?
4. Tell me about your teenager's hobbies, friends, and favorite family activity.
5. In what kind of after-school/summer activities is your teenager involved?
6. What have you discussed so far about house rules, smoking, drinking, drugs, and sexuality?
7. Are you concerned about anyone in the family regarding smoking, drinking, drugs, or behavior problems?
8. Does your teenager follow a reasonable diet, have an exercise program, and get adequate sleep?
9. Does your teenager respect safety issues, such as seat belts, helmets, telephone, and internet safety?
10. Do you have any specific concerns?
11. What one thing would you like me to congratulate your teenager for today?

B. **Questions for the adolescent.** Many of the same questions can be asked of the teenager, with emphasis on the following:
1. Symptoms of depression, isolation, suicidal ideation, and body image distortion.
2. School problems, failure, and vagrancy.
3. Sexual experimentation; sexual, physical, or emotional abuse.
4. Peer group or personal use of tobacco, drugs, huffing, and alcohol.
5. Adequate calcium, iron, B vitamin, and caloric intake.
6. Adequate sleep, exercise, safety equipment use, and personal hygiene.
7. Evidence of personal responsibility (chores), cognitive development (reading, limited television), and good communication (family activities with one or both parents).

II. **Physical Examination**
The physical examination is performed with the parent in or out of the room, depending on the adolescent's preference. If the parent is in the room, the physician should be careful to

respect the adolescent's privacy using appropriate covering. If the parent is not in the room, a chaperone, preferably of the same sex as the adolescent, should be present. Reassuring the adolescent during the examination that physical findings, especially with respect to pubertal changes, are normal is important.

A complete physical should be performed with special attention to the following:

   A. General appearance—well kept, appropriate clothing, mood, interaction with parent.

   B. Blood pressure.

   C. Height, weight, body mass index (BMI).

   D. Skin for acne, moles, warts.

   E. Dental examination—looking for caries, gum disease, malocclusion, molar crowding.

   F. Gynecomastia in males.

   G. Scoliosis.

   H. Tanner staging:
     1. *Breasts and pubic hair in females.*
     2. *Penis and pubic hair in males.*

   I. Pelvic examination and external examination for genital warts (if sexually active female).

   J. Penile examination for genital warts (if sexually active male).

   K. Testicular examination for hernias or masses.

III. Screening Tests

   A. Hearing.

   B. Vision.

   C. Hemoglobin/hematocrit or complete blood count (CBC) with red cell indices to screen for anemia in menstruating females; other adolescents as indicated by the history (experiencing the growth spurt or demonstrating evidence of poor nutrition).

   D. Cholesterol if the family history is positive for hyperlipidemia or early-onset ischemic heart disease.

   E. Tuberculin testing if the adolescent has any of the following risk factors:
     1. *Low socioeconomic status.*
     2. *Residence in areas where tuberculosis is prevalent.*
     3. *Exposure to tuberculosis.*
     4. *Immigrant status.*
     5. *Homelessness.*
     6. *History of incarceration.*
     7. *Employment or volunteer work in health care setting.*

   F. Perform the following if the adolescent is believed to be sexually active:
     1. *Pap smear.*
     2. *Cervical sample* for gonorrhea and chlamydia.
     3. *Wet mount* for trichomonas and yeast.
     4. *Urinalysis for leukocyte esterase* can be used in males as a screen for sexually transmitted disease (STD).

   G. If the adolescent demonstrates high-risk sexual behavior, perform the following:
     1. *HIV serologic examination.*

  2. *RPR serologic examination.*
  3. *Hepatitis B serologic examination* (if not already immunized).
IV. Immunizations
  The immunization record should be examined to ensure that basic immunizations have been given. Special attention should be given to the following:
  A. MMR booster.
  B. HBV vaccine series.
  C. Td booster (if greater than 5 years since last DTaP).
  D. Varicella vaccine (if negative history of clinical disease).
  E. Hepatitis A vaccine (if sexually active, homosexual male).
V. Anticipatory Guidance for the Parent
  A. Communication. Open communication is essential in this age group. Despite their often curt responses, adolescents do like being asked about their day/activities/thoughts. This underscores for the adolescent that the parent is still interested and involved. Communication should be calm, equally interactive, and supportive.
  B. Weapons. The issue of whether weapons should be kept in the home is often a very personal matter to the family. However, parents should know that adolescents usually know where the weapon is stored, where the lock key (if used) is hidden, and where the ammunition is kept. Responsibility should be stressed. The weapon should never be loaded, and ammunition should be kept in a separate area. Serious consideration should be given to removing weapons from a home with a depressed, stressed, or violent teen.
  C. Rule setting. This is very difficult in early adolescence. Limit testing is a major component of this stage, and the parent should be aware that this is normal behavior. Consistency and fairness are key principles. Although anticipating all the necessary rules is impossible, sitting down early on in this stage and reviewing general principles and expectations is helpful.
  D. Privacy issues. Respecting and promoting private time for the teen is important. If possible, teens should be allowed their own room/space (from younger siblings). Early adolescents will become more private with dressing and bathing; sexual self-exploration/masturbation is common (and normal) at this stage.
  E. Increasing responsibility. Graded responsibility is an important goal. Chores should be developmentally appropriate. Significant praise should follow successful completion of a new responsibility.
  F. TV, computer use. Both mediums should be supervised for content. While both resources can provide a wealth of information, access time should be balanced with homework, chores, and exercise.

G. Role modeling. Parents should be reminded that most behavior is learned and that, for better or worse, most is learned in the home. Language, substance abuse, sexual mores, political and social opinions, dress, work ethic, honesty, and cleanliness, to name a few, are all modeled first and foremost after parental behavior, especially at this stage of development.

H. Punishment. Consistency and fairness is key. "Make the time fit the crime." The most effective punishment at this age is loss of privileges. Corporal punishment often reinforces violence and aggression as problem-solving techniques and should be discouraged.

I. Puberty issues. The teen has numerous questions, often unasked, in early adolescence. Parents should be informed of upcoming expected developments, such as the need for deodorant, training bras, and menstrual pads (not tampons) so that they can be prepared to encourage and initiate their use.

J. Personal safety. Parents should review these issues regularly with their teens: good and bad touching, seat belt use, substance abuse, telephone and internet safety, bicycle/skateboard/rollerblade safety, to name just a few items.

K. Confidence building. Parents should seek tasks that will help build confidence in their teens and provide an area for parental praise. Encouraging development in areas of interest to the teen is helpful, whether they are team or independent sports, music, reading, writing, art, computers, or domestic tasks. Parents should identify strengths and weaknesses in the adolescent and help with both.

VI. **Anticipatory Guidance for the Adolescent**
  A. **Health promotion**
    1. *Adequate sleep* (8 to 10 hours per night).
    2. *Regular exercise,* preferably three or more times per week.
    3. *A knowledgeable trainer* for supervision of weight training.
    4. *Balanced diet,* including three meals per day with recommended daily allowances.
    5. *Dental care.* Brushing teeth twice daily, flossing daily, and visiting the dentist every 6 to 12 months.
    6. *Limiting sedentary activities,* such as television, computer games, and internet use.
  B. **Mental health**
    1. *Find a niche.*
    2. *Discuss feelings with someone you trust.*
    3. *Seek help if your safety is in jeopardy.*
  C. **Injury prevention**
    1. *Seat belts.*
    2. *Helmets.*
    3. *Appropriate sports gear.*
    4. *No weapons.*

5. *Conflict resolution.*
6. *Personal safety* by avoiding high-risk physical behaviors suggested by peers (e.g., dangerous skateboarding, gang activities).

D. Substance use
1. *Discourage tobacco use.* Focus on negative physical consequences, such as teeth and finger staining, wrinkles, and bad breath.
2. *Explain hazards of drug and alcohol use.*
3. *Discuss huffing.*
4. *Discourage diet pills.*
5. *Discuss anabolic steroids.*

E. Sexuality
1. *Explain current and expected pubertal changes.*
2. *Encourage open communication with trusted adult.*
3. *Discuss nocturnal emissions and masturbation.*
4. *Encourage and congratulate abstinence.*
5. *Encourage open discussion with parents or health provider if sexually active.* Give explicit instructions on the prevention of STDs and pregnancy, including how and where to obtain birth control and condoms.

VII. Concluding the Adolescent Visit
After the history and physical examination are completed, the primary care provider should sit down with the adolescent and discuss the findings of the examination and laboratory testing (if available; if not, make arrangements to contact the adolescent with the results) and provide anticipatory guidance in areas suggested by the history and physical examination (as noted earlier). This discussion should be unhurried and informal, allowing the adolescent the opportunity to ask questions and to respond to suggestions. Many physicians provide adolescents and parents written information that expands and supplements issues raised during the visit. Finally, follow-up should be arranged and information given to the adolescent and parents regarding how and when to contact the office for appointments, information, or referrals.

ADDITIONAL READING

American Academy of Pediatrics. *Recommendations for preventative pediatric health care (RE9535).* Elk Grove Village, IL: American Academy of Pediatrics; 2000.

American Academy of Pediatrics. *Recommended childhood immunization schedule—United States, January–December 2000* (RE9961). Elk Grove Village, IL: American Academy of Pediatrics; 2000.

Committee on Psychosocial Aspects of Child and Family Health, American Academy of Pediatrics. *Guidelines for health supervision of infants,* 3rd ed. Elk Grove Village, IL: American Academy of Pediatrics; 1997.

Fox CE, III. *Put prevention into practice: clinician's handbook of preventive services,* 2nd ed. Washington, DC: U.S. Department of Health and Human Services; 1998.

Green M, Palfrey JS, eds. *Bright futures: guidelines for health supervision of infants, children, and adolescents,* 2nd ed. Arlington, VA: National Center for Education in Maternal and Child Health; 2000.

McAnarney ER, Kreipe RE, Orr DP, Comerci GD. *Textbook of adolescent medicine.* Philadelphia: WB Saunders; 1992.

Neinstein LS. *Adolescent health care: a practical guide,* 3rd ed. Baltimore: Williams & Wilkins; 1996.

U.S. Preventative Services Task Force. *Guide to clinical preventive services: report of the U.S. Preventative Services Task Force,* 2nd ed. Washington, DC: U.S. Department of Health and Human Services; 1995.

25 ♣ Health Maintenance Visits— Middle Adolescence: 15 to 17 Years

Thomas S. Webb

In middle adolescence, the physical changes of puberty should be nearly complete in females, and at least halfway complete in males. Although physical development is advanced at this stage, cognition is still transitioning from concrete operational to more abstract thinking. In addition, the teen becomes preoccupied with peer identification and acceptance, as well as with independence from parental control. Incomplete understanding of consequences leads to a peak in risk-taking behaviors, especially with sexual exploration, substance and weapons experimentation, and powered-vehicle hazards.

THE MIDDLE ADOLESCENT VISIT

An extended visit is necessary to perform complete interviews with both parent and adolescent and a comprehensive physical examination. The interview should begin with both parent and patient in the room together. If this is the first visit, the physician should introduce himself first to the adolescent and then to the parent. The adolescent is then seen alone for a confidential interview and physical examination. The parent will feel more comfortable knowing the private interview and examination are part of the developmental process in which the adolescent begins an individual relationship with the health care provider. Reassure the parent that any indication of potential harm to the child or others will be relayed and that open communication with the parent will be encouraged.

I. History

The interview process should be performed with the patient remaining clothed. The provider should observe the interaction between parent and child. Is it positive, cooperative, or antagonistic? Does the teenager answer the health provider's questions or turn to the parent for responses? Basic past medical history, family history, social history, medications, and review of systems can be asked of both patient and parent during this time. Parental questions and health concerns can be addressed with both together. If the parent becomes vague or seems uncomfortable, the adolescent can be asked to step out of the room so that the parent can speak freely. The hearing and vision examinations can be performed at this time.

Following the joint interview, the physician should ask the parent(s) to leave and interview the adolescent alone. The confidential interview begins with general questions about school, friends, and hobbies. The physician should assess the patient's cognitive and psychosocial development and ask developmentally appropriate questions. Repeat your assurances and limitations of confidentiality. When possible, conduct the interview with open-ended, nonjudgmental questions. Some clinicians have the adolescent complete a preprinted questionnaire (such as the Adolescent Previsit Questionnaire in Appendix I) that can be reviewed as part of this discussion.

A. Questions for the parent:
1. How is your teenager doing in general? At home? At school?
2. How is everyone getting along?
3. Are there any changes or new stressors in the family?
4. Tell me about your teenager's hobbies, friends, and favorite family activity.
5. Is your teenager dating? Tell me about his/her dates?
6. In what kind of after-school/summer activities is your teenager involved?
7. Does your teenager have an after-school/summer job?
8. What have you discussed so far about house rules, smoking, drinking, drugs, and sexuality?
9. Are you concerned about anyone in the family regarding smoking, drinking, drugs, or behavior problems?
10. Does your teenager follow a reasonable diet, have an exercise program, and get adequate sleep?
11. Does your teenager respect safety issues, such as seat belts, helmets, telephone and internet safety?
12. Do you have any specific concerns?
13. Are there any medical problems, especially somatic complaints?
14. What one thing would you like me to congratulate your teenager for today?

B. Questions for the adolescent. Many of the same questions can be asked of the teenager, with emphasis on the following:
1. Symptoms of depression, isolation, suicidal ideation, and body image distortion.
2. School problems, failure, and truancy.
3. Sexual experimentation; sexual, physical, or emotional abuse.
4. Screening for adequate use and knowledge of contraception and infection control measures if sexually active.
5. Peer group or personal use of tobacco, drugs, huffing, and alcohol.
6. Adequate calcium, iron, B vitamins, and caloric intake.
7. Adequate sleep, exercise, safety equipment use, and personal hygiene.
8. Evidence of personal responsibility (chores, employment), cognitive development (reading, limited television, future plans for after high school), and good communication (family activities with one or both parents).

II. Physical Examination
The physical examination at this age is usually performed without the parents in the room. The adolescent's privacy should be respected using appropriate covering. A chaperone,

preferably of the same gender as the patient, should always be present during the physical examination when the genders of the patient and examiner are different.

A complete physical should be performed with special attention to the following:

A.   General Appearance—well kept, appropriate clothing, mood, interaction with parent.

B.   Blood pressure—both arms at initial visit.

C.   Height, weight, body mass index (BMI).

D.   Skin for acne, moles, warts.

E.   Dental examination—looking for caries, gum disease, malocclusion, molar crowding.

F.   Breast asymmetry, skin changes, or nipple discharge in both sexes; gynecomastia in males.

G.   Scoliosis.

H.   Tanner staging:

1. *Breasts and pubic hair in females.*
2. *Penis and pubic hair in males.*

J.   Pelvic examination with external examination for genital warts (if sexually active female).

K.   Penile examination for genital warts (if sexually active male).

L.   Testicular examination for hernias or masses.

III.   Screening Tests

A.   Hearing.

B.   Vision.

C.   Hemoglobin and hematocrit or complete blood count (CBC) with red blood cell (RBC) indices to screen for anemia for menstruating females; other adolescents, as indicated by history (e.g., experiencing the adolescent growth spurt or demonstrating evidence of poor nutrition).

D.   Cholesterol if there is a family history of hyperlipidemia or early onset ischemic heart disease.

E.   Tuberbulin skin testing if the adolescent has any of the following risk factors:

1. *Low socioeconomic status.*
2. *Residence in areas where tuberculosis is prevalent.*
3. *Exposure to tuberculosis.*
4. *Immigrant status.*
5. *Homelessness.*
6. *History of incarceration.*
7. *Employment or volunteer work in health care setting.*

G.   If the adolescent is sexually active:

1. *Pap smear.*
2. *Cervical sample* for gonorrhea and chlamydia.
3. *Wet mount* for trichomonas and yeast.
4. *Urinalysis for leukocyte esterase* can be used in males as a screen for STD.

H.   If the adolescent demonstrates high-risk sexual behavior:

1. *HIV serologic examination.*
2. *RPR serologic examination.*

3. *Hepatitis B serologic examination* (if unimmunized).

IV. Immunizations

The immunization record should be examined to ensure that basic immunizations have been given. Special attention should be given to the following:

   A.   MMR booster.

   B.   HBV vaccine series.

   C.   Td booster (if greater than 5 years since last DTaP).

   D.   Varicella vaccine (if negative history of clinical disease).

   E.   Hepatitis A vaccine (if sexually active, homosexual male).

V. Anticipatory Guidance for the Parent

   A.   Communication. Open communication is essential in this age group. Despite their often curt responses, adolescents do like being asked about their day/activities/thoughts. This reinforces to the adolescent that the parent is still interested and involved. Routine check-ins that encourage an open, nonjudgmental conversation about school, work, friends, substance use, sexuality, and future plans is important. Communication should be calm, equally interactive, and supportive.

   B.   Weapons. Whether weapons should be kept in the home is often a very personal matter to the family. However, parents should know that adolescents usually know where the weapon is stored, where the lock key (if used) is hidden, and where the ammunition is kept. Responsibility should be stressed. The weapon should never be loaded, and ammunition should be kept separately. Serious consideration should be given to removing weapons from a home with a depressed, stressed, or violent teen.

   C.   Rule setting. As peer identification becomes stronger, continuing fair and consistent enforcement by the parents of house rules is important. As the middle adolescent develops abstract thought, more adultlike negotiations with compromises and consequences can be agreed upon.

   D.   Privacy issues. Although private space and time remain important in middle adolescence, concerns surrounding substance use and dates can challenge privacy issues. Early and open communication and rule setting can resolve these problems before they arise. Having an open-door policy when friends, especially of opposite gender, are visiting is reasonable. Room searches are much more difficult to negotiate and should be substituted, if possible, by other forms of information gathering.

   E.   Increasing responsibility. Graded responsibility remains an important goal. Chores should be escalated appropriately. Rewards should follow successful completion of a new responsibility. A job that does not override school, sports, or useful social commitments provides an excellent opportunity to learn time and money management.

F. TV, computer use. Both mediums should still be supervised for content. Although both resources can provide a wealth of information, access time should be balanced with homework, chores, and exercise.

G. Role modeling. Parents should be reminded that most behavior is learned and that, for better or worse, most is learned in the home. Language, substance use, sexual mores, political and social opinions, dress, work ethic, honesty, and cleanliness, to name a few, are all modeled first and foremost after parental behavior, especially at this stage of development.

H. Punishment. Consistency and fairness are key. The most effective punishment at this age remains loss of privileges, especially if a car or social outings are used. Corporal punishment is ineffective and inappropriate at this age and reinforces violence and aggression as problem-solving techniques.

I. Personal safety. Parents should review safety issues regularly with their teens: drinking and driving, seat belt use, speed limits, substance use, dating safety, telephone and internet safety, and bicycle/skateboard/rollerblade safety.

J. Confidence building. Parents should seek tasks that will help build confidence in their teens. Encouraging development in areas of interest to the teen, whether they are team or independent sports, music, reading, writing, art, computers, or domestic tasks, is helpful. Parents should identify strengths and weaknesses in the adolescent and help with both.

VI. Anticipatory Guidance for the Adolescent
  A. Health promotion
     1. *Adequate sleep* (8 to 10 hours per night).
     2. *Regular exercise*, preferably three or more times per week.
     3. *A knowledgeable trainer* for supervision of weight training.
     4. *Balanced diet*, including three meals per day and recommended daily allowances.
     5. *Dental hygiene*, such as brushing teeth twice daily, flossing daily, and visiting a dentist every 6 to 12 months.
     6. *Limiting sedentary activities,* such as television, computer games, and internet use.
  B. Mental health
     1. *Find your niche.*
     2. *Discuss feelings with someone you trust.*
     3. *Seek help if your safety is in jeopardy.*
  C. Injury prevention
     1. *Seat belts.*
     2. *Helmets.*
     3. *Appropriate sports gear.*
     4. *No weapons.*
     5. *Conflict resolution.*

6. *Personal safety* by avoiding high-risk behaviors suggested by peers (e.g., dangerous skateboarding, gang activities).
D. **Substance abuse**
   1. *Discourage tobacco use.* Focus on negative physical consequences, such as teeth and finger staining, wrinkles, and bad breath.
   2. *Explain hazards of drug and alcohol use.*
   3. *Discuss huffing.*
   4. *Discourage diet pills.*
   5. *Discuss anabolic steroids.*
E. **Sexuality**
   1. *Explain current and remaining pubertal changes.*
   2. *Encourage open communication with a trusted adult.*
   3. *Encourage and congratulate abstinence.*
   4. *Instruct patient in breast and testicular self-examination.*
   5. *Encourage open discussion with parents or health proider if sexually active.* Provide explicit instructions on how to prevent STDs and pregnancy, including how and where to obtain birth control and condoms.
VII. **Concluding the Adolescent Visit**
   After the history and physical examination are completed, the primary care provider should sit down with the adolescent and discuss the findings of the examination and laboratory testing (if available; if not, make arrangements to contact the adolescent with the results) and provide anticipatory guidance in areas suggested by the history and physical examination (as noted earlier). This discussion should be unhurried and informal, allowing the adolescent the opportunity to ask questions and respond to suggestions. Many physicians provide adolescents and parents with written information that expands and supplements issues raised during the visit. Finally, follow-up should be arranged and information should be given to the adolescent and parents regarding how and when to contact the office for appointments, information, or referrals.

ADDITIONAL READING

American Academy of Pediatrics. *Recommendations for preventative pediatric health care (RE9535).* Elk Grove Village, IL: American Academy of Pediatrics; 2000.

American Academy of Pediatrics. *Recommended childhood immunization schedule—United States, January–December 2000* (RE9961). Elk Grove Village, IL: American Academy of Pediatrics; 2000.

American Academy of Pediatrics, Committee on Psychosocial Aspects of Child and Family Health. *Guidelines for health supervision of infants,* 3rd ed. Elk Grove Village, IL: American Academy of Pediatrics; 1997.

Fox CE III. *Put prevention into practice: clinician's handbook of preventive services,* 2nd ed. Washington, DC: U.S. Department of Health and Human Services; 1998.

Green M, Palfrey JS, eds. *Bright futures: guidelines for health super-vision of infants, children, and adolescents,* 2nd ed. Arlington, VA: National Center for Education in Maternal and Child Health; 2000.

McAnarney ER, Kreipe RE, Orr DP, Comerci GD. *Textbook of adoles-cent medicine.* Philadelphia: WB Saunders; 1992.

Neinstein LS. *Adolescent health care: a practical guide,* 3rd ed. Balti-more: Williams & Wilkins; 1996.

U.S. Preventative Services Task Force. *Guide to clinical preventive services: report of the U.S. preventative services task force,* 2nd ed. Washington, DC: U.S. Department of Health and Human Services; 1995.

26 ❧ Health Maintenance Visits—Late Adolescence: 18 to 21 Years

Thomas S. Webb

By late adolescence, the physical changes of puberty are nearly complete. Almost all females have adult body composition, mature secondary sex characteristics, and full reproductive capability. The same is generally true for males (except for the "late bloomer," who should be evaluated); however, some continued height and body mass development can occur during this stage. The developmental focus of this period is in cognitive processes and social independence. The cognitive goal to be attained is Piaget's "formal thought," which includes abstract thought, logic, reason, and deduction. The other developmental goals are adult relationships and independence from family. Higher education, work, long-term intimate relationships, financial independence, and even the adolescent's own children are the predominant focus of the late adolescent.

Unlike the physical changes of puberty, which generally follow a logical progression and continue until completion, cognitive and social development are much more erratic and susceptible to premature arrest. Both cognitive and social development are significantly influenced by socioeconomic background, family support, and gender, with female sex and affluence having a positive effect.

Since independence and intimacy are strong motivations in this patient population when deduction, reasoning, and planning have not yet fully developed, the health provider plays an important role in screening for high-risk behaviors and guiding healthy choices.

THE LATE ADOLESCENT VISIT

Generally, the adolescent is interviewed and seen alone at this age. A brief introduction with an accompanying parent, especially for a new family, may be helpful for an anxious parent or patient. Some background history, family history, and any parental concerns can be addressed at this time, but the majority of the interview and examination should be without the parent (unless there is an obvious developmental problem where the parent needs to assist the patient).

I. History

The adolescent should remain clothed for the interview. Open-ended questions, followed by more specific follow-up questions, should be asked. The health provider should estimate the patient's cognitive development through the quality of his or her answers and should tailor the interview accordingly. During the comprehensive exam, privacy and modesty should be respected, and chaperones should be used appropriately.

While questioning similar to previous adolescent visits is important, the provider should emphasize screening for sufficient financial, nutritional, and housing resources, especially if the patient is living independently. Lack of support in these areas can lead to significant emotional and physical stress, which may manifest in somatic complaints.

A. Questions to include are the following:

1.   Where are you living? With whom? Who is paying the bills and how?

2.   What do you do for income? Working? School?

3.   Are there symptoms of depression, isolation, suicidal ideation, and body image distortion?

4.   Are there school or work problems, failure, or recurrent absences?

5.   Are you sexually active? In a long-term relationship? With whom?

6.   Do you have any plans for marriage or family?

7.   Do you have multiple sexual partners? Male, female, or both?

8.   Are you worried about sexual, physical, or emotional abuse?

9.   If sexually active, what do you use for contraception and infection control?

10.   Are you using tobacco, drugs, or alcohol? Any huffing? From where is the money for these products coming?

11.   Is there adequate calcium, iron, B vitamin, and caloric intake in your diet?

12.   Do you get adequate sleep and exercise, use safety equipment, and attend to personal hygiene?

13.   Do you maintain interest and participation in previous hobbies and recreational activities?

II. Physical Examination

A complete physical examination should be performed with special attention to the following:

A.   General appearance—well kept, appropriate clothing, mood.

B.   Blood pressure—both arms at initial visit.

C.   Height, weight, body mass index (BMI).

D.   Complete skin examination for acne, moles, warts.

E.   Dental examination—looking for caries, gum disease, malocclusion, molar crowding.

F.   Breast asymmetry, skin changes, or nipple discharge in both sexes; gynecomastia in males.

G.   Scoliosis.

H.   Tanner staging:

1.   *Breasts and pubic hair in females.*

2.   *Penis and pubic hair in males.*

J.   Pelvic examination with external examination for genital warts in all females.

K.   Penile examination for genital warts in sexually active males.

L.   Testicular examination for hernias and masses.

III. Screening Tests
   A. Hearing—for first visit and with a history of occupational or recreational exposure to loud noises on a regular basis.
   B. Vision—for first visit, occupational requirement, or history of vision problems.
   C. Hemoglobin/hematocrit or complete blood count (CBC) with red cell indices to screen for anemia for menstruating females or any adolescent demonstrating evidence of poor nutrition.
   D. Cholesterol if family history of hyperlipidemia or early-onset ischemic heart disease.
   E. Tuberculin testing if adolescent has any of the following risk factors:
      1. *Low socioeconomic status.*
      2. *Residence in areas where tuberculosis is prevalent.*
      3. *Exposure to tuberculosis.*
      4. *Immigrant status.*
      5. *Homelessness.*
      6. *History of incarceration.*
      7. *Employment or volunteer work in health care setting.*
   H. All female patients should have a Pap smear by 18 years of age regardless of sexual activity.
   I. If the adolescent is believed to be sexually active:
      1. *Cervical sample* for gonorrhea and chlamydia.
      2. *Wet mount* for trichomonas and yeast.
      3. *Urinalysis for leukocyte esterase* can be used to screen for sexually transmitted disease (STD) in males.
   J. If the adolescent demonstrates high-risk sexual behavior:
      1. *HIV serologic examination.*
      2. *RPR serologic examination.*
      3. *Hepatitis B serologic examination.*
IV. Immunizations
   The immunization record should be examined to ensure that basic immunizations have been given. Special attention should be given to the following:
   A. MMR booster.
   B. HBV vaccine series.
   C. Td booster (if greater than 5 years since last DTaP).
   D. Varicella vaccine (if negative history of clinical disease).
   E. Hepatitis A vaccine (if sexually active, homosexual male).
V. Anticipatory Guidance
   A. Health promotion
      1. *Adequate sleep* (8 to 10 hours per night).
      2. *Regular exercise*, preferably three or more times per week.
      3. *A knowledgeable trainer* for supervision of weight training.
      4. *Balanced diet*, including three meals per day and recommended daily allowances.

    5.   *Dental hygiene*—brushing teeth twice daily, flossing daily, visiting dentist every 6 to 12 months.

    6.   *Limiting sedentary activities,* such as television, computer games, and internet use.

B.   Mental health

    1.   *Find your niche* (school subject or vocation you enjoy).

    2.   *Discuss feelings with someone you trust.*

    3.   *Seek help if your safety is in jeopardy.*

C.   Injury prevention

    1.   *Seat belts.*

    2.   *Helmets.*

    3.   *Appropriate sports gear.*

    4.   *No weapons.*

    5.   *Conflict resolution.*

    6.   *Personal safety* by avoiding high-risk physical behaviors suggested by peers (e.g., unsafe driving practices, gang activities).

D.   Substance use

    1.   *Discourage tobacco use*—focus on negative physical consequences, such as teeth and finger staining, wrinkles, and bad breath.

    2.   *Explain hazards of drug and alcohol use.*

    3.   *Discuss huffing.*

    4.   *Discourage diet pills.*

    5.   *Discuss anabolic steroids.*

E.   Sexuality

    1.   *Encourage open communication with trusted adult.*

    2.   *Encourage and congratulate abstinence or monogamy.*

    3.   *Encourage open communication and questions regarding sexual orientation concerns.*

    4.   *Instruct patient in breast and testicular self-examination.*

    5.   *If sexually active:*

      a.   **Encourage open discussion** with parents or health provider.

      b.   **Give explicit instructions on prevention of STDs and pregnancy**, including how and where to obtain birth control and condoms.

      c.   **Review financial and social responsibilities** if contemplating children.

F.   Social competence

    1.   *Promote community involvement, clubs, church, and peer groups.*

    2.   *Encourage continued parent and sibling involvement.*

    3.   *Help identify other social and community support resources,* where appropriate.

    4.   *Promote continued reading, skill development, and education.*

VI.   Concluding the Adolescent Visit

    After the history and physical examination are completed, the primary care provider should sit down with the adolescent and discuss the findings of the examination and laboratory testing (if available; if not, make arrangements to contact the adolescent with the results) and provide anticipatory guidance in areas suggested by the history and physical examination. This discussion should be unhurried and informal, allowing the adolescent the opportunity to ask questions and respond to suggestions. Many physicians provide adolescents with written information that expands and supplements information given on issues raised during the visit. Finally, follow-up should be arranged and information given to the adolescent regarding how and when to contact the office for appointments, information, or referrals.

ADDITIONAL READING

American Academy of Pediatrics. *Recommendations for preventative pediatric health care (RE9535).* Elk Grove Village, IL: American Academy of Pediatrics; 2000.

American Academy of Pediatrics. *Recommended childhood immunization schedule—United States, January—December 2000 (RE9961).* Elk Grove Village, IL: American Academy of Pediatrics; 2000.

American Academy of Pediatrics, Committee on Psychosocial Aspects of Child and Family Health. *Guidelines for health supervision of infants,* 3rd ed. Elk Grove Village, IL: American Academy of Pediatrics; 1997.

Fox CE, III. *Put prevention into practice: clinician's handbook of preventive services,* 2nd ed. Washington, DC: U.S. Department of Health and Human Services; 1998.

Green M, Palfrey JS, eds. *Bright futures: guidelines for health supervision of infants, children, and adolescents,* 2nd ed. Arlington, VA: National Center for Education in Maternal and Child Health; 2000.

McAnarney ER, Kreipe RE, Orr DP, Comerci GD. *Textbook of adolescent medicine.* Philadelphia: WB Saunders; 1992.

Neinstein LS. *Adolescent health care: a practical guide,* 3rd ed. Baltimore: Williams & Wilkins; 1996.

Pickering LK, ed. *2000 red book: report of the Committee on Infectious Diseases,* 25th ed. Elk Grove Village, IL: American Academy of Pediatrics; 2000.

U.S. Preventative Services Task Force. *Guide to clinical preventive services: report of the U.S. Preventative Services Task Force,* 2nd ed. Washington, DC: U.S. Department of Health and Human Services; 1995.

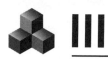

III

Behavioral and Developmental Aspects of the Well-Child Visit

27 ♣ Attention Deficit Hyperactivity Disorder: Evaluation

Claudia Hoffmann

I. Current Concepts of Attention-Deficit/Hyperactivity Disorder (from Barkley, 1997)

A. Attention-deficit/hyperactivity disorder (ADHD) is a developmental disorder characterized by developmentally inappropriate degrees of inattention, overactivity, and impulsivity. Individuals with ADHD appear to have a primary deficit in behavioral inhibition that impairs the development of effective self-regulation. The disinhibition and impulsivity are the characterizing traits of individuals with ADHD/predominantly hyperactive-impulsive type (ADHD/HI) and ADHD/combined type (ADHD/C). ADHD appears to represent the lower end of a continuum of a normal trait or a set of traits that comprise behavioral inhibition and the self-regulation associated with it.

B. Behavioral inhibition makes a fundamental contribution to the effective performance of four executive functions, including the following:

1. *Covert, self-directed sensing* (nonverbal working memory).

2. *Internalization of speech* (verbal working memory).

3. *The self-regulation of affect/motivation/arousal*, or emoting to oneself.

4. *Covert, self-directed behavioral manipulation, experimentation and play* (reconstitution).

C. Each of the executive functions is believed to be derived from its more public, outer-directed, and observable counterparts in human behavior that have become progressively more private, covert, or unobservable (internalized) in form. ADHD delays the internalization of behavior that forms the executive functions and thereby delays the self-regulation they afford to the individual. Research suggests that impairment in behavior inhibition is more characteristic of children with ADHD than of those with academic underachievement, emotional disturbance, conduct disorder, or autism.

D. Behavior is internalized during child development to anticipate change, to prepare for it, and to maximize long-term consequences. ADHD represents a delay in the development of this shift in sources of control. Behavior is more regulated by the immediate context and less by covert executive functions, time, and the future. Children with ADHD often have the skills and know what they should do, or should have done, in a given situation, but this provides little influence over their behavior.

1. *Accident prone.* Studies have found that hyperactive-impulsive children are more prone to accidents than normal children, yet they are not deficient in their knowledge of safety or accident prevention.

2. *Driving.* Teens and young adults with ADHD have significantly more motor vehicle accidents and other driving risks (speeding) but demonstrate no deficiencies in their knowledge of driving, safety, and accident prevention.

E.   The hyperactivity and inattentiveness demonstrated by children with ADHD result from their disinhibition and delayed self-regulation. With the child's development, the delay in these executive functions may no longer appear as hyperactivity but as deficiencies in working memory, private speech, rule-governed behavior, and emotional/motivation self-regulation. Later, deficiencies may be noted in problem solving, behavioral flexibility, sense of time, and behavioral self-management.

F.   In Attention Deficit Hyperactivity Disorder, Barkley suggests that individuals with the ADHD/ predominantly inattentive type (ADHD/I) do not have significant difficulties with disinhibition and should be thought of as having a qualitatively different condition. In a study comparing groups of children with ADHD/HI and ADHD/I:

1. *Children with ADHD/HI* were characterized by less self-control, great impulsivity; increased risk for serious aggressive or oppositional behavior and antisocial conduct; and difficulty with sustained attention or maintaining the motivation and effort to complete a task.

2. *Children with ADHD/I* were characterized by poor focus of attention; deficient speed of cognitive processing of information (i.e., input analysis and retrieval of stored information); daydreaming and sluggish, lethargic behaviors; more anxiety and shyness; and more depression.

3. *Families of ADHD/HI* children were characterized by more aggression and substance abuse, and families of ADHD/I children had more anxiety.

4. *More ADHD/I than ADHD/HI children were nonresponders to Ritalin* (24% vs. 5%), and more of them (35%) responded best to the low dose, whereas more ADHD/HI children responded best to the high dose (71%).

G.   The prevalence of ADHD is estimated at 3% to 5% in school-aged children. Higher levels of activity and impulsivity are seen in young children; the activity level normally decreases in adolescence. The disorder is much more frequent in males than in females, with male-to-female ratios ranging from 4:1 in the general population to 9:1 in clinic settings. Preliminary studies of ADHD/I show that the predominance of males to females is lower, with a ration of 2:1.

II.   Development of the Individual with ADHD

A.   Significant problems associated with ADHD during development:

1. *Infancy*—sleep problems and crying.
2. *Preschool age*—gross motor overactivity.
3. *School age*—restlessness, inattention, and impulsiveness.
4. *Adolescence*—rebelliousness and antisocial behaviors.
5. *Adulthood*—core symptoms persist for 50% to 80%.

B. **Common problems associated with ADHD:**
1. *Conduct problems*—oppositional, hostile/defiant behavior (60% to 65%); temper tantrums, anger outbursts; destructiveness; verbal and physical aggressiveness; antisocial behavior/conduct disorder (20% to 30% in childhood; 40% to 60% in adolescence).
2. *Academic performance problems*—underachievement (90%); excessive variability in performance; learning disabilities (20% to 50%); lowering of IQ over time.
3. *Social skills problems (50%)*—self-centered; rejected by peers, intrusive/disruptive; little regard for social consequences; immature; less reciprocity in social interactions.
4. *Emotional immaturity (higher than 50%)*—exaggerated responses to situations (overreaction); low frustration tolerance; poor self-esteem.
5. *Developmental/medical problems*—immature motor coordination (30% to 60%); enuresis (43%); encopresis (18%); sleep disturbances (56%); accident prone (46%).

III. **Biological and Neurologic Development in ADHD**
A. **ADHD clusters among biological relatives of children with adults with the disorder strongly imply a hereditary basis.** Research shows that if a parent has ADHD, the risk to the offspring is 57%. Twin studies indicate a greater concordance in monozygotic than in dizygotic twins for different components of the ADHD syndrome. Twin studies on symptoms of ADHD indicated that the average inheritability is 0.80 for the symptoms of this disorder (range = 0.50 to 0.98).
B. **Research suggests that maternal smoking, maternal alcohol consumption, and other risk factors during pregnancy, as well as significant prematurity of birth and smallness for gestational age, may play some contributory role beyond that of genetic factors alone.** Such nongenetic, nonshared factors would appear to play only a small though significant role in the expression of ADHD in a child, perhaps accounting for 15% to 20% of the differences among individuals in the traits comprising ADHD.
C. **Research has been conducted into the genetic mechanisms involved in the transmission of ADHD.** The association of ADHD and genes related to dopamine is currently being studied.
D. **Neuroanatomically, the frontal lobe, particularly the prefrontal and striatal areas, clearly plays an important role in ADHD.** Neurotransmitters such as norepinephrine, dopamine, and (to a lesser degree) serotonin are

clearly important. However, that no one area or neurotransmitter will adequately explain the neuropathology or neurophysiology of this condition is also clear.

E.   Multiple reviews of psychological and cognitive literatures have concluded that ADHD children show greater variability in central and autonomic arousal pattern. Much of this evidence implicates frontal lobe underactivity, particularly underactivity to events. Stimulant medications (e.g., methylphenidate and dextroamphetamine) are structurally similar to certain brain neurotransmitters and are used to increase the arousal or alertness of the central nervous system.

IV.   Differential Diagnosis and Comorbidity

Concerns regarding inattentiveness, overactivity, and impulsivity are commonly reported by parents and teachers. The initial goal of the evaluation is the determination of the presence or absence of ADHD, as well as the differential diagnosis of ADHD from other childhood developmental, psychiatric, and/or medical disorders (Table 27.1).

A.   The Classification of Child and Adolescent Mental Diagnoses in Primary Car (DSM-PC), published by the American Academy of Pediatrics, provides an excellent, comprehensive coding system to facilitate the recognition and management of common behavioral and developmental symptoms in primary pediatric care.

1.   *Severity.* Information is provided regarding the spectrum of severity of the child's presenting problems, as well as stressful environmental situations.

2.   *Diagnosis.* The differential diagnosis section includes alternate causes for specific behaviors, including general medical conditions; substances, legal and illegal, that could cause behavioral manifestations (i.e., hyperactivity, impulsivity, inattention); or mental disorders that may present with similar behavioral symptoms.

a.   ***General medical conditions.*** These include any disease that acutely affects central nervous system (CNS) functions, including meningitis, encephalitis, head injury, CNS tumor, cerebrovascular accident, lupus with CNS inflammation, CNS chemotherapy, iron deficiency anemia, and lead poisoning. (Since the treatment of ADHD behaviors is the same whether or not there is an associated neurologic disorder, the accepted practice is to consider these disorders comorbid conditions.)

b.   ***Chronic medical conditions.*** Any chronic medical condition that increases anxiety or depression may result in hyperactive/impulsive and/or inattentive behaviors, including insulin-dependent diabetes, chronic renal disease, and serious physical injury.

c.   ***Substances.*** These include any medication that affects CNS function or produces anxiety or depression,

Table 27.1. Differential diagnostic tips for distinguishing other mental disorders from ADHD

ADHD, Predominantly Inattentive Type
Lethargy, staring, and daydreaming more likely than in ADHD, combined type
Sluggish cognitive tempo/slow information processing
Lacks impulsive, disinhibited, or aggressive behavior
Possibly greater family history of anxiety disorders and learning disabilities
Makes significantly more errors in academic work
No elevated risk for oppositional defiant or conduct disorder

Oppositional Defiant Disorder and Conduct Disorder
Lacks impulsive, disinhibited behavior
Defiance primarily directed toward mother initially
Able to cooperate and complete tasks requested by others
Lacks poor sustained attention and marked restlessness
Resists initiating demands, whereas ADHD children may initiate but cannot stay on task
Often associated with parental child management deficits or family dysfunction
Lacks neuromaturational delays in motor abilities

Learning Disabilities
Has a significant IQ/achievement discrepancy (+1 standard deviation)
Places below the 10th percentile in an academic achievement skill
Lacks an early childhood history of hyperactivity
Attention problems arise in middle childhood and appear to be task or subject specific
Not socially aggressive or disruptive
Not impulsive or disinhibited

Anxiety/Affective Disorders
Likely to have a focused, not sustained attention deficit
Not impulsive or aggressive; often overinhibited
Has a strong family history of anxiety disorders
Restlessness is more like fretful, worrisome behavior, not the "driven," inquisitive, or overstimulated type
Lacks preschool history of hyperactive, impulsive behavior
Not socially disruptive; typically socially reticent

Thought Disorders
Shows oddities/atypical patterns of thinking not seen in ADHD
Peculiar sensory reactions
Odd fascinations and strange aversions
Socially aloof, schizoid, disinterested
Lacks concern for personal hygiene/dress in adolescence
Atypical motor mannerisms, stereotypes, and postures
Labile, capricious, unpredictable moods not tied to reality
Poor empathy, cause–effect perception
Poor perception of meaningfulness of events

(continued)

Table 27.1.   *Continued*

Juvenile-Onset Mania or Bipolar I Disorder

Characterized by severe and persistent irritability

Depressed mood exists more days than not

Irritable/depressed mood typically punctuated by rage outbursts

Mood swings often unpredictable or related to minimal events

Severe temper outbursts and aggression with minimal provocation (thus, ODD is often present and severe)

Later onset of symptoms than ADHD (but comorbid early ADHD is commonplace)

Press of speech and flight of ideas often present

Psychotic-like symptoms often present during manic episodes

Family history of bipolar I disorder more common

Expansive mood, grandiosity of ideas, inflated self-esteem, and high productivity (goal-directed activity periods) often seen in adults with bipolar disorder are usually not present; children more often have the dysphoric type of disorder

Requires that sufficient symptoms of bipolar disorder be present after excluding distractibility and hyperactivity (motor agitation) from bipolar symptom list in DSM-IV before granting bipolar I diagnosis to a child with symptoms of ADHD

Suicidal ideation is more common in child (and suicide attempts more common in family history)

Source: Barkley RA. *Attention deficit disorder,* 2nd ed. New York: Guilford Press; 1998. Reproduced with permission.

including theophylline, antihistamines, phenobarbital, and systemic steroids.

   d.   ***Mental disorders.*** Those presenting with ADHD-like symptoms may include autistic disorder, major depressive disorder, generalized anxiety disorder, panic disorder, posttraumatic stress disorder, avoidant personality disorder, panic disorder, dysthymic disorder, separation anxiety disorder, and social phobia.

 B.   Comorbidity of ADHD with other disorders is frequently diagnosed. The same disorders that were present in the differential diagnoses may all occur simultaneously. In addition, children with Tourette syndrome or mental retardation often have comorbid ADHD disorders.

   1.   *Suggested rates of comorbidity in ADHD from epidemiologic and clinical studies* (rates are typically higher in clinic-referred than in non–clinic-referred individuals):

   a.   Thirty percent to 50% for conduct disorder.

   b.   Thirty-five percent to 60% for oppositional defiant disorder.

   c.   Twenty percent to 30% for anxiety disorders.

   d.   Thirty percent for mood disorders.

   e.   Twenty percent to 25% for learning disabilities.

2. *Increasing multiple comorbidity awareness.* Biederman et al. found that 20% of ADHD individuals were comorbid for two or more conditions. The number, type, and particular combination of comorbid conditions are likely to have significant implications for etiology, course, and treatment.

In a study by Hoffmann et al (preliminary data; study in progress) of 60 ADHD children (ages 6 to 14), 72% were diagnosed with at least one comorbid disorder. Children with ADHD and comorbid diagnosis of either learning disabilities or oppositional defiant disorder were significantly more likely to show a positive response when treated with dextroamphetamine than when treated with methylphenidate.

a. ***Anxiety and depression.*** Symptoms of significant anxiety and depression may be a predictor of poor response to stimulant medication.

b. ***Bipolar disorder.*** Presence of high levels of irritable mood, severely hostile and defiant behavior, and periodic episodes of serious physical aggression and destructive behavior may be early markers for later bipolar disorder in children.

V. Guidelines for Conducting ADHD Evaluations

A. The American Academy of Pediatrics has recently published clinical practice guidelines for the diagnosis and evaluation of the child with ADHD that contain the following six recommendations:

1. *Evaluation.* The primary care clinician should initiate an evaluation for ADHD of a child 6 to 12 years of age who presents with inattention, hyperactivity, impulsivity, academic underachievement, or behavior problems.

2. *Diagnosis.* The diagnosis of ADHD requires that a child meet DSM-IV criteria (Table 27.2).

3. *Assessment and parental input.* The assessment of ADHD requires evidence directly obtained from parents or caregivers regarding the core symptoms of ADHD in various settings, the age of onset, duration of symptoms, and degree of functional impairment.

4. *Assessment and educator input.* The assessment of ADHD requires evidence directly obtained from the classroom (teacher or other school professional) regarding the core symptoms of ADHD, the duration of symptoms, the degree of functional impairment, and coexisting conditions. Any school-based multidisciplinary evaluations should be reviewed.

5. *Coexisting conditions.* Evaluation of the child with ADHD should include assessment for coexisting conditions.

6. *Additional screening.* Other diagnostic tests (e.g., screening of thyroid function, brain imaging studies and electroencepthalography, continuous performance tests) are not routinely indicated to establish the diagnosis of ADHD.

Table 27.2.   Diagnostic Criteria for Attention-Deficit/Hyperactivity Disorder

A. Either (1) or (2):

(1) Six (or more) of the following symptoms of inattention have persisted for at least 6 months to a degree that is maladaptive and inconsistent with developmental level:

Inattention

(a) Often fails to give close attention to details or makes careless mistakes in schoolwork, work, or other activities
(b) Often has difficulty sustaining attention in tasks or play activities
(c) Often does not seem to listen when spoken to directly
(d) Often does not follow through on instructions and fails to finish schoolwork, chores, or duties in the workplace (not due to oppositional behavior or failure to understand instructions)
(e) Often has difficulty organizing tasks and activities
(f) Often avoids, dislikes, or is reluctant to engage in tasks that require sustained mental effort (such as schoolwork or homework)
(g) Often loses things necessary for tasks or activities (e.g., toys, school assignments, pencils, books, or tools)
(h) Is often easily distracted by extraneous stimuli
(i) Is often forgetful in daily activities

(2) Six (or more) of the following symptoms of hyperactivity–impulsivity have persisted for at least 6 months to a degree that is maladaptive and inconsistent with developmental level.

Hyperactivity

(a) Often fidgets with hands or feet or squirms in seat
(b) Often leaves seat in classroom or in other situations in which remaining seated is expected
(c) Often runs about and climbs excessively in situations in which it is inappropriate in adolescents or adults (may be limited to subjective feelings of restlessness)
(d) Often has difficulty playing or engaging in leisure activities quietly
(e) Is often "on the go" or often acts as if "driven by a motor"
(f) Often talks excessively

Impulsivity

(g) Often blurts out answers before questions have been completed
(h) Often has difficulty awaiting turn
(i) Often interrupts or intrudes on others (e.g., butts into conversations or games)

B. Some hyperactive–impulsive or inattentive symptoms that caused impairment were present before age 7 years

(continued)

Table 27.2. *Continued*

C. Some impairment from the symptoms is present in two or more settings (e.g., at school [or work] and at home)

D. There must be clear evidence of clinically significant impairment in social, academic, or occupational functioning

E. The symptoms do not occur exclusively during the course of a pervasive developmental disorder, schizophrenia, or other psychotic disorder and are not better accounted for by another mental disorder (e.g., mood disorder, anxiety disorder, dissociative disorder, or a personality disorder)

Source: *Diagnostic and statistical manual of mental disorders,* 4th ed. Copyright 1994 American Psychiatric Association. Reproduced with permission.

B. Figure 27.1 depicts a detailed clinical pathway for the diagnosis and evaluation of ADHD and highlights the implementation of the six recommendations.
C. The use of ADHD-specific rating scales by parents and teachers is recommended as a clinical option when evaluating children for ADHD. The ADHD specific questionnaires and rating scales have been found to distinguish children with ADHD accurately.

1. *The Vanderbilt Teacher Behavior Evaluation Scale* is an ADHD-specific rating scale that consists of the DSM-IV criteria for ADHD (18 items) and also screens for comorbid DSM-IV disorders of oppositional defiant disorder and conduct disorder (10 items) and symptoms of anxiety and depression (seven items). (This scale is in the public domain and is printed in pad form for physicians as a service by Shire Richwood, Inc. It is also available on the internet at: http://peds.mc.vanderbilt.edu/cdc/VTBES.html.)

2. *The Disruptive Behavior Rating Scale* consists of the DSM-IV criteria for ADHD and oppositional defiant disorder. This ADHD-specific scale and the norms for clinical cutoff scores for the ADHD items for boys and girls, ages 5 to 13, for both parent and teacher rating are available with purchase of the *Clinical Workbook.*

3. *The Connors Parent Rating Scale* (1997) and *the Connors Teacher Rating Scale* (1997) are widely used by primary care physicians to quantify the behavioral characteristics of ADHD in boys and girls from 6 to 17 years of age. These scales differentiate children with ADHD from peers with a specificity greater than 94%.

D. The use of broad-band scales is not recommended in the diagnosis of children for ADHD, although they may be useful for other purposes. Broad-band measures such as the Behavior Assessment System for Children

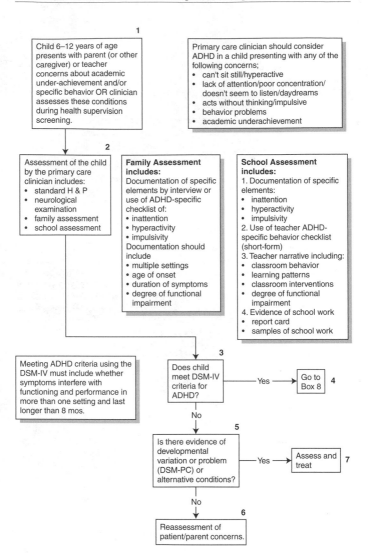

1

Child 6–12 years of age presents with parent (or other caregiver) or teacher concerns about academic under-achievement and/or specific behavior OR clinician assesses these conditions during health supervision screening.

Primary care clinician should consider ADHD in a child presenting with any of the following concerns;
• can't sit still/hyperactive
• lack of attention/poor concentration/doesn't seem to listen/daydreams
• acts without thinking/impulsive
• behavior problems
• academic underachievement

2

Assessment of the child by the primary care clinician includes:
• standard H & P
• neurological examination
• family assessment
• school assessment

Family Assessment includes:
Documentation of specific elements by interview or use of ADHD-specific checklist of:
• inattention
• hyperactivity
• impulsivity
Documentation should include
• multiple settings
• age of onset
• duration of symptoms
• degree of functional impairment

School Assessment includes:
1. Documentation of specific elements:
• inattention
• hyperactivity
• impulsivity
2. Use of teacher ADHD-specific behavior checklist (short-form)
3. Teacher narrative including:
• classroom behavior
• learning patterns
• classroom interventions
• degree of functional impairment
4. Evidence of school work
• report card
• samples of school work

Meeting ADHD criteria using the DSM-IV must include whether symptoms interfere with functioning and performance in more than one setting and last longer than 8 mos.

3
Does child meet DSM-IV criteria for ADHD? —Yes→ Go to Box 8 **4**

No

5
Is there evidence of developmental variation or problem (DSM-PC) or alternative conditions? —Yes→ Assess and treat **7**

No

6
Reassessment of patient/parent concerns.

Adapted from: Committee on Quality Improvement, Subcommittee on ADHD, American Academy of Pediatrics. Clinical Practice Guideline: Diagnosis and Evaluation of the Child with ADHD. *Pediatrics.* 2000;105:1158–1170. Reproduced by permission.

Figure 27.1.   Clinical algorithm for the diagnosis and evaluation of the child with attention deficit/hyperactivity disorder.

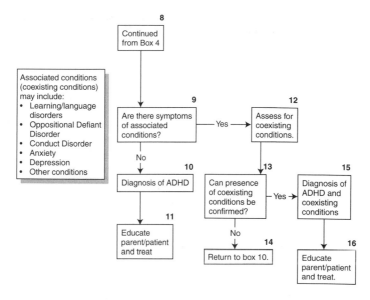

Adapted from: Committee on Quality Improvement, Subcommittee on ADHD, American Academy of Pediatrics. Clinical Practice Guideline: Diagnosis and Evaluation of the Child with ADHD. *Pediatrics.* 2000;105:1158–1170. Reproduced by permission.

Figure 27.1. *Continued*

(BASC) and the Child Behavior Checklist (CBCL) assess the main dimensions of child psychopathology, and these rating scales are often included in evaluations by psychologists.

    1. *The BASC has scales rating the following:*

    a. ***Internalizing problems*** (i.e., anxiety, depression, somatization).

    b. ***Externalizing problems*** (i.e., hyperactivity, aggression, conduct problems).

    c. ***School problems*** (i.e., attention problems, learning problems).

    d. ***Other problems*** (i.e., atypicality, withdrawal).

    e. ***Adaptive skills*** (i.e., adaptability, leadership, social skills, study skills).

    f. ***Indexes of validity and response set.***

    2. *Scale scores in the "At-Risk" range are between one and two standard deviations from the mean.* A score in the "At-Risk" range may indicate the following:

    a. ***The presence of significant problems*** that, although they require treatment, may not be severe enough to warrant a formal diagnosis.

b. *Potential or developing problems* that need to be monitored carefully.

3. *Scale scores in the "Clinically Significant" range are usually two standard deviations from the mean and denote a high level of maladaptive behavior.*

4. *BASC scales can be hand or computer scored.* The interpretation of the BASC requires specific training that most physicians do not have. Physicians can consult with psychologists regarding test interpretations. According to the American Guidance Service, plans to develop a new version of the BASC results designed to meet the needs of physicians who may have limited training in psychopathology are in the works.

E. **Clinical interview**

1. *Explore current concerns, including history and pervasiveness of problems.* (Why was evaluation for ADHD initiated at this time? Is the family experiencing any other stressors? Do parents agree about the nature of the child's problems?)

2. *Inquire about any family history of ADHD, learning disabilities, mental illnesses, and substance abuse.* (Is the child's temperament and/or problem similar to anyone else's in the family?)

3. *Review the child's developmental and medical history and educational progress in detail.* Explore the child's functioning within the family, in school, and with peers. (When were signs of hyperactivity and/or distractibility first noted? Is the child aggressive?)

4. *Interview parents about whether their child meets the DSM-IV criteria for ADHD (Table 27.2)—oppositional defiant disorder, conduct disorder, anxiety disorders, depressive disorders, and/or pervasive developmental disorders.* As previously noted, familiarity with developmental variations for common behavioral and developmental symptoms, as presented in the Classification of Child and Adolescent Mental Diagnosis in Primary Care (DSM-PC), is invaluable in ascertaining whether a child is presenting with significant problems.

5. *Review results of psychological evaluation, if available, to assess the child's level of intellectual functioning and the presence of any developmental disorders.* Be aware that children can have significant developmental delays that may be impeding their academic functioning but that may not qualify for learning disabilities services.

F. **Medical examination.** It is essential that children being considered for a diagnosis of ADHD have a complete pediatric physical examination, with a focus on differential diagnosis of ADHD from other medical conditions.

1. *Seizure disorders and ADHD.* As many as 20% of children with a seizure disorder may have ADHD as a comorbid disorder, and approximately 30% may develop ADHD-

like symptoms or have them exacerbated by the use of phenobarbital or phenytoin as anticonvulsant. Changing to a different anticonvulsant may reduce these symptoms.

2. *Asthma treatment.* Theophylline, used in the treatment of asthma, may affect attentiveness.

3. *Cardiovascular difficulties.* A history of high blood pressure or cardiac difficulties may be a contraindication to a trial of psychostimulant due to the known presser effects of these drugs on the cardiovascular system.

4. *Family and personal history.* Children with a family or personal history of tic disorders or Tourette syndrome may develop or increase the severity of their tic disorder when treated with stimulants.

5. *Additional screenings.* Hearing, vision, and blood pressure should be screened.

6. *Medication levels.* Blood assays of levels of stimulant medications, such as methylphenidate, D-amphetamine, and Adderall, have not been useful in determining appropriate dosage; accordingly, they are not recommended.

G. Based on the results of the total evaluation, diagnostic impressions are formulated, and the types of interventions needed to address impairments can be considered.

1. *If the child has been diagnosed as ADHD, would he or she benefit from a stimulant trial?* Standardized rating forms can be used to monitor the child's response to the medication. A rating of possible side effects to the stimulant should be completed by the parent before the initial trial and following a 1-week trial or any change in the dosage level.

2. *Determine whether additional psychological and psychiatric evaluations are necessary to rule out problems associated with the following:*

a. **Learning disabilities related to developmental disorders.**

b. **Pervasive developmental disorders or atypical behaviors.**

c. **Anxiety and/or depressive disorders.**

d. **Adjustment disorders reflecting family problems or other stressors.**

VI. Treatment of ADHD

A. Treatment with stimulant medication or other psychopharmacologic agents can result in improvement or normalization of the underlying neuropsychological deficit in behavioral inhibition and of the executive functions dependent on such inhibition. Research shows that clinical improvement in behavior occurs in as many as 75% to 92% of those with the hyperactive-impulsive form of ADHD and results in normalization of behavior in approximately 50% to 60% of these cases. It is the only treatment known to date to produce such improvement and normalization rates.

B.   The most useful behavioral treatments will be those that are in place in a natural setting at the point of performance where the desired behavior is to occur. Since internalized, self-generated forms of motivation are weak at initiating and sustaining goal-directed behavior, behavior modification strategies can be used to externalize sources of motivation. Token systems provide one of the best means for creating an artificial reward program for children 5 years of age and older in an effort to promote goal-directed behavior.
C.   Behavior modification programs using artificial rewards can be reduced in their frequency and immediacy, over time, as the ADHD child's neurologic maturation results in an increase in ability to self-motivate. Nevertheless, at any age at which one is working with an individual with ADHD, such external sources of motivation must still be relied upon more than is normal for the child's age.
D.   Individuals with ADHD are now eligible for special education services and/or appropriate adaptations and intervention in their regular classroom program under Part 3 ("Other Health Impaired") of the Individuals with Disabilities Education Act (IDEA) or Section 504 ("Handicapped Person") of the Rehabilitation Act of 1973. Section 504 of the Rehabilitation Act is not new or recently passed. The U.S. Department of Education has recently issued a policy memorandum to the individual states regarding specifically how individuals with ADHD are included under Section 504 provisions.

ADDITIONAL READING

Achenbach TM. Child Behavior Checklist-Cross-Informant Version, 1991. (Available from Thomas Achenbach, Ph.D. University of Vermont, 5 South Prospect Street, Burlington, VT 05401.)

American Academy of Pediatrics. Clinical practice guideline: diagnosis and evaluation of the child with attention-deficit/hyperactivity disorder. *Pediatrics* 2000;105:1158–1170.

American Psychiatric Association. *Diagnostic and statistical manual of mental disorders,* 4th ed. Washington, DC: American Psychiatric Association; 1994.

Barkley RA. *ADHD and the nature of self-control.* New York: Guilford Press; 1997.

Barkley RA. *Attention deficit hyperactivity disorder,* 2nd ed. New York: Guilford Press; 1998.

Barkley RA, Murphy KR. *Attention deficit hyperactivity disorder, a clinical workbook.* 2nd ed. New York: Guilford Press; 1998.

Biederman J, Faraone SV, Lapey K. Comorbidity of diagnosis in attention deficit hyperactivity disorder and attention deficit disorder. *Child Adolesc Psychiatr Clin N Am* 1992;2:335–361.

Green M, Wong M, Atkins D, et al. *Diagnosis of attention deficit/hyperactivity disorder. Technical review 3.* Rockville, MD: U.S. Department of Health and Human Services, Agency for Health Care Policy and Research; 1999. AHCPR publication 99-0050.

Greenhill LL, Osman BB, eds. *Ritalin: theory and patient management.* Larchmont, NY: ML Liebert; 2000.

Miller KJ, Castellanos FX. Attention deficit/hyperactivity disorders. *Pediatr Rev* 1998;19:373–384.

Reynolds C, Kamphaus, R. *Behavioral assessment system for children,* 1994. (Available from American Guidance Service, 4201 Woodland Road, Circle Pines, MN 55014.)

Wolraich ML, ed. *The classification of child and adolescent mental diagnoses in primary care.* Elk Grove Village, IL: American Academy of Pediatrics; 1996.

Wolraich, ML. *Vanderbilt Teacher Behavior Evaluation Scale.* Nashville, TN: Vanderbilt Child Development Center; 1999.

Weiss G, Hechtman LT. *Hyperactive children grown up: ADHD in children, adolescent and adults,* 2nd ed. New York: Guilford Press; 1993.

Books for Parents

Barkley RA. 1995;. *Taking charge of ADHD: the complete authoritative guide for parents.* New York: Guilford Press.

Boyles NS, Contadino D. *Parenting a child with attention deficit/hyperactivity disorder.* Los Angeles, CA: Lowell House; 1996.

Dornbush MP, Pruitt SK. *Teaching the tiger: a handbook for individuals involved in the education of students.* Duarte, CA: Hope Press; 1995.

Forehand R, Long N. *Parenting the strong-willed child.* Chicago: Contemporary Books; 1996.

Greene R. *The explosive child.* New York: Harper Collins; 1998.

Ingersoll B. *Your hyperactive child.* New York: Doubleday; 1988.

Web Sites

http://www.chadd.org/ (Children and Adults with ADHD)

http://www.focusonadd.com/ (Resources for parents, children, educators)

http://peds.mc.vanderbilt.edu/cdc/VTBES.html (Vanderbilt Teacher Behavior Evaluation Scale)

28 ♣ Attention Deficit Hyperactivity Disorder: Management

Nancy E. Lanphear

I. Overview

The treatment of attention deficit hyperactivity disorder (ADHD) is threefold and includes (a) changes and adaptations at home, (b) support and modifications in the school, and (c) for some individuals, medication. As with all chronic disorders, physicians need to maintain optimal continuity, remain current on treatment possibilities, and stay open to the input and expertise of the family. Treatment should be individualized and multimodal. Too often physicians simply prescribe stimulants only. This may address the core symptoms of impulsivity, hyperactivity, and inattention while the child is on medication but will not affect many other areas of difficulty that will affect long-term functioning. Finding ways to address organizational strategies, social skills, homework routine, and consistent discipline and follow-through at home and school is important for the future. Parents should be directed to appropriate literature, websites, and local and national support organizations. At times, parents also require the guidance of a child-oriented therapist who is knowledgeable about ADHD.

Children with ADHD frequently also need outlets for exercise and group activities. These should be carefully chosen to allow for the greatest success. Typical activities tend to be for the individual or a small group and to be structured, adult directed, and responsive to the child's interest or strength.

In the school setting, having the "best fit" in selection of school and teacher is helpful. Modifications in the school setting may include such things as a signal system between the child and teacher, a communication notebook between home and school, regular meetings between school personnel and parents, and help with organization and use of a planner for assignments. In the younger school-aged child, the system will need to be closely monitored and adapted by the teacher and parent. If a child has significant learning issues, evaluation for a concomitant learning disability should be sought. Students may require either an Individualized Education Plan (IEP) or an accommodation plan called a 504. These are documents created with input from both the parent and the school.

II. Medications

Stimulants (methylphenidate/Ritalin, dextroamphetamine/Dexedrine, and more recently, Adderall) have been and remain the medical treatment of choice to address most symptoms of ADHD with or without hyperactivity. Regularly in the lay media, articles warn of the significantly negative risks and side effects. These reports are often alarmist and anecdotal. Discussing with families the true risks and benefits is important. Medications in the young child should be used cautiously and preferrably under the guidance of physicians with behavioral expertise. Primary care physicians will likely feel more at ease with the school-aged child.

Starting with a low dose is best; for methylphenidate, this is typically 0.3 mg/kg, or 5 mg. The maintenance dose is typically 0.3 to 1.0 mg/kg daily. Dextroamphetamine is not dosed the same as methylphenidate, and the total daily dose is frequently lower. The starting dose for dextroamphetamine is 2.5 mg/dose. The total number of doses per day ranges from one to three, depending on individual needs and activities. Medication is increased to address desired goals of attention, impulse control, and decreased activity, while watching for side effects. Typical side effects may include anorexia, insomnia, headache, abdominal pain, and irritability. Titrating the dosage will be necessary for maximal effectiveness and minimal side effects. Information from both parent and school is helpful to guide adjustments. During the period of adjustment of medication, frequent contact is necessary between the physician and the parent and child.

Adderall, the newest psychostimulant for use in children with ADHD, should generally be used when the medications discussed above do not result in an adequate response as it is more expensive. In addition, less information is available about its use in ADHD. The starting dose of Adderall is 2.5 to 5.0 mg/dose. This medication is usually effective when given once or twice a day with a somewhat longer interval (4 to 6 hours) between doses than for either methylphenidate or dextroamphetamine.

Once a satisfactory dose has been determined, regular follow-up visits to monitor and fine-tune the medication regimen are indicated; usually these occur every 3 to 6 months, depending on child's age and response to a treatment regimen. At these visits, the history should focus on the psychobehavioral response in the school and at home, educational progress as reported by the teacher and parents, and side effects of the medication. Blood pressure and growth parameters, including height and weight, should be obtained on these visits. Children should be included in the evaluation and discussion, and explanations for intervention strategies should be developmentally appropriate to ensure the child's understanding and cooperation.

Using medication that addresses the child's core symptoms is important. Some children will be on medication on a daily basis; others are treated only on school days. Parents must be able to see the child's response to medication, as they will be most sensitive to negative side effects. Drug-free summers and medication holidays are indicated for children who do not require medication for behavioral control in the home or child care setting or who have poor weight gain through the school year.

Alternative medications may be necessary for a child who does not respond or has negative side effects to stimulants. In this circumstance, it would be appropriate to revisit the accuracy of the diagnosis and consider guidance from a specialist.

ADDITIONAL READING

American Academy of Pediatrics. Clinical practice guideline: diagnosis and evaluation of the child with attention-deficit/hyperactivity disorder. *Pediatrics* 2000;105:1158–1170.

Barkley RA. *Attention deficit disorder,* 2nd ed. New York: Guilford Press; 1998.

Greenhill LL, Osman BB, eds. *Ritalin: theory and patient management.* Larchmont, NY: ML Liebert; 2000.

Miller KJ, Castellanos FX. Attention deficit/hyperactivity disorders. *Pediatr Rev* 1998;19:373–384.

Books for Parents

Barkley RA. *Taking charge of ADHD: the complete authoritative guide for parents.* New York: Guilford Press; 1995.

Ingersoll B. *Your hyperactive child.* New York: Doubleday; 1988.

Web Sites

http://www.chadd.org/ (Children and Adults with ADHD)

http://www.focusonadd.com/ (Resources for parents, children, educators)

29 ♣ Behavior Management and Discipline

Janet R. Schultz

As many as half of all families in the United States consult their primary care provider at some point about mental health and behavioral issues in their children. With the gatekeeping role of primary care physicians growing, this number is likely to increase in the future. This chapter addresses the overall principles of behavior management in children and offers the primary care provider some suggestions and guidelines for managing and counseling parents about behavioral issues commonly encountered in the pediatric primary care setting.

I. **Barriers to Uncovering Behavior Problems During Well-Child Care**
   A. **Parents may try to communicate their concerns, but they are not acknowledged by the health care provider.**
   B. **Parents may not mention these concerns.** Some studies have indicated that about one-third of the time, parents do not express their greatest concern about their child's health and development, behavioral or otherwise. Primary reasons parents may not express their concerns to the physician are the following:
      1. *Perception.* They perceive physicians as "too busy," "not interested," or not qualified to be of assistance with the problem.
      2. *Personal feelings.* They are embarrassed or afraid that they will be blamed for the problem.

II. **Methods Physicians Can Use to Elicit Behavioral Concerns from Parents**
   A. **Be supportive of the parents, not critical.**
   B. **Be empathic to the parents and show interest in their child as a person.**
   C. **Ask about behavioral and emotional concerns directly.**
   D. **Pay particular attention to the parent while he or she is talking about behavioral concerns by maintaining eye contact and being verbally responsive** (phrases and reflections that show you are listening) **during the interaction.** Good listening by physicians has been shown to elicit more detailed illness-related information, disclosure of a larger number of patient concerns, greater parent satisfaction with office visits, reductions in parental concern, and increased compliance with the physician's recommendations.

III. **Goals of Behavior Management**
   A. **Prevention of behavior problems.** Accomplish with parent education and intervention by addressing development and temperament of the child.

B. Detection of early signs. Notice growing behavior problems or the development of mild but bothersome behavior patterns in which the physician can competently intervene.

C. Detection and identification of psychopathology or behavioral problems warranting referral to a specialist. Many pediatric behavioral problems are best addressed by the joint efforts of the primary care physician and the consulting specialist. General criteria for referral might include the following:

1. *Effect on daily life.* The behavior(s), relationship(s), and/or emotional state(s) interfere with everyday life in a recurrent, substantial way, or the quality of family interactions has become predominantly negative.

2. *Type and severity of problem.* The type or severity of the concerns is outside the range of expertise of the primary care physician (which depends on individual training, experience, and confidence).

3. *Lack of resources.* The type or severity of the problem(s) is within the range of expertise of the physician, but resources, such as time, ready availability, back-up, and perhaps desire or interest to treat these problems, is not present.

IV. Context of Behavior

Behavior occurs in a complex context that needs to be considered when attempting to change behaviors. The following are important factors that impact management:

A. Temperament of the child.

B. Developmental level of the child.

C. Personality and general functioning of parents.

D. Developmental level of the family (first child, last child, settled marriage, etc.).

E. Composition of and relationships within the family.

F. Subcultural and cultural values.

G. Particular life events for the family, including stressors and helpful occurrences.

Conclusion: *No one right way to raise a child exists. Different ways work for different families, but reliable themes for successful behavior management have been identified.*

V. General Principles of Behavior Management

A. Child behavior is usually maintained by its consequences.

1. *Immediacy.* The sooner the consequence (positive or negative) follows the action, the more impact it will have.

2. *Specificity.* Praise works best when it is specific (e.g., *"Every piece of dirty clothes is in the hamper, and all your books are back on the shelf! That's what I call a good job cleaning up!"* is more instructive than *"Nice job"* or *"Good girl"*).

3. *Appropriate.* A punishment should "fit the crime" in magnitude and logic (e.g., a child who rides his bike in the

street when he has been forbidden to do so might lose use of his bicycle for 3 days rather than losing television for a day).

4. *Outcome-oriented.* Whether a consequence is positive or negative should be defined by the outcome, not by an *a priori* judgment. Some behaviors can be maintained by a parent's scolding because the child gets attention, even though the content is not positive.

5. *Consistent.* Consistency is very important. Consistency must be maintained from parent to parent (e.g., if mother does not allow a snack just before dinner, the father should not allow it, even if the period just before dinner is the first opportunity he has had to play with the child); situation to situation (e.g., a temper tantrum at the grocery should be handled the same way as a temper tantrum at home); and time to time (e.g., name calling should be handled the same way Monday afternoon, when the family is alone, as it is on Sunday afternoon, when the clergyman is visiting). Sometimes what parents do matters less (within broad limits) than that it is employed consistently.

B. Child behavior tends to be governed by the actions of parents, not their words (e.g., parent spanking child and saying, *"This will teach you to hit someone smaller than yourself!"* or father smiling while discussing his son's aggression problem on the playground). Threats are not effective in managing behaviors and tend to leave parents feeling frustrated.

C. Children learn much of their behavior by the examples set around them. The more important the model, the bigger the impact. This includes the behaviors of parents, other adults, other children, and television characters.

D. Behavior occurs in a relationship. If the relationship is positive, the child will behave better to please the adult (if the adult shows his or her pleasure) than he or she will if the relationship is negative. Often before any major behavioral change can occur, some positive activities must be implemented. Suggestions often include 15 to 20 minutes per day of playtime with the child during which the child directs the play rather than the parent. The parent should avoid demands or questions and should simply make descriptive comments on the child's play during that special time (e.g., *"The car crashed into the blocks"*).

E. In general, punishment, especially physical punishment, tends to suppress behavior briefly, not to eliminate the undesirable behavior (*"I spank him; and 15 minutes later, he's back doing the same thing!"*). Punishment alone rarely conveys what behavior is expected from the child. Explanation (not complex reasoning or persuasion) and positive reinforcement (praise, tangible reward, hug, attention) for the desired behaviors are far more instructive.

VI. Discipline

A. Definition. The word *discipline* comes from the Greek word meaning "to lead." Discipline is a teaching process, not a synonym for punishment. It is the process by which a child learns values, limits on behaviors in specific settings, general rules of interaction, and other familial, cultural, and societal expectations and rules. It can be thought of as the process of "civilizing" or socializing children. The process is lifelong, and with the right parental direction, children develop "self-discipline," internalized controls on their own behavior in the absence of externally provided structure or reaction to long-delayed consequences.

B. Age. Even as a newborn, the child begins to learn that crying has an impact on events, that certain things bring discomfort, and that others result in comfort and satisfaction. The process of discipline changes with the developmental age of the child, parents, and family.

C. Aspects of developmentally targeted discipline.

   1. *Environmental "engineering"*—structuring the environment to be conducive to good behavior (e.g., removing breakable figurines from a child's reach).

   2. *Matching behavior management techniques to development.*

   3. *Recognizing normal developmental trends that affect behavior* (e.g., growing need for autonomy and accommodating that need).

   4. *Consistency of rules across settings*—or at least clear discrimination between settings (*"That may be okay at Grandma's but at home, we don't eat candy before dinner"*).

D. Effects of positive management. The more positive behavior management methods are, the more positive the parent/child relationship.

E. General approach to behavioral problem solving.

   1. *Identify the patterns.* To do so, parents need to keep a chart of whenever the designated problem behavior occurs by date, time, location, activity going on, persons present, and outcome of the behavior.

   2. *Analyze the pattern.* Identify associated events and consequences.

   3. *Generate alternatives.* These include changing consequences, addressing associated events (e.g., changing nap times to avoid overfatigue), or teaching new, more desirable behaviors.

   4. *Implement alternatives and evaluate their effectiveness.* Continue to chart behaviors.

F. Specific techniques that can be used across developmental ages.

   1. *Positive reinforcement is a powerful force for shaping desired behaviors.*

   2. *Differential attention is a powerful technique for managing undesirable behaviors that do not hurt anyone else.* Parents often feel that ignoring undesirable behavior is not enough or that other parents will judge them harshly. If the interest is in outcome, many small infractions of rules

are best treated by ignoring them, as long as desirable behavior reliably receives positive attention. This includes temper tantrums, nonphysical struggles with siblings, noise-making activities, and so on.

G. Time out

1. *Time out (TO) can be introduced after 2 years of age—* age varies, depending on verbal development.

2. *TO should be used only for specific behaviors.* In the preschool range only a few important behaviors should be followed by TO—namely, when a child in this age range does something significantly out of bounds (e.g., hits a sibling or parent).

3. *The purpose of TO is to remove the child from opportunities for positive consequences, to break into the flow of behavior, and to teach the child limits to behavior.*

4. *Parents should decide on a somewhat isolated place where the child cannot see television or play with toys, but can be supervised by the parent.* Sitting on a specified couch, chair, or stairstep is often successful. The child should be placed there *calmly* by the parent with the words *time out* used in some way to label the event (e.g., *"When you hit, you get a time out"*). The parent should not threaten (e.g., *"Do you need a time out?"* or *"If you do that again, you'll have to go to time out"*). After the first introduction of the rule, the TO should just be carried out without delay and without bargaining.

5. *The child should sit in the designated place for about 1 minute per year of chronological age.* Most parents make it for too great a length of time. A mechanical timer, either digital or old-style baking timer, is useful because it makes the timing more objective for both parties.

6. *A common pitfall is* **interacting with the child during the TO.** During the period of TO the child should be ignored. The parent should not be engaged (in conversation, body gesture, or glance) by the child during this period (e.g., *"But, Mom, why do I have to sit here?"* *"Because you misbehaved; that's why."*).

7. *When the TO is over, the parent should restate in a positive fashion the rule that was broken* (e.g., *"We are gentle with each other"* or *"We use words to show what we want"*).

8. *What should the parent do with the child who won't stay in TO?* Often children who have been taught TO at an early age will learn to take "good" TOs. But some children introduced to the concept later, or those involved in more defiance regardless of age of introduction, may refuse to stay in the designated TO spot. Sometimes refusal is a direct result of parental inconsistency with TOs or mishandling (e.g., talking to the child). Three options are suggested for the child who refuses to sit in TO:

a. **The best is having a toy-free, hazard-controlled room prepared as back up.** If the child does not stay in a properly administered TO spot, he or she should be told, *"Since you did not stay in the chair, you'll have to be by yourself."* The parent should then lead the child to the room and leave the lights on and the door closed. All child behavior is ignored and 60 seconds later, the child is led by the hand back to the chair for a full TO. If you (or the parents) feel discomfort about this particular child being left alone with the door shut, then a sheet of plywood slid across the open door and held in place by the parent is a good alternative. The rest of the procedure is carried out the same way. The parent must *not* interact with the child. If the child makes a mess, he or she must return to the TO chair and finish TO and must then be led back to the room to clean up the mess.

b. **The child can be held in the TO chair.** The parent should say, *"Since you didn't stay in time out, I'll have to help you."* The child is returned to the chair in a businesslike fashion. The parent should be behind the chair reaching around to hold the child's wrists firmly crossed in front of him. If the TO chair has arms, the adult's arm can simply cross in front of the child, grasping the chair arm firmly to essentially create a seat belt. When the child's struggling decreases, the parent releases the hold with the statement, *"Now finish your time out."* This is repeated as necessary.

c. **The least desirable of the three (but better than not having any effective behavior control) is a spanking.** The parent should say, *"Since you did not stay in time out, I'll have to spank you."* The parent then spanks the child twice with open hand on the clothed buttocks and returns him or her to the TO chair with the statement, *"Now finish your time out."* This may need to be repeated. **This recommendation should only be made with careful consideration of the family and parental anger control.**

Usually several trials of any of the preceding will teach the child to stay in the TO chair. In turn, applied correctly, TO will be a portable, safe way of teaching children when they have violated a major rule.

H. Spanking. Spanking is controversial and, as addressed earlier, tends to suppress behaviors; it does not teach desired behaviors. Nonetheless, the estimation is that more than 60% of parents spank their children. Primary care physicians who recommend spanking for behavior control are not uncommon. Sometimes addressing how to spank with parents is a better idea than pretending spanking does not occur. The child should be spanked only on the clothed buttocks and never on the head (face). An open hand should be the only thing used, never paddles, extension cords, wooden spoons, or other objects. One stern spank is more effective than multiple light taps. Spanking works best (if at all) when saved for major infractions. The parent should wait until he or she calms down rather than spanking the child in anger. Actually, the parent leaving the room to cool down can be thought of as a sort of TO equivalent and may be just as effective without the spanking.

VII.   Discipline Guidelines by Age of Child

   A.   Toddlers and preschoolers. In the early years, much of discipline is environmental engineering. This includes baby-proofing for the safety of the child and belongings, thereby reducing the frequency of frustration-producing, "No-no's." Behavior management also includes attending to the physical needs of the infant or toddler to reduce the trouble times of fatigue and hunger. Physicians can often help parents identify what they are already doing, praise them for their specific behaviors, and help them generalize the concept to problem-solve for their own specific family needs.

   1. *Under 18 months.*

   Teaching tasks: To teach the child that the world is a safe, pleasant, and reliable place where the child's needs will be met. To teach that some behaviors have different consequences than others.

   For parents: The physician should help parents recall that developmentally, the child cannot possibly do things to "get" the parents. Toddlers are cognitively incapable of that kind of sophisticated analysis of a situation, including putting themselves in the place of the parent. Things a child does may "get" the parent or "push his or her buttons" but that is not why the child does them. When parents attribute this kind of intent, they almost inevitably feel the child must be punished to teach him or her not to defy parental authority. This attitude is not helpful and may set the stage for long-term power struggles. The physician should help parents not expect too much. Instead, environmental planning becomes key so that the child is safe to explore without unnecessary frustration on the part of adult or child.

   Physical punishment should be avoided with children this age because the behaviors being punished are generally a result of normal development (e.g., the urge to explore, a tendency to mouth objects, experimentation with the world, including throwing things). Redirection of the child's activity or physically moving the child away from the forbidden object or activity (distraction) is more educational and effective.

   Language is not yet controlling for toddlers, so parents should be given the anticipatory guidance that "No, no" will be a temporary deterrent at best. At around 18 months of age, a point in development occurs where some children respond to any sort of linguistic command by speeding up the behavior rather than stopping it. This reaction is related to neuropsychological development of language functioning in which language may facilitate rather than inhibit behavior.

2. *Eighteen to 36 months.*

   Teaching task: The child begins to learn that rules and limits exist that the child can learn and do for himself. The child begins to learn to use words and to modulate self-expression. The child begins to learn independence.

   Language is developing, but frustration tolerance is very limited. Children this age can only delay for a minute or so. When dealing with the rigidity and inflexibility of this age ("*I want what I want when I want it*"), parents should avoid head-on confrontation. Instead, environmental engineering is helpful. Parents should simplify routines, not offer too many (or too complex) choices, and allow the child to express the growing urge to be independent through self-help skills.

   Positive statements of rules are more effective than negative ones (e.g., "*We walk in the house*" rather than "*No running!*"). Frequent disciplinary issues include temper tantrums and physical aggression, especially hitting and biting. Both are almost inevitably linked to frustration of the child with something else, such as the adult, the child's own limitations, a toy, or another child (see later).

3. *Three- to 5-year-olds.*

   Teaching task: To help the child learn to use words to delay gratification, avoid physical aggression, and meet their own needs.

   Prevention of behavior problems becomes more verbal at this level of development. Children can say not just *no,* but also *yes,* and *we* instead of just *me.* Rituals are less necessary. Language is very powerful, so behavior can be influenced by words like *new, different, help, guess,* and so on. Many preschoolers love to please and to conform as far as they are capable. They can attend to spoken directions but need them to be specific (e.g., "*We sit quietly in church*") rather than general (e.g., "*Be good*").

   This is a "me too" age and children are motivated by the behavior of others, especially if they see the other child being praised for desirable behaviors. Reasoning now enters into discipline but cannot be depended on. Fantasy is big at this age, and parents can use it to get the child's cooperation by entering into the game (e.g., "*Can the engineer drive the train all the way back to the toy box?*"). Indirect approaches often work well. For example, a parent might get a child this age to take off his outer clothing by guessing what color his socks are (of course, guessing all the wrong colors first). Whispering or exaggerating can be helpful too. The parent will be more effective if he/she avoids asking the child to do something if the intent is a command.

   Especially when a child is more than 4 years of age, firm limits, consistently and fairly administered, are important to help him limit his actions and keep him safe. Because their own feelings and actions may scare them in their intensity, many children feel far more secure with clear limits at this age. Clear, specific expectations should be announced before entering new situations. TOs should be used through this age period but should be seasoned with a heavy allotment of praise, rewards, and affection. Star charts and public admiration are attractive at this age. Heroes are important too, so parents should consider their exposure carefully. Children at this age will model their hero's behaviors.

If a preschool child does something wrong, having the "punishment fit the crime" is especially helpful (e.g., if a child leaves the toys all over the playroom, he or she not only has to clean up the room but cannot use the toys for 1 day). Similarly, a child who damages the belongings of another should make up for it in some way. Besides "making sense" to the child, this kind of approach allows the child to regain some dignity through restitution.

Preschool children who do not readily comply with the requests and commands of adults are at greater risk for the development of behavior disorders during the school years. This observation does not mean preschoolers should always be obedient little automatons. However, parents should be able to get their preschoolers to do what they need them to do with a minimum of repetition and TOs.

B. School-aged children

Teaching task: To help children learn the behavioral expectations outside the home and to channel their energy for learning, working, socializing, and having fun into constructive directions.

The same behavioral principles apply, but because of the child's developmental level, the child has a greater capacity to delay gratification. Praise and punishment can also be a little further removed in time from the behaviors that earned them. Unfortunately, typical parents tend to use praise less often with school-aged children than with younger ones. Parents also have a tendency to praise outcomes more than the behaviors that led to the outcomes. For example, good grades may be praised more than the studying and working that led to the grades.

TOs may lose their effectiveness after 8 years of age. Removal of privileges becomes more powerful for older children as they acquire more privileges and opportunities to venture outside the family. Although money becomes a more powerful positive reinforcer for school-aged children, parental time is often equally or more effective. For example, the child makes his bed every day for a week to earn an extra amount of time with parents or a special activity with them, such as playing Monopoly or another game that a parent might not otherwise play.

Anticipatory guidance at this age should include the warning against assuming that since children always seem busy and tied up with friends, they no longer need positive time with parents. The child needs to interact with the parent at play and at work. Doing tasks together cooperatively rather than in a parallel fashion will help keep the relationship positive. This, in turn, helps the child want to please the parent. Communication without criticism or judgment threat is also imperative. Asking questions generally is the least effective way of learning about the child's life. Rather, having quiet, positive times together when the child can offer up small reports without criticism is more likely to help keep communication open.

School-aged children still need supervision. Clear evidence suggests that children, especially ones who already have a history of acting out, will engage in far more frequent unacceptable and aggressive behaviors if left unsupervised at this age.

Preteens continue to need praise and generally respond to it more than punishment or threats of punishment. Praise has to be meaningful and not empty words. Genuine praise for an accomplishment that the young person feels required effort is a very positive act from the parent. Recognizing his or her particular struggles makes for powerful praise (e.g., a C in math that required hard study may be much more praiseworthy than the A in social studies). The values of friends become increasingly important, and the presence of a constant set of parental values is an important balance. However, values that are not lived, but just spoken, will be very rapidly seen as hypocritical. Parents and their own behaviors remain very important to their children throughout development.

ADDITIONAL READING

American Academy of Pediatrics. *Report of the Task Force on Education.* Elk Grove Village, IL: American Academy of Pediatrics; 1978.

Barkley R. *The defiant child: a clinician's manual for parent training.* New York: Guilford Press; 1987.

Campbell SB. *Behavior problems in preschool children.* New York: Guilford Press; 1990.

Schmitt B. *Your child's health,* rev. ed. New York: Bantam Books; 1991.

Wissow L, Roter D, Wilson M. Pediatrician style and mothers' disclosure of psychosocial issues. *Pediatrics* 1994;93:289–295.

Books for Parents

Carey WB, Jablow M. *Understanding your child's temperament,* New York: Macmillan; 1997.

Clark L. *SOS: help for parents.* Bowling Green, KY: Parents Press; 1985.

Sloane HN. *The good kid book: how to solve the 16 most common behavior problems.* Champaign, IL: Research Press; 1988.

Crary E. *Without spanking or spoiling: a practical approach to toddler and preschool guidance.* Seattle: Parenting Press; 1979.
Leach P. *Your baby and child.* New York: Knopf; 1978.

Websites for Parents

www.new-life.net/discipln.html (Christian orientation)
www.happy-kids.com (General)

Website for Physicians

www.dbpeds.org/links/behavior.html (Pediatric Development and Behavior Online)

30 ♣ Biting

Kathleen Burklow

Biting behavior in young children is quite common and distressing for parents. Not only is biting painful and of some health risk (e.g., infection) to the child who is bitten, but it also has negative social implications for the child who bites. It can lead to ostracism from a peer group and to being labeled as aggressive by adults. Biting is especially problematic when the child is required to interact socially with other children in unstructured free play situations, as is common in day care and preschool settings. Depending on the tolerance and skill level of the day care or preschool setting, the consequences for the child who bites chronically can be significant. In some situations, biting behavior may result in the child being suspended or expelled from the setting altogether until the behavior is resolved.

I. Developmental Considerations

Children bite for reasons that can vary with the age of the child. In infants, biting may be in response to the child's efforts to relieve the sensitivity and discomfort associated with teething. In toddlers and preschoolers however, biting behavior may reflect the child's feelings of anger, excitement, and/or frustration, especially if the child does not have adequate language skills to express his or her feelings. Although young children developmentally are unaware of the pain that their biting inflicts upon others, parents should address the biting behavior immediately to avoid further biting and other aggressive behaviors.

II. Prevention

The key to reducing biting behaviors in children is **prevention**.

A. Determine patterns of and triggers for the biting. Parents and caretakers should be encouraged to watch for patterns in the child's biting behavior. As parents and caretakers become more aware of the situations that trigger biting, they will be able to intervene earlier to prevent the biting from occurring. Because feelings of frustration or excitement, common triggers for biting, are more likely to occur in unstructured situations, parents and caretakers should attempt to structure and closely monitor social interaction opportunities for their young children before conflicts escalate enough to initiate biting.

B. Teach, reinforce, and model appropriate social behaviors. Parents and caretakers should teach, enforce, and regularly review rules of social play, including how to take turns and share objects and activities with others. Adults are important models of behavior for young children. Therefore parents and caretakers themselves should avoid using aggressive behaviors, such as yelling or throwing objects, when they are angry or frustrated. Similarly, adults who bite the child back to demonstrate how much biting hurts the other person are more likely to model hurtful behaviors than teach the child not to bite.

III. Intervention

When a young child has already begun to engage in biting behavior, parents should implement immediate interventions based on general child behavior management techniques. These techniques involve setting consistent behavioral expectations and limits as well as establishing firm consequences for displays of inappropriate behavior.

A. Observe the patterns of biting. Parents should pay attention to observed patterns of biting behaviors. For example, if a child tends to bite when in larger groups, then parents and caretakers should make attempts to reduce the play group size. If the child tends to target one child specifically (such as an older or bigger child who may be teasing or bullying the child), then parents and caretakers should decrease the opportunities for these two children to be together.

B. Intervene immediately. When the child bites, he or she should experience immediate consequences. Parents should verbally reprimand the child (e.g., "*No biting!*") and then place the child in time out (see "Time Out" in Chapter 29).

C. Teach alternative behaviors. Children who bite need to be provided with alternative behaviors. When the child returns from time out, parents and caretakers can say, "*When you are angry, you should ask for help or walk away instead of biting.*" Then the parent and caretaker should help the child practice these alternatives through a simple role-play of a similar situation leading up to the biting.

D. Comfort the child who was bitten. To avoid inadvertently reinforcing the child who bites through the social attention provided during the disciplinary action, parents and caretakers should ensure that they give extra attention and comfort to the child who was bitten. If the biting resulted in a conflict over an object or activity, the child who was bitten should receive access to the object or activity, not the child who was the biter. By providing most of the attention to the child who was bitten, parents and caretakers will help the child who bites learn better ways to get positive social attention.

E. Seek professional help. If the biting persists despite consistent efforts to intervene and reduce the frequency of biting behaviors, parents and caretakers should seek professional help from a psychologist or counselor to eliminate these behaviors.

When parents and caretakers intervene immediately and consistently manage biting behaviors as outlined in the preceding list, children usually learn quickly that biting will get them into trouble as they are banished to the time-out chair and the bitten child gets all the attention. A clear connection is made between the biting and the negative consequence. At the same time, as children make developmental gains and improve their ability to express their emotions in more positive ways, they learn to replace the biting behavior with more effective language expression. This also acts to decrease the biting behavior.

ADDITIONAL READING

Brayden RM, Poole SR. Common behavioral problems in infants and children. *Prim Care* 1995;22:81–97.

Brazelton TB. *Touchpoints: your child's emotional and behavioral development.* Reading, MA: Perseus Books; 1992.

Turecki, S. *The difficult child.* New York: Bantam Books; 1989.

31 ♣ Bullying and Teasing

Kathleen Burklow

Nationwide, newspaper headlines have described the negative consequences of school violence and aggression within the school and classroom setting. The most extreme and devastating consequence of school violence has been the recent increase in the reports of the number of school shootings and other hate crimes. Often the perpetrators of these crimes are students who are or who have been the victims of bullying and teasing by other students.

Although being teased or bullied is regarded as a universal experience common to childhood, these encounters can have a long-lasting impact upon an individual's emotional and social development. For instance, most adults can vividly recall instances in childhood during which they were involved in some degree of teasing or bullying, either as the instigator or as the recipient. Given the emotional impact of their own past experiences with teasing and bullying, parents often want to respond quickly to bullying and teasing issues, especially when their child is the victim.

Previous research has demonstrated that the most common topics that children tease and bully others about and the topics that they are teased and bullied about themselves are related to physical appearance and unusual behavior. Children's responses to teasing can differ. Most children acknowledge that their usual response to teasing is to ignore the teasing or to tease back. Yet when specifically asked to rate the effectiveness of different responses to teasing, children rate responding to teasing in a humorous manner as more effective than responding with ignoring or hostility.

Unfortunately, because of the emotional volatility characteristic of such encounters, not all children are able to respond to teasing or bullying in a humorous manner. Even most adults are unable to generate an immediate verbal comeback in response to teasing, much less ensure that the response contains humorous elements. Therefore a child's inability to come up with a witty "zinger" in response to another child's teasing or bullying in the heat of the moment is not unexpected. Fortunately, however, most children tend to be teased for the same issues repeatedly (e.g., the way they dress, the unusual color of their hair, a characteristically odd laugh). Some children are teased repeatedly simply because they react or behave in a manner that encourages more teasing. Pediatric primary care providers and parents can help the child who is being teased and bullied by generating several verbal and nonverbal strategies ahead of time to deal with the teasing and bullying.

I. Strategies to Help the Recipient of the Teasing and Bullying

A. **Ask the child to provide more details.** Parents should try to find out *who* is doing the teasing, *when* the teasing is happening (e.g., during recess, on the bus ride home from school), *where* the teasing is occurring (e.g., in the neighborhood, at school), *how* their child reacts (e.g., laughs, cries, becomes angry), and *what* the bully's response is to the child's reaction (e.g., laughs, teases more, leaves the child alone). Parents should encourage their children to talk with them about the episodes so that the frequency and characteristics of such encounters can be recorded. While they obtain information from their child, parents should carefully monitor their own feelings and avoid overreacting. When children see extreme reactions from their parents, some will hesitate to tell their parents that they are being bullied or teased because they do not want their parents to think less of them or to get involved. By obtaining information in a nonjudgmental manner, parents may be able to determine patterns to the teasing and bullying episodes and to decide upon the most appropriate approach to the problem.

 B. Help the child to respond appropriately. There are two strategies that parents can help their children use to respond to teasing.

 1. *Ignore it and walk away.* According to general behavior theory, if a behavior is not reinforced, the behavior is less likely to recur. Teasing follows this same behavioral principle in that if the recipient of the teasing does not attend to (i.e., if he or she ignores) the teasing, then the teaser will be less likely to tease him or her again. Thus teaching the child to ignore and to walk away from the teasing and bullying without reacting can be a powerful tool for decreasing the verbally aggressive behaviors over time. Children need to be warned, however, to anticipate a brief increase in the teasing as the teaser intensifies efforts to get a reaction. The child needs to remain calm, to stand firm, and to show no reaction if such a situation occurs. As the teaser begins to realize that the recipient of the teasing is not going to respond, he or she will typically give up his or her efforts.

 2. *Come up with verbal comebacks ahead of time.* Parents need to work with their child to develop a set of appropriate verbal and behavioral responses to teasing. As described earlier, children judge humorous responses to teasing as most effective. Therefore helping children to generate witty responses to teasing may help to diffuse a potentially volatile situation and may distract the teaser from persisting in his or her teasing. The reply must be free from hostility and can not involve or invite teasing back. Although generating their own response is most effective for children, younger children may have difficulty doing so. Parents may need to provide a list of options to help the child discover a reply that matches his or her personality style. Some examples include the following:

"So?"
"Let me know when I'm supposed to laugh."
"And your point is?"

Sometimes a child finds providing a response that seems, on the surface, to agree with the bully's teasing remarks helpful. For example,

Bully: *You waddle like a duck! Quack, Quack!*
Child: *Yeah, I can see what you are saying.*

Such replies frequently take the momentum from the bully, enough to stop the teasing from continuing. If a child chooses to use such replies, however, parents and the child must discuss the importance of not believing everything that other people say about him or her, especially if the comments are negative and hurtful.

3. *Practice, practice, practice.* Parents need to help their child practice using the replies comfortably in the face of actual teasing. Thus parents should role-play a typical teasing episode with their child and should encourage the child to reply using the responses generated. To keep the interactions playful and humorous instead of emotionally charged, parents should laugh with the child each time the response is given. For example:

Parent: *Now, let's practice! I am going to pretend that I am* [**bully's name**] *at the* [**typical location of teasing**]. *You need to practice using your comebacks and not to let it seem like it bothers you. Get ready. You laugh like a donkey and look like one too!*
Child: *So?*
Parent: *That's great! I like that answer. Let's try another one.*

Typically, the teaser will issue another teasing statement when the individual who is being teased responds back for the first time. Therefore children need to be prepared for additional teasing by having several potential responses ready. Eventually the teaser will likely exhaust the number of teasing statements that he or she can generate and will stop.

4. *Keep checking on the effectiveness of the strategy.* Parents should continue having discussions with their child to determine the effectiveness of the responses. Parents should reinforce the child's attempts to use the strategies, whether or not the techniques succeed initially. Parents also should try to assess the frequency of the teasing. In most cases, the frequency of teasing will decrease over time in response to the effective use of predetermined strategies.

5. *Do not encourage violence or aggressive retaliations.* Children should never be encouraged to bully the bully by fighting back or using revenge. Not only can the child get hurt (and get into trouble), but such parental messages also teach the child to use violence to deal with violence.

C. When and how should parents get involved? Parents always should stay involved when their child reports that he or she is being bullied or teased. The level of involvement, however, depends on the level of teasing or bullying that is occurring. In most circumstances, children benefit from openly discussing the bullying and teasing episodes and problem-solving together with their parent as described earlier. In other, more extreme instances, however, bullying and teasing can have a significant impact on the recipient's behaviors and emotional well-being and require more intensive parental involvement.

1. *Common characteristics of a child who is being bullied severely include children who exhibit the following:*

a. **Sudden declines in schoolwork.**

b. **Less interest in schoolwork than before.**

c. **School avoidance or frequent headaches and stomachaches on school days.**

d. **Preferences for taking out-of-the-way routes to common locations.**

e. **Missing books, money, or other belongings without adequate explanation.**

f. **Increases in requests for extra money; stealing.**

g. **Unexplained injuries or torn clothing.**

2. *Parents whose children exhibit such emotional and behavioral characteristics should request a private meeting as soon as possible with the teacher to discuss the matter.* Parents should not confront the bully or the bully's parents because doing so may escalate the problem. Frequently, children who are severely teased and bullied do not wish to be seen as tattletales for fear of retaliation from the bully. Parents, however, need to remember that bullying should not be tolerated. By failing to take action against the bullying, the parent can send a message that he or she implicitly condones violence and aggressive behavior.

3. *Because the victim of the bullying can feel vulnerable to the aggression and intimidation of the bully, parents (and teachers) need to put systems into place to protect the child who is bullied or teased persistently.* Therefore, the following steps should be taken:

a. **Parents should encourage school personnel to impose disciplinary action on the bully.** This sends the message to the bully as well as to other students that bullying, teasing, violence, and aggression are not tolerated.

b. **Parents and teachers should closely monitor and limit the interactions between the bully and victim.** The bully should be told explicitly that he or she is not allowed within 20 feet of the child whom he or she has been bullying. The bully should be penalized immediately if he or she gets closer than this distance to the victim. These guidelines will not only reinforce to the bully that aggression is wrong, but will also show the victim that he or she was correct in telling an adult about the bullying.

They will also demonstrate to the victim that he or she will be protected.

c. ***Parents need to teach their children appropriate assertion skills.*** Bullies use intimidation. Therefore coaching children how to be assertive and how to say "*No!*" when a bully tries to force them to do something they do not wish to do is important. As described earlier, practicing assertion skills in role-plays can be very helpful with teaching the child to be comfortable in intimidating situations. Children who are confident and resourceful are less likely to be bullied.

d. ***Parents should encourage their child who is teased to surround himself or herself with friends.*** Parents may need to discuss these possibilities with the child's teacher. Because children who are teased are often the same children who are isolated socially and lack social skills, they may need additional supports from parents and teachers to arrange for positive opportunities to interact with a group of friendly, compassionate peers.

e. ***If the situations occur on the bus or the walk home from school, parents should consider temporarily picking the child up from school or making alternative arrangements for the child after school.*** As the systems for addressing the bullying and teasing become better established, children should be encouraged to return to their previous routines. Parents who continue to make alternative arrangements with the intent of protecting their child even after systems have been effectively initiated, maintained, and monitored may inadvertently teach and reinforce avoidant behaviors to their child. Therefore children who are encouraged to return to previous routines after protective mechanisms and consequences for bullying have been established learn that positive changes can occur when they are assertive and speak up for their rights.

II. Strategies to Help Parents Whose Child Is Identified as the Bully.
Some parents discover that their child is not the one who is being teased but the one who is doing the bullying and teasing. Many parents are not even aware that their child is bullying another child and do not find out about it until they are called to the school to discuss such issues with their child's teacher or principal.

A. Characteristics of bullies.
1. *Typically, bullies are physically stronger than their peers.* They often will seek out children to tease who seem vulnerable (e.g., smaller stature, younger, physically weaker, quiet, emotionally sensitive).

2. *Bullies have several peers who do not usually start the teasing and bullying but who enjoy following and laughing about the bullying and teasing.*

3. *Bullies have difficulty seeing things from someone else's perspective.* As a result, they may have different interpretations of situations to justify their aggressive behavior.

4. *Bullies frequently misread social cues and often perceive provocation in situations where others do not.* This misperception increases the likelihood that a bully will respond with aggression and intimidation during ambiguous social interactions with other children.

B. Ways parents can intervene with a child who bullies.

1. *Talk to the child about the reports of the bullying.* Parents need to be matter-of-fact when discussing the reports of bullying with their child. They must anticipate that the child might try to deny or minimize the teasing and bullying behavior. Nonetheless, parents need to send the clear message that bullying is wrong and will not be tolerated.

2. *Establish strict rules to prevent the bullying.* Parents should inform the school that they are aware of the situation and are putting guidelines into place to intervene within settings outside of school. School personnel should responsible for monitoring the child's behaviors during the school day. Examples of rules that parents of a child who bullies can make include the following:

a. **The bullying child needs to stay away (20 feet minimum) from the child whom he or she has been bullying.**

b. **If the child gets too close to the child whom he or she has been bullying, he or she will be penalized.** (See "Disciplinary Strategies" later.)

c. **The child is not allowed to do anything on the way to school or on the way back home from school.**

d. **The child is not allowed to play at other children's houses unless the parent knows the family and the other child's parents or guardians are at home to supervise and monitor directly.**

3. *Establish disciplinary strategies when the child violates the rules.* Parents need to assess consistently their child's adherence to the rules. Each time the child has opportunities to interact socially with other children, parents should always check in with the supervising adult to determine whether or not the child has engaged in bullying or aggressive behaviors. If the child violates the rules however, parents need to apply immediate consequences for the rule violations.

a. **Parents first need to tell the child what behavior the child engaged in that is in violation of the rule.** (For example, "*You went near* [the child who has been bullied] *in the park. You are supposed to stay away from him because you have been teasing him.*")

b. **Parents then need to implement a penalty.** Penalties can involve restriction of favorite or planned activities or taking away a favorite activity or toy for a specified period of time. (For example, *"Because you went near him when you weren't supposed to, you will not be allowed to watch TV tonight."*)

c. **Parents must enforce the penalty without holding a grudge against the child.** Parents need to give the child an opportunity to learn from the mistake and change the behavior positively.

d. **Parents should never use physical punishment (i.e., hitting or spanking) to penalize the child who breaks a rule.** Parents who use physical punishment can send a mixed message to the child. The child may become confused if they are being punished with the same kind of aggressive behaviors for which they are being disciplined.

4. *Parents should watch for and praise their child when he or she exhibits positive prosocial behaviors.* Parents need to "catch" their child being kind to others and reinforce this behavior (For example, *"I saw how you helped that little girl. I like it when I see you doing something so kind. Keep it up!"*) Through such reinforcement for their prosocial behaviors, children can learn the types of social behaviors that please their parents.

III. When to Seek Professional Help

Some children and families will need to seek additional help when their efforts to manage the behaviors do not produce positive results. Regardless of whether their child is the instigator or victim of the bullying and teasing, parents who see an increase in the behaviors (despite efforts to intervene) and significant changes in their child's emotional and social well-being should seek additional help from a psychologist or other mental health professional.

ADDITIONAL READING

Frankel F. *Good friends are hard to find: help your child find, make and keep friends.* Glendale, CA: Perspective Publishing; 1996.

Miller P. Teasing: a case study in language socialization and verbal play. *Q News Lab Comp Hum Cogn* 1982;4:29–32.

Olweus D. *Bullying at school: what we know and what we can do.* Cambridge, MA: Blackwell Publishers; 1993.

Scambler D, Harris M, Milich R. Sticks and stones: evaluations of responses to childhood teasing. *Soc Dev* 1998;7:234–249.

32 ♣ Children Exposed to Domestic Violence

Barbara W. Boat

I. Exposure to Violence in the Home

Domestic violence is a major health concern, with as many as 10% to 40% of women disclosing abuse by their partners when screened by physicians in primary care settings. An estimated 95% of children in violent homes are either present or in an adjoining room during violent incidents.

Children of abused women can experience a variety of effects. Direct effects include physical danger to the child (thrown objects, child attempting to intervene), emotional and behavioral coping problems (sleeplessness, depression, school problems, numbing with alcohol or drugs), and learned aggressive behaviors in conflict situations. Indirect effects include deprivation of maternal support because of the mother's stress level, exposure to parental anger and irritability, and inconsistent or overly harsh discipline. Some children live under high levels of stress because of fear of injury to self or parent. In children who have developed posttraumatic stress disorder (PTSD), smaller intracranial and cerebral volumes relative to matched controls have been documented on MRIs. In addition, children who grow up where violence is present are

- Six times more likely to commit suicide.
- Twenty-four times more likely to be sexually assaulted.
- Sixty times more likely to engage in delinquent behavior as an adult.
- One thousand times more likely to be abusers themselves.

Recognizing these profound effects, the American Academy of Pediatrics has recommended that all pediatricians incorporate screening for domestic violence as a part of anticipatory guidance and active child abuse prevention.

II. Factors Determining Impact of Domestic Violence on Children

A. Age and developmental level of the child (Table 32.1)

1. *Infants to 5 years of age.* These children are the most exposed and vulnerable. Infants especially are extremmly susceptible to physical harm. Young children cannot self-soothe or regulate their responses to the violence and frequently develop somatic and behavioral problems.

2. *Ages 6 to 12.* At these ages, children may have access to more resources outside the home to help with coping. However, they are more likely to use violence, become hypervigilant, blame themselves for events, and worry about the welfare of their siblings and mothers. Their shame and embarrassment may lead to social isolation.

3. *Adolescents.* Teens are even more prone to engage in violent behaviors (the highest number of paternal homi-

Table 32.1. Possible effects of exposure to domestic violence

Infants	Preschool	School Age	Adolescent
Attachment needs not met as mother less available	World perceived as unsafe and unstable	Aggressive behaviors	Feelings of rage, shame, betrayal
Routines disrupted; eating and sleeping problems	Signs of terror: yelling, hiding, stuttering	Blames self for violence at home	High-risk behaviors: school truancy, early sexual activity, substance use/abuse, delinquency, runaway
Increased risk of physical injury	Somatic complaints and regressive behaviors	Feelings of shame and embarrassment	
Decreased responsiveness to adults	Anxious attachment behaviors: whining, crying, clinging, stranger anxiety	Traumatic arousal symptoms: distracted, avoidant, hypervigilant	Impaired or diminished recall of childhood events
Increased crying		Limited range of emotional responses	Short attention span; unresponsive
	Insomnia, sleepwalking, and nightmares	Psychosomatic complaints	Defensive
		Uncooperative, suspicious, guarded	

Adapted from Jaffe PG, Wolfe D, Wilson S. *Children of battered women.* Newbury Park, CA: Sage; 1990; and from Wolak J, Finkelhor D. Children exposed to partner violence. In: Jasinski JL, Williams LM, eds. *Partner violence: a comprehensive review of 20 years of research.* Thousand Oaks, CA: Sage; 1998.

cides are committed by teenaged boys who witnessed their mothers being battered), to attempt to escape or run away, and to engage in high-risk behaviors. They frequently try to parent younger siblings.

B.   Nature, severity, and frequency (a single episode or chronic occurrence) of event. In one study, 100% of the children who witnessed a parental homicide developed PTSD.

C.   Direct maltreatment of the child either during the violent event or at other times.

D.   Availability of support from others, such as extended family or community resources.

III.   Screening for Exposure to Violence in the Home

A.   Parent screening. Talk to the mother alone, preferably in an office setting. Assure her that the conversation is confidential and that resources are available for help (if violence is identified). A few states require that medical professionals report suspected domestic violence. The screening will require 5 to 10 minutes.

Some suggested questions for mothers follow. These should be preceded by a statement such as, *"We are concerned about the health effects of domestic violence, so we now ask a few questions of all our children's mothers."*

1. *"Do you ever feel unsafe at home?"*

2. *"Has anyone at home hit you or tried to injure you in any way?"* (This question and question 1 have a sensitivity of 71% and a specificity of 85% in detecting domestic violence.)

3. *"Has anyone ever threatened or tried to control you?"*

4. *"Have you ever felt afraid of your partner?"* (This question and question 3 assess for controlling behavior and threats from the batterer.)

5. *"Has your partner ever hurt, or threatened to hurt, any of your children?"*

6. *"Do you have pets? If so, has your partner ever hurt or threatened to hurt your pets?"*

7. *"Are there any guns in your house?"*

B. Child screening: talk to the child alone. Ask permission from the mother to speak to the child. Ask about pets because frequently a batterer also abuses pets or threatens them with harm; in addition, children are more likely to talk about their pets than about themselves.

Some suggested questions for children follow. They should be preceded by a statement such as, *"I have a few questions to ask about your family. Your mother said it was okay for me to talk to you."*

1. *"What happens in your house when your mother and* **[father figure or partner]** *get angry with each other?"*

2. *"Is there any hitting at your house?"*

3. *"Does anyone get hurt? Have you or* **[siblings]** *ever been hurt?"*

4. *"What do you do during the fights?"*

5. *"Do you have pets?"* *"Has anyone ever hurt or threatened to hurt your pet?"*

6. *"Do you worry about bad things happening to your pet?"*

C. Issues to consider before you screen

1. *Reserve the necessary time.* Asking the questions and responding appropriately to a disclosure takes time.

2. *Formulate a policy on chart documentation.* Do not document disclosures in the child's chart, as this may place mother and children at risk if the batterer has access to the chart. In some settings the chart is flagged with a special sticker.

3. *Update training.* Adequate training on reporting guidelines and domestic violence resources as well as on safety issues for the child and parent is needed to aid the family effectively. If you suspect the child is at risk for abuse or neglect, you are mandated to report to your chil-

dren's services agency. Domestic violence programs offer hotline assistance. Know your local resources well!

4. *Understand that even though you ask, you may not uncover the fact that violence is present.* When family violence is chronic, both parent and child may deny or minimize as a general coping style.

5. *Remain culturally sensitive.* Willingness to disclose domestic violence may depend on several multicultural issues, such as religious beliefs.

IV. "Red Flags" for Physicians to Screen for Domestic Violence

Ideally, all mothers and children would be screened yearly. Minimally, any child or mother presenting with any of the following symptoms should be screened for exposure to domestic violence.

A. Child's symptoms

1. *Heightened arousal, overactivity, problems with concentration.* These symptoms may look like attention-deficit/hyperactivity disorder but can be a fear-induced reaction.

2. *Developmental delays.* Children with disabilities are overrepresented in abuse statistics.

3. *Changes in eating or sleeping habits.*

4. *Increased physical aggression.*

5. *Self-destructive behaviors.*

6. *Gastrointestinal, urinary, or bowel problems.*

B. Maternal Symptoms

1. *Pregnancy.* Pregnant women are at greater risk for domestic assault.

2. *Overt signs of depression or, in some cultures, somatic symptoms.*

3. *Suspicious marks on face or arms.*

ADDITIONAL READING

Eisenstat SA, Bancroft L. Domestic violence. *N Engl J Med* 1999; 341:886.

Jaffe PG, Wolfe D, Wilson S. *Children of battered women.* Newbury Park, CA: Sage; 1990.

Knapp JF. The impact of children witnessing violence. *Pediatr Clin North Am* 1998;45:355.

Siegel RM, Hill TD, Henderson VA, Ernst HM, Boat BW. Screening for domestic violence in the community pediatric setting. *Pediatrics* 1999;104:874–877.

Wolak J, Finkelhor D. Children exposed to partner violence. In: Jasinski JL, Williams LM, eds. *Partner violence: a comprehensive review of 20 years of research.* Thousand Oaks, CA: Sage; 1998.

33 ♣ Developmental Delay: Evaluation and Management

Nancy E. Lanphear

Developmental delay is a term typically reserved for the young child who has failed to meet expected developmental milestones. This term implies that the delays are not permanent and that the child will "catch up." This assumption is accurate in the young child, where significant and rapid gains can be made over time. Continuing to use the term *developmental delay* in an older child would be inappropriate and euphemistic, when a more specific diagnosis, such as mental retardation or a learning disability, would be more appropriate.

When development lags outside the expected range, careful consideration of the cause is important. The cause of developmental delay can be significant and due to real pathology, or it can be correctable with limited intervention. For example, now that the recommendation is to place infants on their backs to sleep, they spend less time on their abdomens and may exhibit mild gross motor delays (e.g., head control, rolling, crawling). These apparent delays can be avoided or at least minimized by specifically recommending that parents place their infants in the prone position while awake. On the other hand, a child may have similar motor delays due to hypotonia and may eventually be diagnosed with cerebral palsy.

The World Health Organization estimates that worldwide, 15% to 20% of children have a developmental disability. The estimate in the United States is 5% to 20%. A developmental disability is any type of disorder present from a young age and continuing into adulthood that affects the functioning status of an individual. (Table 33.1) illustrates the possible causes of developmental delay.

The approach for a child with developmental delay is based on the age of onset and the severity of the delay. Primary care physicians should use a model of developmental surveillance at all well-child checks. Implementation requires (a) physician knowledge of the normal sequence of acquisition of developmental and behavioral milestones, (b) a routine practice by the physician of eliciting parental concerns about development at each well-child visit, and (c) consistent, routine questioning of parents about the child's current developmental skills. If either the parent or the physician finds areas of concern, further evaluation for determining etiology and treatment must be considered.

The primary care physician is in a unique position to observe children over time as they grow and develop. They can provide education, guide the parents by addressing developmental and behavioral concerns, screen for potential difficulties, and refer as appropriate for concerns. The primary caregiver of the child is in the unique position to observe a child's day-to-day functioning and behavior. Obtaining a history from this primary caregiver is essential in assessing for developmental abilities, as the physi-

Table 33.1.   Potential causes of developmental delay*

Prenatal Causes
Chromosomal (including syndromes)
Metabolic
Physical abnormalities (e.g., spina bifida, cleft lip and palate, limb anomalies)
Effects of intrauterine environment
Prenatal exposure to substances, such as alcohol and illicit drugs
Maternal toxemia
Intrauterine infections, such as cytomegalovirus (CMV), rubella, toxoplasmosis
Disruption of maternal/placental/fetal circulation
Multiple gestation

Perinatal Causes
Birth asphyxia
Jaundice
Infection

Postnatal Causes
Infection
Injuries, such as traumatic brain injury
Chronic health conditions
Exposure to such substances as lead and mercury

*The most common cause of developmental delay is idiopathic or unknown. Listed above are potential causes for difficulties that later may be categorized as mental retardation, developmental delays, cerebral palsy, attention deficit/hyperactivity disorder, learning disabilities, language disorders, and behavioral difficulties. These terms are more descriptive of the symptoms that have been noted rather than a specific cause for the symptoms. Often a specific cause for developmental concerns cannot be identified. This list is not all-inclusive but illustrates the large differential that is possible for the underlying etiology of developmental delay.

cian's time with the child is limited. Furthermore, children often "act different around other people" and are anxious in the office setting; this may make the brief period of observation by the physician less effective and reliable. Primary care physicians must listen carefully to parental concerns, as again and again these concerns have been found to be an appropriate marker for true developmental difficulties in children.

In the young child with developmental delay, a wait-and-see attitude is only appropriate if the physician has considered the many possible causes of the delay and has screened for other aspects of developmental delay. Each child should be viewed in an individual manner, taking into consideration risk factors, environmental stimulation, and current health status. Development should be considered in all areas: gross motor, fine motor, cognitive, language, and social/emotional. The physician needs to consider the appropriate screening tools to use in the office (and methods for administering and interpreting them) and know the community resources that are available for further evaluation. A careful overall physical examination, a comprehensive neurologic examination, an evaluation for the presence or absence of primitive and pathologic reflexes, and a hearing and vision screening are essential in the initial evaluation of the developmentally delayed child. Diagnostic medical tests should be considered based on the differential diagnosis resulting from the history, physical, and developmental assessment.

I.   Birth to 3 Years of Age

Children who are newborn to 3 years of age with developmental delay may be eligible for an early-intervention (EI) program. This program is federally mandated and is included as an amendment to the Individuals with Disabilities Education Act (IDEA). The criteria and eligibility for services vary from state to state, and the programs may differ somewhat in each county. In many areas the public health department should be able to identify the appropriate system in the area.

In addition, some communities have intervention programs designed for the children who do not yet have identifiable developmental delay but who are at high risk because of biological or environmental risk factors. Risk factors for developmental delay include known risk factors, such as trisomy 21, fetal alcohol syndrome, or spina bifida. Biological risk factors include prematurity or drug and alcohol exposure. Examples of environmental risk factors include poverty, inadequate stimulation, and postnatal exposure to lead.

EI programs are supposed to reach all eligible children (without cost to the patient), to include a comprehensive and multidisciplinary approach, and to emphasize the family. In some areas referral to the EI program would provide the primary care physician with confirmation of developmental concerns and some assessment of developmental abilities. This information can help the physician to arrive at a medical diagnosis. EI programs, however, do not typically include a medical component. Therefore, although children with autism and cerebral palsy, for example, may qualify for services, the EI program and its providers cannot diagnose a specific developmental disability. This diagnosis must come from the physician or a subspecialist to whom the patient has been referred.

II.   Three to 5 Years of Age

Children with delay at 3 to 5 years of age can be managed in a way similar to that of the younger child. The physician should obtain a detailed history, inquire about parental concerns, and either screen in the office or refer the child for further assessment to address the area or areas of concern. As in the younger child, careful physical examination and an extended neurodevelopmental assessment are needed. Specific medical diagnostic tests should be considered in light of history, examination, and extent of the developmental issues. For example, if the in-office assessment reveals global issues (concerns in several developmental areas, such as motor, cognitive, and speech), a comprehensive evaluation would be necessary. If the area is specifically that of speech and language, proceeding with a speech and language assessment may be appropriate.

For the 3- to 5-year-old child with significant developmental issues, the local school district will have a mechanism to assess and provide services. The parent can self-refer for this evaluation. Again, the physician needs to remember that the school will not provide a medical assessment or attempt to diagnose the cause for the delay.

The older child with delay is assessed similarly to the age groups described earlier (see Chapter 39, "School Failure").

The primary care physician can guide a family through the often difficult process of assessment, understanding of a diagnosis, and development of an intervention plan. Developmental issues can and do significantly affect overall family functioning. The family will need an advocate with the expertise to help overcome obstacles, to provide moral support and encouragement, and to act as a "sounding board" for intervention strategies.

ADDITIONAL READING

Batshaw ML. *Children with disabilities,* 4th ed. Baltimore: Paul H. Brookes; 1997.

Bennett FC, Guralnick MJ. Effectiveness of developmental intervention in the first five years of life. *Pediatr Clin North Am* 1991; 38:1513–1528.

Blasco PA. Pitfalls in developmental diagnosis. *Pediatr Clin North Am* 1991;38:1425–1438.

Capute AJ, Accardo PJ. *Developmental disabilities in infancy and childhood: neurodevelopmental diagnosis and treatment,* 2nd ed. Baltimore: Paul H. Brookes; 1996.

Coleman WL, Taylor EH. Family-focused behavioral pediatrics: clinical techniques for primary care. *Pediatr Clin North Am* 1995; 16:448–455.

Klein SK. Evaluation for suspected language disorders in preschool children. *Pediatr Clin North Am* 1991;38:1455–1468.

Roizen NJ, Diefendorf AO. Etiology of hearing loss in children: nongenetic causes. *Pediatr Clin North Am* 1999;46:49–64.

Shelov SP, Hannemann RE, DeAngelis CD. eds. *Caring for your baby and young child: birth to age 5,* rev. ed. New York: Bantam Doubleday Dell; 1998.

34 ♣ Managing Difficult Interactions with Parents

Lisa M. Vaughn and Kathleen Burklow

Primary care providers inevitably encounter difficult parents at some point in their careers. Such interactions can be especially challenging because the provider/parent encounters typically occur at a time of stress when parents are concerned about their child's health and well-being. When approaching a difficult parent interaction, providers should consider three major factors that contribute to the situation. These factors include (a) the provider, (b) the parent, and (c) the environment. Difficult interactions are often caused by an interplay of these factors and rarely by one of the three factors exclusively.

I. **Provider Issues**
   A. **Before approaching the difficult parent, primary care providers must consider their own contribution to the encounter.** All providers have biases, triggers, and stressors related to particular parents. If providers can recognize these individual "hot buttons" in themselves, they will be able to handle difficult parents better by understanding their own contribution to the problem.
   B. **Knowing one's limits of expertise and skill in managing difficult parents is equally important.** Many primary care providers have not been trained to address the more subtle aspects of negative social interactions, including resolving conflicts, communicating nondefensively, building relationships during difficult situations, and diffusing volatile situations.
   C. **On occasion, a basic mismatch exists between the styles and personalities of the provider and parent that contributes to a potentially negative situation.** In such cases, providers must identify the mismatch and consider referring the parent and child to a colleague with a different, more compatible style.

II. **Parent Issues**
   A. **Although primary care providers should resist the urge to blame the parent for difficult interactions, in some cases, the parent may actually be an individual who is interpersonally challenging.** Sufficient literature exists that suggests that patients can be the major contributor to difficult provider/patient interactions. Because the parent is the primary vehicle to the child, the difficult parent (rather than the difficult patient) can impede successful intervention with children. One of the first steps in managing the difficult patient/parent is to understand those parental factors that lead to the problematic behaviors.
   B. **Previous studies have identified many parental characteristics that lead to a difficult encounter.** The most common characteristics identified by health care pro-

viders are stressed and anxious, demanding and controlling, angry, and challenging behaviors and also difficulty with understanding explanations. Additional, less common characteristics are untruthfulness, intimidation by the physician, manipulative and indecisive behaviors, drug or alcohol dependence, abusiveness (to the child), disorganization, religious or alternative medicine issues, and psychiatric disorders. Providers have reported that the most difficult types of parents to manage are those who are abusive to their child; who are manipulative, demanding, and controlling; and who have psychiatric disorders or drug and alcohol dependence. The least difficult parents to manage are those who are intimidated easily, indecisive, or disorganized or who have alternative medicine or religious issues.

III. Environmental Issues
   A.   Parents and children in the primary care setting may have experienced considerable stress or difficulty before their arrival at the medical facility. For example, families who are dependent on public transportation may have been in transit for a long time or may have had to bring several siblings in addition to their ill child to the doctor because no babysitter was available or they could not afford one.
   B.   Previous experiences that parents have had with medical care in other settings may have shaped their perceptions of the health care system. If these perceptions are negative, that will impact their subsequent interactions with their care provider. An example is a family who perceives it has been denied certain services because of its dependence on state-funded medical assistance.
   C.   Cultural influences can also contribute to difficult interactions. Health care providers and parents may not understand or identify with each other's sociocultural environment and background; this leads to misunderstandings and misperceptions. For example, grandmothers in some cultures have a very matriarchal and pivotal role in rearing grandchildren, which a physician might interpret as interfering.

IV. Strategies to Assist with the Management of Difficult Parents
       Just as difficult provider/parent interactions culminate from a variety of factors, a variety of strategies are helpful to manage the challenging situation. The following strategies are intended to help the health care provider address these difficult parent interactions within the primary care office setting.
   A.   Explore the Interaction for a "Hidden Agenda." Parents' frustrations often build when they perceive that their care provider is not accurately addressing the true concern that they have for their child. However, for a variety of reasons, as described earlier, parents often have difficulty articulating these concerns to their care provider. In many instances, the parents may need some assistance from the care provider to uncover their true concern.

For example, a mother may arrive for a health care visit to discuss her toddler's failure to potty-train. The care provider conducts a physical examination and assures the parent that the child is in good physical health and that no physiologic reason exists for the child's inability to potty-train successfully. Despite the care provider's discussion, the mother continues to express concern that her child is not demonstrating an interest in toilet training and appears to have difficulty understanding and accepting the physician's explanation. In reality, the mother felt that her care provider "missed the boat" and failed to address her true concern—that her child was developmentally delayed. Had the care provider attended to the mother's emotional persistence with the toilet-training matter and continued to explore the issue, the care provider might have uncovered this "hidden agenda," allowing a discussion of normal developmental milestones and variations from normal.

Uncovering this important information would have changed the content and direction of this visit dramatically. Thus for the care provider, exploration with the parents of their underlying concerns is important instead of making assumptions about what diagnostic and management information to share with the parents. In most cases, asking the parent directly what issues they are most concerned about for their child and why they are concerned about them can help to establish the goals and agenda of the health care visit to the satisfaction of both provider and parent.

B.   Don't underestimate the value of listening. By the time some parents reach the care providers' office, they may be feeling so frustrated that the only emotion they can express is anger. Although the care provider may feel that the parents are directing the negative feelings explicitly at him or her (legitimately or not), the parents may simply need to vent their negative emotions to anyone who will listen. In such circumstances, the care provider easily could become defensive and offer an unsolicited opinion, walk away from the situation, or ignore the parents' complaints. However, this reaction tends to escalate the negativity that the parent is already feeling. Instead the care provider should take the time to listen to the parent and demonstrate an understanding of the parent's concerns. Such reflective listening skills can be both nonverbal and verbal.

  1. *For example, the care provider can communicate nonverbal support by doing the following:*
     a.   maintaining eye contact with the parent;
     b.   nodding in understanding;
     c.   maintaining an "open," relaxed body posture (i.e., not crossing his or her arms in front of the body); and
     d.   sitting down with the parent(s) instead of standing during the interaction.

2. *Verbally, the care provider should avoid being confrontational with the parent.* Rather, the care provider should verbally acknowledge the parent's concerns (e.g, "*I can tell that you are angry/frustrated/worried.*" or "*This situation sounds like it has been difficult for you.*"). Thus by first **listening** to the parent's concerns and then **acknowledging** the negative emotions, the care provider can defuse a potentially volatile situation.

C. **Respect the parents' role.** Throughout training, primary care providers learn a prescriptive model of health care. They frequently prescribe medications to address illness, provide guidance for parents regarding child-rearing issues, and make referrals to other medical subspecialties. Throughout this entire process, care providers often overlook the unique perspective of the parents who are, in most cases, most familiar with their child's temperament and personality. To parents, such an oversight might seem as if the care provider does not respect their knowledge of and familiarity with their child, thereby creating psychological distance between the parent and provider. To avoid fostering negative encounters, the care provider should solicit the parents' input whenever appropriate. For example, for the care provider to ask a parent his or her opinion on which antibiotic to prescribe is not appropriate, but the provider can and should ask parents whether they think the child would prefer a pill or liquid form. Only parents would know which form of medication their child would best accept. Although this is a basic example and most care providers follow such practices when prescribing medications, it illustrates the importance of valuing the parents' exclusive knowledge of their child when determining a care plan.

D. **Establish clear guidelines.** Parents who exhibit challenging and controlling behaviors regarding the care of their child may overstep boundaries and make demands of their care provider that are beyond typical and acceptable health care practices.

1. *As a general rule, health care providers should discuss the fundamentals of their medical practice during the parents' first visit.* At this visit, basic information should be discussed, including office hours, methods for making appointments, fees, insurance, prescription information, use of antibiotics, calling in case of a medical emergency, and definition of a medical emergency. Establishing clear guidelines regarding the parent/provider interaction is important for the provider in order to prevent circumstances in which parents might try to overstep appropriate boundaries.

2. *Some parents, however, may have difficulty following such instructions, may fail to see how these guidelines apply to them and their child, and/or may become hostile when the medical staff does not respond immediately or appropriately (in their opinion) to their demands.* In such cases, the care

provider should review the guidelines of the office practices and emphasize that such rules are in place to establish the conditions necessary to provide optimal care for their child. Care providers should remind the parent that when he or she reacts negatively or fails to comply with established guidelines, the care of their child might be compromised because emotional energies are being directed toward their demands rather than at the medical care of their child.

   3.   *When reviewing such office guidelines, care providers should communicate the information in a calm, matter-of-fact manner, avoiding a defensive posture, which only tends to aggravate the interaction.* Moreover, when the challenging parent adheres to the established guidelines in the future, the care provider should recognize, express appreciation for, and commend the parent's efforts to cooperate.

E.   Know when to refer. Regrettably, in some instances, some barriers to providing optimal care may be too wide to overcome. For the care provider recognizing the limits of their efforts and competence is important. In some circumstances, a "mismatch" in provider/parent personality styles exists in which conflicts are predictable and frequent despite efforts to address the apparent problems. In other instances, fundamental differences (e.g., race, culture, religion) between provider and parent may be so extreme that they interfere with the care provider's ability to provide optimal care for the child.

   Although working through such differences can establish the groundwork for invaluable self-discovery and learning for the care provider as well as the parent, this process tends to consume time and energy. When this is not possible, referring the family to a different care provider is better than compromising the care of the child.

   Rather than viewing a difficult interaction with parents as one to avoid, primary care providers should view the circumstance as a challenge that, if appropriately managed, may eventually result in a better relationship with parent and child. Not resolving a difficult interaction with a parent can result in frustration, dissatisfaction, noncompliance, and lack of cooperation for both parent and provider that in the end only compromises the health and well-being of the child. Ultimately, if providers can understand and better manage potentially difficult interactions with parents, they will be better equipped to provide optimal care to children.

ADDITIONAL READING

Anstett R. The difficult patient and the physician-patient relationship. *J Fam Pract* 1980;11:281–286.

Grove J. Taking care of the hateful patient. *N Engl J Med* 1978;10:280.

Jackson JL, Kroenke K. Difficult patient encounters in the ambulatory clinic: clinical predictors and outcomes. *Arch Intern Med* 1999;159:1069–1075.

Korsch B. Difficult encounters with parents. In: Parker S, Zuckerman B, eds. *Behavioral and developmental pediatrics.* Boston: Little, Brown; 1995.

Korsch B. Do you know these patients? High-risk pediatric encounters. *Pediatr Rev* 1988;10:101–105.

Merrill J, Laux L, Thornby J. Troublesome aspects of the patient-physician relationship: a study of human factors. *South Med J* 1987;80:1211–1215.

Quill TE. Recognizing and adjusting to barriers in doctor-patient communication. *Ann Intern Med* 1989;111:51–57.

Rogers DE. On trust: a basic building block for healing doctor-patient interactions. *J R Soc Med* 1994;87:2–5.

Smith S. Dealing with the difficult patient. *Postgrad Med J* 1995; 71:653–657.

Sunde ER, Mabe PA, Josephson A. Difficult parents. From adversaries to partners. *Clin Pediatr (Phila)* 1993;32:213–219.

Vaughn LM, Baker RC. The difficult parent. *Abstracts of the Combined Pediatric Academic Societies and American Academy of Pediatrics Meeting,* May 1–5, 2000, Boston, MA.

35 ♣ Eating and Mealtime Behavior

Janet R. Schultz and Kathleen Burklow

How a child grows and thrives is often viewed as a public statement of how well parents are doing their job of nurturing their babies. When feeding problems, actual or perceived, emerge, parents often become quite anxious and question their competence as parents. Sometimes these feelings leave parents hesitant to raise real questions that they may have about their child's eating. Primary care providers can open communication with parents by asking about both the child's food intake and mealtime behaviors. Anticipatory guidance can be especially helpful because many feeding problems in young children are related to parents' inadequate understanding of how feeding skills, behaviors, and attitudes develop. Early feeding behavior is controlled by reflexes and distress induced by hunger. Since babies communicate their hunger (and almost everything else!) by crying, parents sometimes misinterpret their child's messages. This leads some parents to use feeding as the "solution" to manage most aspects of their child's distress when other strategies could be just as effective.

During the first months of life, nighttime feedings are the rule. These feedings normally fade as the infant learns to sleep through the night. Nighttime feedings, however, may unnecessarily linger beyond the first months if feeding becomes associated with sleeping and the child does not learn the skills needed to fall asleep on his or her own (see Chapter 43, "Sleep and Bedtime Behaviors"). Commonly, young children feed on demand during the day until table food is introduced and mealtimes become predictably established. Another common error is that many parents believe that solids or table foods are more satisfying and appetizing to their children. This belief may lead to early introduction of solids, before the child has the oral/motor skills to manage these textures. In general, children should be introduced to various foods at the following ages:

- *Birth to 4 months.* Infants should be fed exclusively a liquid diet, preferably breast milk with formula used as an alternative. Cow's milk should be avoided until the age of 12 months.
- *Four to 6 months.* Infant cereal and pureed foods can be introduced.
- *Six to 10 months.* When teeth begin to erupt, selected chopped table food can be added. In this age range children usually begin to feed themselves with their fingers.

Spoon use follows at around 12 months. By 15 months, most children can independently feed themselves. (See also Chapter 7, "Nutrition," and Chapter 8, "Breast Feeding.")

Weight gain is most rapid during the first year of life (about 12 to 15 pounds). As children grow older, the growth curve becomes more gradual, and children gain only 5 to 6 pounds over the next few years. After the first year of life, children tend to eat less and to express their personal tastes, preferences, and behavioral inclinations more. That feeding problems most frequently emerge between 1 and 2 years of age is no surprise. Estimates of feeding problems in children range from 20% to as high as 60%, even though the problems in most cases are related more to the parents' frustration and concerns than to the child's health status. Parents, often concerned about some of the normal changes in their child's eating behavior and diet, benefit from hearing from their physician that their child is growing at a normal rate. This reassurance will reduce the pressure that parents impose on their children to eat and will make mealtimes more pleasant and less likely to result in major power struggles. The more that food becomes part of a power struggle, the more frustrated everyone becomes, and children will be less likely to eat the quantity or selection of food that their parents desire.

I. Toddler and Preschoolers

During the toddler years, children often go on "food jags" during which they want to eat only a narrow range of foods over and over. Many parents may interpret this behavior as being a "picky" eater. The parent, to show the importance of a healthy diet, must model good eating habits by offering a wide variety of nutritious (not junk) foods during this time. Over time, if offered nutritious food options, most healthy children will not only eat an adequate amount of food, but will also have a relatively balanced diet. During the preschool years, snacks remain an important source of calories and nutrition. Appropriately chosen foods, offered at times and in quantities that do not interfere with structured mealtimes, should be considered healthy additions.

If parents do not acquiesce to their child's food fads and do not make a big deal out of "pickiness" in general, their child will continue to grow well. Even though eating itself is usually a positive experience for most healthy children, mealtime behaviors remain subject to the normal principles of behavior. An estimated 45% of normally developing children have problem mealtime behaviors. In preschoolers these can include failing to sit at the table for meals, dawdling or refusing to eat meals (and yet often wanting snacks), crying, throwing tantrums, and throwing or spitting food. Parents should take into consideration the following strategies for addressing their young child's mealtimes:

A. Parents should not insist that preschoolers remain at the table more than 15 to 20 minutes. Doing so may make mealtimes unpleasant and may inadvertently increase the likelihood that the child will begin to avoid eating. However, once the child leaves the table, parents should not allow the child to take additional bites of food or return to the table to eat under most circumstances (bathroom trips are sometimes an exception).

B. Parents should present small portions of food that do not overwhelm a child. Children may also be more interested in eating when food is served on child-attractive dishes. Young children often eat more when allowed to feed

themselves. Suggest that parents facilitate this independence by serving finger foods, providing child-sized utensils,
and cutting difficult-to-manage foods (e.g., meat, spaghetti)
ahead of time.

C. A child should not be forced to eat. If the child
chooses not to eat, no snack or other foods should be made
available until the next time food would normally be offered,
whether that be a planned snack time or a meal. While particular dislikes can be respected, parents often find expecting
the child to take a "hello" bite of a new or infrequently offered
dish can help.

D. Coaxing children to eat can backfire. Children may
eat even less and learn that the way to guarantee their parents' intense involvement (attention) with them is to avoid
eating. Coaxing a "few last bites" can undo the whole attempt
to encourage eating. Prompting children to eat may increase
their intake but usually only by getting them to eat faster,
which may not be desirable in the long run.

**E. The behavioral equivalent of verbal coaxing should
be discouraged as well.** Sometimes parents become very
invested in this problem and spend unusual amounts of time
trying to make delectable and visually tempting food. Then,
when the child doesn't eat the "elephant" that the parent so
cleverly crafted out of an orange, the parent is more likely to
feel angry, frustrated, or even worse, hurt and/or rejected.

**F. Mealtimes should be pleasant times, without un-
due emotional arousal.** Thus children should not be able
to watch television programs or to play with toys during
meals. At the same time, mealtime is a good time for children
to share information about their day's activities, such as
school and reading. With several children of different ages,
taking turns may be necessary to ensure everyone, including
the youngest, gets a chance to talk.

**G. Parents should focus on the desired mealtime be-
haviors of the child rather than on the negative mealtime behaviors.** Mealtime is an especially good time for parents to use "differential attention" in which they pay more
attention to the child when he or she eats and behaves in the
desired fashion and pay less or no attention to the child during the periods when he or she does not. Parents should focus
on praising positive mealtime behaviors rather than on
praising the amount of food eaten.

**H. Allowing children to help choose and prepare
foods can increase intake.** Even healthy but marginally
attractive foods (e.g., bran muffins) tend to be eaten with
more zest if the child has been the chef and perhaps has
added his or her own special touches.

**I. When possible, parents should be discouraged
from using food as rewards, punishment, or threats**
(e.g., *"If you don't eat this spinach, you won't get any dessert"*).
Especially in families where food has become an issue, this

extra emotional baggage tends to make matters worse. Food should not be linked to "good" or "bad" behavioral status.

J. Most preschoolers are purists. They do not care for foods that are combined as much as they do ones they can identify and separate. Hence casseroles, stews, and other combination textured foods may be less appetizing than serving all the food components separately. Adults, recognizing this, should purchase and prepare foods accordingly as they have significant control over the content of the preschoolers' diets (young children cannot buy their own snacks and generally must choose from the food that is served).

K. If a child is disruptive during the meal, parents can use time outs (see Chapter 29). After the second time out is implemented, parents should consider the meal over. No additional food should be offered until the next planned snack or meal.

II. School Age Children.
Older children often have different issues with eating. Strong evidence exists suggesting that some boys and many girls develop concerns about being overweight while in the third to fifth grades. Often this fear originates with their parents who share some of their own fears, emphasize not getting "fat," and model strong concerns for their own weight. Pressure to meet model standards of appearance surround the child but are particularly meaningful if pressure exists within the home. Additionally, "emotional eating" patterns can be well established by 9 or 10 years of age. If obesity is a problem from the perspective of the health care provider, reducing television viewing (a sedentary occupation that tends to be associated with snacking) and the availability of "junk" food and increasing physical activity is probably a better plan than "dieting" (except in unusual cases). Emphasizing good eating and exercise habits as a general health promotion effort is better than overemphasizing appearance. If being underweight is the problem, careful behavioral and food intake records need to be examined, since school aged children may develop eating disorders. Similarly, family dynamics and general attitudes about appearance, body type, and child performance should be considered relevant factors in children who are underweight or overweight.

In addition to the family view of food, parental mental health status makes a difference in children's eating. Children of substance abusers have been found to eat more fast food and other high-fat foods, whereas children whose parents, especially mothers, are depressed eat less of all types of food.

ADDITIONAL READING

Birch LL, Mailin DW. I don't like it: I never tried it: effects of exposure on two-year old children's food preferences. *Appetite* 1982; 3:353–360.

Frank D, Silva M, Needleman R. Failure to thrive. Mystery, myth, and methods. *Contemp Pediatr* 1993;10:104–113.

Reau NR, Senturia YD, LeBailly SA, Christoffel KK. Infant and toddler feeding patterns and problems: normative data and a new direction. *Develop Behav Pediatr* 1996;17:149–153.

Satter EM. Childhood eating disorders. *J Am Diet Assoc* 1986;86: 357–361.

Satter EM. The feeding relationship. *J Am Diet Assoc* 1986;86: 352–356.

Striegel-Moore RH, Morrison JA, Schreiber G, Schumann BC, Crawford PB, Obarzanek E. Emotion-induced eating and sucrose intake in children: the NHLBI Growth and Health Study. *Int J Eating Dis* 1999;25:389–398.

Books for Parents

Satter EM. *How to get your child to eat . . . but not too much.* Emeryville, CA: Publishers Group West; 1987.

Websites

http://www.parenttime.com/sears/home/index.html(Ask Dr. Sears)
http://www.sneakykitchen.com/All_about/picky_eaters.htm (All About Picky Eaters)

36 ♣ Homework

Janet R. Schultz

Teaching task: **To help the child learn the responsibility and organizational skills to work independently on tasks that may not be immediately and intrinsically rewarding to him or her.**

Homework is an area of recurrent tension in many homes. If parents handle homework issues appropriately, the completion of the homework will serve two purposes: the child will learn the academic material, and the child will learn about responsibility and organization. Several principles of homework management follow.

I.   Responsibility for Homework

Homework is the child's problem, not the parents' problem. Hence parents should not do the homework or take primary responsibility for ensuring it is done.

II.   Routines for Homework

After school, the parent and child should look over papers and materials sent home from school together. This is a good time for parents to praise, or at least to encourage, whenever possible. With younger children, parents may find joining in to estimate how much time assignments will take and to set an order in which they will be done useful. Some families feel homework should be done right after school so that the rest of the evening is clear. Others feel the child should have a break after a day of scholastic activity. **The choice of when homework is done is less important than ensuring that *consistency* and an *established routine* for doing homework exist.**

III.   Feedback on Homework

With many younger children, homework goes better if parents ask to see each assignment as it is finished. Feedback on accuracy and neatness can be given, if it communicated in a positive way, with praise wherever possible. Older children who generally do their homework without parental intervention can choose whether or not they need parental review.

IV.   Development of Study Habits

Emphasis should be on the development of good study habits for the students. This can be stressed by taking pride in their work, providing a quiet (television-free) place to study that is equipped with what they need, and learning ways to organize work, set priorities, and check for accuracy. For some children, developing good study habits includes learning how to break down assignments into manageable pieces that they complete unit by unit. Reviewing notes when no examination is imminent can be introduced at the junior high level unless the school indicates otherwise.

V.   Involvement by Parents

Children generally do more homework and do better in school if their parents are in contact with the teachers and know what the expectations for the student are. A student tends to have better achievement and enhanced self-esteem with more parental involvement in the school and its activities (e.g., PTA/PTO, open house, musical performances, sports activities).

VI.   Communication with Teachers

If an older child routinely has no homework, a phone call to the teacher may be appropriate. If a child does not do homework when it has been assigned, then the teacher and parents (and often the child) need to be in communication. Some teachers prefer that the problem of incomplete homework should be handled between the teacher and the student only. This often serves to take the aspect of rebelling against parents out of the struggle. This method of handling also emphasizes that the homework is the child's responsibility, not the parents'.

Other times, especially with younger students, parents may want to establish an assignment book that goes between the teacher and parent. The child records the assignments, which the teacher initials to confirm accuracy at the end of the day. Parents read the notebook and initial the list of assignments as each is finished. A reward system is useful here. In general, rewards are more helpful if they focus on short-term work rather than on end-of-quarter grades. Children do better when the emphasis is placed on learning for the sake of knowledge and pleasure rather than for stars, stickers, candy, or money. Some children though ultimately need extrinsic rewards if the intrinsic ones do not motivate them adequately.

Most children who do not do homework are operating in an avoidance paradigm. The reward for not doing homework is the avoidance of the task itself, plus the freedom available to do other things. Sometimes the avoidance is based on anxiety about or dislike for the work, especially if the child does not understand it. Sometimes the child's failure to complete work signals academic problems rather than being the cause of them. Parental (or sometimes physician) contact with teachers may help clarify this. (See also Chapter 39, "School Failure" and Chapters 27 and 28, which deal with attention deficit hyperactivity disorder.)

ADDITIONAL READING

Durlak JA. School problems of children. In: Walker CE, Robert MC, eds. *Handbook of clinical child psychology,* 2nd ed. New York: John Wiley & Sons; 1992.

Books for Parents

Canter L. *Homework without tears: a parent's guide for motivating children to do homework and to succeed in school.* New York: Harper Collins; 1993.

Radencich MC, Schamm JS, Esepeland P, eds. *How to help your child with homework: every caring parent's guide to encouraging good study habits and ending the homework wars.* Minneapolis, MN: Free Spirit Publishers; 1997.

Rosemond, J. *Ending the homework hassle.* Kansas City: Andrews and McMeel; 1990.

Sloane HN. *The good kid book: how to solve the 16 most common behavior problems.* Champaign, IL: Research Press; 1988.

Websites for Parents

http://www.nslsilus.org/Kids/hmwrk.html
http://www.parentsplace.com/family

37 ♣ Lying

Kathleen Burklow

Lying, a common behavior in children, emerges in the preschool years and continues throughout adolescence. Parents, when they discover that their child has lied, frequently become alarmed, question their child's level of truthfulness in other situations, and wonder whether the child has a chronic problem or if that was an isolated incident. The primary care provider plays a critical role in helping parents understand this behavior and in determining the most appropriate strategy for intervention.

I. Developmental Perspectives

Parents need to be aware that the underlying reasons that children lie coincide closely with their level of development.

A. Preschoolers frequently lie because they have not yet understood that lying is unacceptable or deceitful. In addition, at this age, young children have active fantasy lives and are learning the difference between makebelieve and reality. As a result, some children may make up stories that are not true or that are greatly embellished or exaggerated. In some instances, however, children may lie to get something that they want or to avoid something that they perceive as negative. Typically, preschoolers tell two kinds of lies that should be addressed differently:

1. *Tell an exaggerated story.* If the child exaggerates the details of a story, parents should listen but not respond at all to the embellishments. As an alternate choice, they may choose to listen and respond with a dose of reality. For example, when a child says, "I can run faster than a car," a parent may say, "Wow, it is fun to pretend that you can run quickly!"

2. *Lie to get what he or she wants.* Children who tell these types of lies frequently do not realize that telling such lies is wrong. An added factor at this age, however, is that children want to please their parents and make them happy. Thus parents need to teach their preschoolers that lying is wrong and dishonest. Parents also should calmly and matter-of-factly explain that lying makes the parents unhappy and telling the truth makes them happy.

B. Children 5 to 8 years of age frequently lie for the same reasons as preschoolers: they may try to get what they want, or they may want to avoid potential punishment. In contrast to the preschool years, however, children at this developmental level now can understand that lying is unacceptable and that it has an impact on others. Children at this age have begun to understand the importance of obeying rules and can think in terms of fairness. Thus parents should explain to the child (a) that lying hurts the feelings of the person who is lied to and (b) the ways in which such dishonesty directly impacts family and friends because it develops patterns of distrust, cheating, and disappointment. These discussions should be followed with punishment for the dishonesty. Parents need to be cautious, however, in determing the intensity and frequency of the punishment for lying. Overly intense or too frequent punishments may inadvertently increase the child's lying in an effort to avoid harsh punishment.

C. Children 8 to 12 years of age lie for reasons similar to those of younger children. At this age, however, they also have heightened social awareness and concerns regarding interactions and relationships with peers. Although children at this age continue to want to please their parents, the conflict they may feel between the social pressures they experience with their peers and their parents' expectations can result in lying behaviors. As a result, in addition to using lying to avoid punishment or to get something that they want, children between 8 and 12 years of age will lie to boost their self-image, to seek approval, and to conform to and/or win admiration from their friends. Because children at this age are aware that dishonesty is wrong, parents should implement punishments and consequences for such behaviors, such as removal of privileges and possibly paying restitution for the consequences of the lying. Parents should also address their child's concern with self-image and help them understand that lying can impact reputation negatively.

D. Adolescents (12 years and older) possess better-developed abstract reasoning skills that allow them to understand the broader impact of lying on a community or societal level. Therefore teens begin to understand abstract concepts, such as loyalty and the consequences of loss of trust within relationships. The social influence of peers peaks during adolescence. As a result, during this developmental period, parents may find that they have less influence on their teenagers than do members of their teenager's peer group. This developmental shift reinforces the importance and necessity of teaching honesty and truthfulness when the child is young, while parents still have the most influence on their child's attitudes and behaviors. When parents discover that their teenager has lied, they should avoid angry interrogation. Instead, parents need to ask questions in a calm, matter-of-fact manner to avoid causing the teen to react defensively and to resort immediately to lying to protect themselves. Parents should implement consequences when they discover that their teenagers have engaged in dishonest behaviors. As mentioned previously, disciplinary actions should include the removal of privileges and possibly restitution for the consequences of the lying and dishonesty.

II. Other General Strategies

A. Establish clear rules and expectations regarding lying. Parents need to establish clear rules so that the child is aware of when he or she has engaged in behaviors that can be considered lying. They should teach children the factors that constitute lying and the direct consequences for engaging in such behaviors. Parents need to begin teaching these concepts when the child is young; such discussions should take into consideration the developmental maturity and perspectives on lying as described earlier.

B.   Serve as positive role models for truthfulness. When children see their parents using lying and dishonesty to avoid or to get out of something that they do not want to do, they begin to learn that lying has positive benefits. This positive outcome may overshadow the consequences for failing to tell the truth. Parents therefore need to model honesty and telling the truth in front of their children.

C.   Reinforce children when they tell the truth. Parents need to recognize and praise children when they tell the truth, especially if the situation could have easily invited lying. Children who are praised for their honesty will be more likely to engage in such truthful behaviors in the future.

D.   Carefully determine the punishment for the lying. Children should not be made to feel that they are bad individuals when they lie. Instead, they should be made to understand that their lying behavior is wrong, unacceptable, and dishonest. Consequently, severity of discipline for lying should closely parallel the magnitude of the lie. For example, if the child lies to get something that he or she wants, then parents may implement a harsher punishment than for a situation in which the child lies to protect a family member or friend out of feelings of loyalty. Whereas the latter situation may feel more admirable than the first situation, parents nonetheless need to be consistent with following through with consequences for lying. If clear rules and consequences for lying have been established, then consistently enforcing them with the punishment emphasizes their importance. In addition, parents need to apply specific disciplinary measures for the targeted lying behavior rather than to institute a general disciplinary action for overall misbehaviors. Through specifically targeted interventions, children can learn the expectations for appropriate and inappropriate behaviors, including lying.

E.   Ensure that children do not get reinforced for lying. This strategy is especially true if the child lies to get something that he or she wants. In such instances, parents need to make sure that the child does not get what he or she wants.

F.   Look for patterns to the child's lying. Parents need to monitor the types of lies told and the circumstances surrounding the lying. If, for example, the child seems to be telling lies to avoid punishment, then the parent may need to reexamine the disciplinary measures used (i.e., whether the punishments are too harsh and inconsistent with the level of misbehavior) or to establish clear consequences for specific misdeeds. If, however, the child seems to be lying to impress and to get attention from others, then the parents need to consider that their child may be experiencing feelings of low self-esteem. Children who lie for these reasons may benefit from engaging in activities that promote positive self-concepts.

III. Underlying Emotional and Behavioral Problems

For some children, frequent lying may be indicative of underlying emotional and behavioral problems. If the child's lying persists, parents may benefit from seeking professional help from a psychologist or counselor to address these issues further.

ADDITIONAL READING

Brazelton TB. *Touchpoints: your child's emotional and behavioral development*. Reading, MA: Perseus Books; 1992.

Ekman P. *Why kids lie: how parents can encourage truthfulness*. New York: Penguin Books; 1991.

38 ♣ School Avoidance

Janet R. Schultz

I. Definition

School avoidance, also called *school refusal,* is a term for a disorder previously called school phobia. The terminology has changed, since *school phobia* implies a limited etiology (fear of school), whereas *school avoidance* (or *refusal*) implies that children avoid school for reasons other than fear. The term does not include occasional deliberate acts of truancy. Truancy is distinguished from school refusal by where the child stays when not at school as he should be. School refusers tend to be at home or in the care of family friends or relatives. Children who are truant are out on the street or in the homes of friends, usually without benefit of adult supervision.

II. Etiology

School refusal is, in most respects, a problem of avoidance. The child avoids the unpleasant or anxiety-provoking situations of leaving home (and usually the parent) and/or of attending, performing, and socializing in school. Chronic refusers usually avoid some combination of those situations. Sometimes the parental nurturing that accompanies any physical symptoms displayed maintains or reinforces the pattern, but avoidance still remains the most powerful force acting in school refusal.

III. Presentation

School avoiders often present to the primary care physician's office, not with the complaint of school refusal, but with physical symptoms, such as stomachaches, headaches, or general malaise. Often the symptoms are vague, varying from day to day and recurring on Sunday evenings or Monday mornings after disappearing over the weekend. If certain classes engender more anxiety than others, a variation often exists, which can be matched to the class schedule. This pattern tends to be more characteristic of older children. Children who avoid school may attend school initially only to leave after a major emotional storm in the morning, or they may leave early, "going home sick."

IV. Prevalence and Patterns

The incidence of school refusal is difficult to establish because many school refusers are not diagnosed as such. The current estimation is 1% to 2%. Unlike many childhood behavior problems, school refusal is not identified in boys primarily. Some studies indicate equal incidence by gender; others suggest it may be more frequent in girls. No clear socioeconomic correlations or difference in occurrence by birth order have been established. School refusers have intelligence and achievement scores that do not differ from those of their schoolmates. The data are somewhat unclear, but probably three peaks exist: (a) age 5 or 6 years (beginning elementary school), (b) around 11 years (often middle school or junior high transition), and (c) around 14 years (beginning high school). Generally, the older the child, the more difficult the problem is to treat and the more significant the associated family problems.

V. **Significance**

A. **The problem of school avoidance results in considerable distress for the child and parents.** Parents' anxiety may become intense, equaling their reluctance to believe that the physical symptoms they may see are not related to a significant organic disorder.

B. **Chronic absence may contribute to poor academic performance.** Some districts have a policy of mandatory retention in a grade if the child misses a specified percentage of days of school.

C. **School refusal sets children apart from their peers, and the accomplishment of typical developmental milestones may be impeded by the disorder and its associated anxieties.**

D. **School refusal often reflects other anxieties and family dysfunction, especially in older children and chronic refusers.**

E. **Children with severe or chronic school refusal are at risk for being more "neurotic" as adults and tend to have significant adjustment and social problems.** Adults with agoraphobia have a particularly high rate (retrospectively) of school avoidance.

VI. **Onset**

Although separation anxiety is a well-known contributor, other sources of school refusal should be routinely considered.

A. **The onset may be linked to a clear precipitant for the family or child.** Examples of precipitants may include death, separation, or divorce of parents; the birth of a sibling; or the change of teacher. Given the apparent association of transition times with peaks of symptoms, new school routines with unclear expectations and social challenges may be involved. Older school refusers often come from families with a significant level of dysfunction that is not always apparent in well-child visits.

B. **There are "reality-based" considerations as well.** For example, a child may be a target of an intimidating child (the class "bully") or adult and may fear for his safety. Similarly, children who have their lunches or lunch money stolen regularly or who must walk to school through neighborhoods with intimidating people (or animals) may develop aversions and fears. Other children may have motion sickness from the bus ride or may dislike the lengthy or unruly school bus ride with older children.

C. **Especially in younger children, a "personality clash" with the teacher or a feeling that the teacher does not like the student may contribute to school refusal.**

D. **The first time school avoidance becomes evident, it may remit on its own within a week.** Many researchers do not define children as substantially school avoidant until the behavior persists beyond the second week.

VII.   Detection of School Refusals

   A.   Sometimes the diagnosis of school refusal is clear because the child says outright that he refuses to go to school and clings to the parent when the time to go arrives.

   B.   Other times physical symptoms predominate; the physician must rule out physical illness first and then consider school-related problems. The latter may be suggested by patterns of symptoms relative to school attendance and questions about school directed to the parent (e.g., *"Does your child's illness usually keep him home from school?" "How many days has he missed in the last month?" "Is he usually better on weekends until Sunday evening?"*). If other occurrences of mild illness have resulted in school absences, especially associated with Mondays or the day of return to school after holidays, the index of suspicion is raised. Many cases of recurrent abdominal pain include a component of school refusal.

VIII.   Management of School Refusal

   A.   The most important part of the treatment of school refusal is to return the child to school as soon as possible. Sometimes doing so involves intervention in the fear-inducing events, especially if they are able to be clearly identified. If the fear or avoidance is more generalized, returning the child to school may take one of several forms.

   1.   *Sometimes just hearing from the health care provider that the child should be in school will motivate the parent to get the child there.* The physician should make clear, though, that the child is not "faking" symptoms so that no punitive edge is assigned to the parents' actions. This is most successful when the child has not missed much school yet.

   2.   *Often the parent, and at times the physician, should contact the school personnel to inform them that the child is well enough to attend school and to enlist their assistance.* Many schools, especially elementary schools, have dealt with such problems previously and have a protocol. These plans usually involve having the parent hand the resisting child over to the teacher and leaving promptly. The school personnel then take over with reassurance and firmness.

   3.   *If the school does not have a protocol, a good proposal, if the child has been out for several days already, is to have the child arrive late for part of the day and then always to have him or her leave with the other children.* (This is much better than repeating what has often happened already—namely that the child goes to school with the children in the morning and leaves early.) Over a week, the child's school day should be gradually extended until the child is present all day. The school should be told by the parent or physician that the child should not be sent home from school. If the child is "too sick" to stay in class, the child should remain at the school, preferably in the nurse's or first-aid office (without TV or positive reinforcement from a well-meaning nurse or secretary). The physician should set an objective rule with

the school (e.g., temperature over 100.4 or vomiting) for sending the child home. If the parent is not sure if the child is too sick to attend school, the same or a similar objective rule should be enforced to avoid ambivalence. Sometimes keeping breakfast light (but making sure the child does eat something) helps prevent the child's nausea or motion sickness.

B. The child will need follow-up appointments for monitoring for several weeks. These should not be scheduled during school. The parent must also clearly understand that the purpose is to monitor progress, not to make sure that "nothing organic was missed."

C. Although the child may resume school attendance, the physician should explain to the parent that school refusal occurs for a reason, which may still exist. To prevent recurrence and to deal with what is behind the development of the symptom, the parent needs to be in contact with the school and to consider the home situation to determine major stressors and contributions.

D. If the physician and the parent together cannot identify the source of the problem and figure out how to address it, a referral to a psychiatrist, psychologist, or other therapist who addresses biobehavioral issues may be indicated. (Depression and anxiety are frequently involved in school refusal.) If the child does not resume regular attendance promptly, then a referral, sometimes to an intensive treatment setting, is indicated. The longer the child is out of school, the harder getting the child to return is. Similarly, children, especially older ones, who have a history of repeated episodes of school refusal are difficult to treat and should be referred.

E. Cognitive behavior therapy has the best empirical support for its efficacy in treating chronic school refusal, but a variety of approaches may also be helpful, including intensive day treatment and family therapy. Cognitive behavior therapy is a type of therapy in which the therapist attempts to change the thinking processes, belief systems, and self-evaluation of the patient in order to influence emotions and behaviors.

ADDITIONAL READING

Durlak JA. School problems of children. In: Walker CE, Robert MC, eds. *Handbook of clinical child psychology,* 2nd ed. New York: John Wiley & Sons; 1992.

Kearney CA, Tillotson CA. School attendance. In: Watson ST, Gresham FM, eds. *Handbook of child behavior therapy.* New York: Plenum Press; 1998.

Last CG, Francis G. School phobia. In: Lahey B, Kasdin AE, eds. *Advances in clinical child psychology.* New York: Plenum Press; 1988.

Websites for Parents

www.apa.org/monitor/sep97/define.html
http://schools.eastnet.ecu.edu/wilson/psycweb/schphobia.htm

39 ♣ School Failure

Nancy E. Lanphear

School is the "work" of children 5 to 18 years of age in the United States, and their sense of competence will be largely influenced by their ability to succeed in school. Without success in a school situation, expertise in other areas, such as athletics, is necessary for a child to gain self-esteem. School failure may affect and may be affected by overall family functioning. Furthermore, school failure is likely to have long-term effects beyond the school years.

Primary care physicians can play a valuable role in helping a family understand learning styles, differences, and disabilities. Physicians can assess how the child has integrated into the school environment, identify children at risk, and advocate and assist in an evaluation if school failure occurs. School failure has been estimated to occur at a rate of 10% to 15% of students per year in the United States. This rate may vary, depending on the demographic and socioeconomic makeup of the pediatric practice.

Success in school hinges on child, family, and school factors. Child-related factors include learning style, temperament, and inherent abilities. Learning style is defined as how a child learns most effectively and efficiently and is based on the child's personal strengths and weaknesses. Family support of educational achievement is an important element in a child's success in school. This support includes involvement of one or both parents in school choice, homework, and parent/teacher meetings, and the structure incorporated into the family's day-to-day activities to help the child establish good learning patterns. While the educational level of the parents is important, it is not the only factor. School factors include the educational environment, the teacher's ability and enthusiasm, the availability of resources, and community support of the school.

Often at the suggestion of the school, children who underachieve in school are seen by their primary care physician to determine the cause. Occasionally a simple cause, such as poor vision or mild hearing difficulties, is found. More commonly however, the problem is more complex (e.g., a learning disability or a significant emotional problem). Significant learning difficulties and school failure usually require referral to other professionals to provide a diagnostic evaluation and an intervention plan.

I. Causes of School Failure

Because many causes of school failure exist, the primary care physician needs to keep a broad differential in the initial work-up. Frequently more than one cause is present. For example, a child may have both ADHD and a learning disability. School failure is only a symptom, not a specific diagnosis. Some of the causes of school failure follow.

   A. Attention-deficit/hyperactivity disorder and learning disabilities.

   B. Cognitive deficits.

C. Emotional disorders (e.g., child abuse, depression).
D. Disorders of communication (hearing, speech, or language).
E. School phobia (avoidance).
F. Unrealistic parental or teacher expectations.
G. Poor school attendance.
H. Lack of motivation (often without parental involvement to encourage the child).
I. Environmental circumstances (e.g., unsupportive, chaotic home; child not permitted to do homework due to babysitting or work responsibilities; malnutrition).
J. Poor teaching.
K. Poor school/teacher and child fit.
L. Acute or chronic health problems (e.g., sleep apnea, asthma).

II. **Evaluation**

The evaluation of a child's poor school performance should begin before actual school failure. The primary care physician's role, depending on interest level, could include involvement in the investigation for causes and in the development of an intervention plan.

A. A careful history is necessary, including birth history, significant past medical history, early developmental history, family history of school achievement and mental abilities, psychosocial and environmental history, and a review of systems.

B. A detailed physical examination should include a careful neurologic examination with a search for soft neurologic findings and difficulties in communication. Vision and hearing testing are mandatory. Other medical tests are ordered only as indicated from the history and physical examination (e.g., complete blood count [CBC] to rule out anemia, electroencephalogram [EEG], urinalysis, blood chemistries, thyroid studies, urine chromatography, and chromosomal analysis). In most cases few medical diagnostic studies are needed.

C. Information must be obtained from the child's school to determine the school's primary concerns, results of previous testing, available resources, and suggestions for improvement. These would include the following:

1. *The child's report cards.*
2. *Group standardized achievement tests,* including proficiency tests.
3. *Behavioral ratings scales and any specific diagnostic evaluations* administered by the school psychologist to evaluate learning issues.

An example of a form designed to obtain specific educational and behavioral information from the school is indicated in Table 39.1. Standardized tools, such as the Connors Teacher Report form, are available but should be interpreted in conjunction with the other information that has been found.

(*text continues on page 270*)

Table 39.1.   School Performance Record

<u>SCHOOL PERFORMANCE RECORD</u>   Date _____

Name _____
Date of Birth _____   Grade _____
School _____   Homeroom Teacher _____
School Phone # _____   Visiting Teacher _____
                         Principal _____

Achievement:

Reading Level

Subject	Very Good	Average	Barely Passing	Failing

Reading Method

Subject	Very Good	Average	Barely Passing	Failing

Do you think this child is working up to his mental capacity? _____
What special placement or help has he had? _____
What special provisions would you recommend? _____
Is this special help or placement available? _____

<u>PLEASE CHECK MAJOR AREAS OF CONCERN IN BLOCK TO RIGHT OF ITEM</u>

LANGUAGE:

A. Difficulty following verbal directions	
B. Difficulty following written directions	
C. Difficulty following the child's conversation	
D. Difficulty understanding the child's words	

REVERSALS

A. Difficulty determining right & left in games	
B. Tends to reverse printing letters, numbers	
C. Tends to reverse reading letters, numbers, words	
D. Tends to draw or read from left to right	
E. Other	

Table 39.1. *Continued*

BEHAVIOR:

A. Disrupts classroom with aggressive behavior	
B. Difficulty coping with frustration	
C. Difficulty establishing peer relationships	
D. Poor self-image	
E. Poor group participation	
F. Other	

ATTENTION CENTER FUNCTIONS:

A. Overactive	
B. Underactive	
C. Distractible	
D. Overreacts to touch and/or noise	
E. Poor attention span	
F. Unable to organize independent work	
G. Other	

MOTOR SKILLS:

A. Gross motor—skipping/playground activities	
B. Fine motor (writing)	
C. Hesitant to participate in physical games and activities	
D. Clumsy—poor body coordination	
E. Other	

FORM & SPACE PERCEPTION

A. Difficulty with puzzles, etc	
B. Poorly spaced & messy papers	
C. Difficulty recognizing shapes, letters, words	
D. Poor sense of direction	
E. Poor awareness of self in space	
F. Poor math concepts (larger than, smaller than, etc)	
G. Difficulty with spelling	

Poorly established hand dominance (switches hands)	
Poor eye tracking (skips letters, words, lines in reading)	

Have psychological studies been done? _____
If so, may we please have a copy? _____

Impression of home situation _____
_____
_____
_____

D.   Behavioral information should also be sought from parents to understand the child's behavior in the home and to compare that appraisal with behavioral and educational information from the school. There are standardized tools to collect this information, such as the Connors Parent Symptom Questionnaire.

E.   To evaluate academic failure or specific learning disability fully, a multidisciplinary evaluation is needed. This would include a measure of intelligence, such as the Wechsler Intelligence Scale for Children (WISC-3), and tests of academic achievement in areas of reading, writing, mathematics, general knowledge, and possibly processing skills. If language deficits are present, speech and language testing should be incorporated into this broad assessment. If fine motor problems are present, tests of graphomotor abilities, possibly by an occupational therapist, may be needed.

By law, children have the right to be assessed for learning deficits by their school district. This process is started at the request of the parent or the recommendation of the schoolteacher. Parental permission is necessary and must be in writing. If a parent wishes to request an evaluation, this request should be made in writing and delivered to the school principal. As part of a school-based intervention or diagnostic team, the school psychologist typically performs the testing. Results are shared with the family (and the family has legal access to these records). If obtaining this evaluation through the school is impossible or if a second opinion is necessary, the primary care physician should be aware of community resources to obtain this type of evaluation.

After an evaluation has been completed, the primary care physician should arrange a time to discuss the findings with both parents. If the child has been found to have a learning disability or other significant impairment, he or she may be eligible for special education services through the school district. The family and occasionally the pediatrician would work with the school to develop an Individualized Education Plan, or IEP, to address the areas of deficit. In some instances, an Accommodation Plan, called a 504, is also created if specific educational criteria are not met for an IEP.

Finding a specific cause for a child's academic difficulties not only directs intervention but also allows greater understanding of a child's strengths and weaknesses. It also may link these children's families to others who are working with the same issues in a community.

School retention without testing or without a plan to address the area of weakness is seldom indicated and may be detrimental to the long-term achievement and self-esteem of the child. Children who are retained will typically do better in the initial portion of the retained year but will continue to struggle later on and will fail to make the appropriate gains without additional support for their learning needs.

The physician, family, and school must work as a team and allow the child to draw on strengths to compensate for weaknesses.

Strategies may include appropriate class placement, tutoring, speech and/or language therapy, or medication and counseling for the child with ADHD. The primary care physician should coordinate the educational, therapeutic, consultative, and counseling services necessary as the evaluation and treatment programs progress. In this way, the physician not only acts as advocate for the child and the family in the community but also provides specific medical treatment.

ADDITIONAL READING

Connors CK. Parent Symptom Questionnaire. *Psychopharmacol Bull* 1985;21:835–822.

Connors CK. Teacher Questionnaire. *Psychopharmacol Bull* 1985;21:823–827.

Dworkin P. School failure. *Pediatr Rev* 1989:10:301–312.

Jordan NC, Levine MD. Learning disorders: assessment and management strategies. *Contemp Pediatr* 1987;4:31–62.

Levine MD. *Developmental variation and learning disorders.* Cambridge, MA: Educators Publishing Service; 1987.

Levine MD, Jordan NC. Learning disorders: the neurological underpinnings. *Contemp Pediatr* 1987;4:16–43.

Levy HB, Harper CR, Weinberg WA. A practical approach to children failing in school. *Pediatr Clin North Am* 1992;4:895–928.

McInerny TK. Children who have difficulty in school: a primary pediatrician's approach. *Pediatr Rev* 1995;9:325–332.

Wechsler D. *Wechsler Intelligence Scale for Children—3 Manual (WISC-3).* New York: Psychological Corporation; 1989.

Website

http://www.naspweb.org (National Mental Health and Education Center for Children and Families)

40 ♣ School Readiness

Janet R. Schultz and Nancy E. Lanphear

The primary care physician is in a unique position to aid a family with decisions about school readiness and about the appropriate school fit for an individual child. Ideally, the physician has been the child's primary care provider over time and has monitored the child's ongoing development, allowing anticipation of possible problems and problem-solving interventions when needed. When a child is found to have significant delay before kindergarten, referral for appropriate therapeutic intervention should be instituted when the delay is noted rather than waiting until the time arrives for the child to enter the school system. If a child has developmental delay or is at high risk for delay, placement in a preschool program, as early as 3 years of age, is needed. Specialized preschool services are available by law in the United States for children who qualify and may include specialized therapies, such as speech, occupational, or physical therapy (Public Law 94-142). Many school districts have also developed 2-year "developmental kindergartens" for children who are not quite ready for the typical, more academic kindergarten setting.

I. School Entry

The timing of school entry is shifting in the United States. Before the 1970s, children tended to start school at kindergarten age or around 5 years of age. This was generally the child's first out-of-home experience. As Head Start programs began, more children were enrolled in these programs and in day care, so first entry into the school system became more frequent in the preschool years. Readiness for preschool is largely dependent on the child's and parent's ability to separate for a period of approximately 2 hours. The experience of preschool can help a child gain socialization skills, improve language skills, and increase exposure to preacademic tasks, such as learning colors, numbers, letters, and puzzle-solving abilities.

II. Family Expectations

Inquiring about the family's expectations of a school and for their child's performance is also important. Realistic goals and parental expectations can make the transition and choice of placement more satisfying. Many parents feel that children must be prepared to compete early and place great weight on school achievement. Some families even consider holding a child back so that he or she will be more advanced or larger than their peers, a strategy that has not proven effective after the early school years. Other parents are embarrassed by the idea of holding a child an extra year in preschool, feeling it reflects on how "bright" the child is.

III. School/Child Match

The best approach to helping families with school entry decisions is to review the child's development and maturity and then to discuss with the family the best fit of school placement for the individual child. For example, an immature child who has not had preschool exposure and who is just turning 5 years of age may benefit from a preschool year or a prekindergarten class if it is available in the school district. A child with significant delay may require a specialized school placement. A child who is shy may do best in a smaller school, which has the ability to individualize the child's experience. Knowing the community resources in each school district, including available private schools, is important for the primary care physician.

IV.   Assessing Readiness for School
Readiness for school requires cognitive abilities, emotional maturity, gross and fine motor skills, and peer individual and group social skills. Intelligence is only one part of the equation.

When parents ask physicians about the readiness of their children for school, the opinion should be based on several sources of information:

A.   Physician's observation of the child and his or her relationship with the parent(s). Specific things to watch for include the following:

1.   *Ease of separation of child from parent.*

2.   *Speech development and articulation,* including the initiation and sustainability of conversation.

3.   *Understanding of and ability to follow multistep directions.*

4.   *Preacademic skills,* such as knowledge of at least four colors; ability to count to 10; knowledge of age and first name, last name, address, and phone number; ability to copy a circle, cross, and triangle; and ability to print or copy first name.

5.   *Motor skills,* including ability to skip, stand on one foot, catch a bounced ball with hands, tie shoe laces (maybe), and dress and undress without assistance.

B.   The parent's opinion and observations at home or at other caregivers.

1.   *Can the child play well with other children?* Does the child share, take turns, and generally use words to resolve conflicts and have needs met?

2.   *Does the parent trust the child in the backyard alone, with the parent occasionally monitoring from inside the house?* Is the child trusted to stop at a street corner or curb and wait for an adult? Can the child be trusted to cross a low-traffic, good-visibility street on his or her own?

3.   *Has the child shown interest in books or letters and numbers?*

4.   *Can the child sustain attention to quiet activities?*

5.   *How frequent are toileting "accidents" and how good are the child's self-help skills?*

6.   *Does the child still really need a nap?*

C.   Child's history of separation from parents and success in preschool settings. This should include the opinion of the child's preschool teacher.

D.   The child's chronological age and gender. While the relationship between school readiness and these demographics is not perfect, children do better in kindergarten if their fifth birthday is at least 4 to 6 months before the beginning of school. In addition, girls are usually ready earlier than boys.

E. The child's developmental history. Has the child generally been in the average range or in the slower range?

F. Knowledge of the proposed program for the child. Very academic kindergartens demand greater readiness than specially designed developmental programs or more traditional kindergarten programs. School readiness is in part a question of fit or match.

V. Screening Devices Available

An easy screening device for parents to perform is the Child Development Inventory, which is a series of true/false questions requiring about 30 minutes or less to complete. Many other instruments have been created and typically include the same type of skills as described earlier. The primary care physician must realize that few of these inventories are well normed and only serve as screening devices, not as diagnostic tests with clear outcomes based on scores. Specific learning disabilities will not be picked up on these general developmental screens. In addition, many schools have their own screening for potential incoming kindergartners.

VI. Consequences of Inadequate Readiness

A child needs some success in school to enjoy it and learning in general. Pushing a child into an environment for which he or she is not prepared can contribute to problems, such as school refusal, lack of enjoyment of school, poor school achievement for both early and later grades, and behavioral problems. Holding a child back for reasons of developmental delay in the false hope that the child will catch up can lead to the same type of problems. In general, holding a child back for reasons of immaturity after first grade is not recommended.

ADDITIONAL READING

Bredekamp S, Copple C., eds. *Developmentally appropriate practice in early childhood programs*, rev. ed. Washington, DC: National Association for the Education of Young Children; 1997.

Casey PH, Evans LD. School readiness: an overview for pediatricians. *Pediatr Rev* 1993;1:4–10.

Dixon S, Stein M. *Encounters with children*. St. Louis: Mosby Year Book; 1992.

Golant S, Golant M. *Kindergarten: it isn't what it used to be*. Los Angeles: Lowell House; 1990.

Graue ME. *Ready for what? Constructing meanings of readiness for kindergarten*. New York: SUNY Press; 1993.

Books for Parents

Brazelton TB. *Touchpoints: the essential reference*. Reading, MA: Addison Wesley; 1992.

Elovson A. *The kindergarten survival handbook: the before school checklist & a guide for parents.* Cambridge, MA: Parent Education Resources; 1993.

Walmsley SA. *Kindergarten: ready or not? A parent's guide.* Portsmouth, NH: Heinemann Press; 1996.

Websites for parents

http://readyweb.crc.uiuc.edu/ (Ready Web)

http://www.aea11.k12.ia.us/ec/readiness/defining%20readiness.html (Heartland Area Education Agency)

http://www.nauticom.net/www/cokids/index.html (Western Instructional Support Center)

41 ⚙ Sexuality in Well-Child Care

Nancy E. Lanphear

A pedantic definition of sexuality is a state characterized and distinguished by sex or interest in and concern with sexual activity. Many primary care physicians would readily agree that sexuality is an important area for discussion in an adolescent well-child check, but they may not consider it a component in the younger years. This view unfortunately reduces the complex nature of sexuality to the physical changes that occur with the onset of puberty. Sexuality in its full context includes gender identification and socialization and the development of beliefs and behaviors that will allow an individual to have intimate human relationships. Seeing sexuality as another component of the developmental maturation of a child and therefore as a process that begins at birth and continues into adult life is helpful. Pediatricians can benefit families and, eventually, the patient, by providing education in typical sexual development. This could include addressing areas with parents that can be concerning. Some such areas include early physical exploration by the infant, masturbation in the young child, "playing doctor" in the preschool-aged child, the emergence of early pubertal changes, counseling for prevention of premature sexual activity, and counseling for pregnancy or use of contraceptives. Initiating a discussion about some of the "less weighty" topics in early childhood may ease the transition for discussions necessary in the more intense adolescent years.

I. Infancy

Gender typing frequently begins at birth but, with the increasing identification of the baby's sex before birth, may begin during pregnancy. This typing commonly influences choice of colors for the infant's nursery decor, clothing, toy selection, and the preceptions of early behaviors. Sharing these influences with the parents may help the family improve consciousness of the ways that they may unconsciously shift perceptions of children based upon gender.

As in all areas of development, the family and parents are the initial key influence. A child's sense of bonding comes from the initial bond made with a parent or primary caregiver. Infants require their needs for food, stimulation, sleep, and physical contact to be met. The sense of trust that develops with the caregiver allows a child to feel safe and secure and to develop a sense of connectedness to another human being.

Infants will self-explore all body parts, including genitalia. This self-exploration during diaper changes or bathtime may be a source of discomfort for the parent. The primary care physician should discuss this normal behavior and curiosity at early well-baby visits in anticipation of the activity.

Many families will also discuss sleeping arrangements, especially cosleeping. Though this is dependent on cultural practices, the physical environment, and personal choice, the best approach for the primary care physician is simply to ask about current sleeping practices and to investigate the reasons for specific choices, such as cosleeping. Both cultural sensitivity and a nonjudgmental style are important. Establishing separate sleeping arrangements allows children their own space and begins the process of autonomy and individuation.

II.   Toddler and Preschool Years

As the child grows and matures, the need for autonomy and independence from the caregiver becomes more important. This stage, accompanied by temper tantrums and increased use of the word *mine*, can also include the wish to be independent in toileting and dressing. As toilet training occurs, the child should learn appropriate words for genitalia, including *penis* and *vagina*. The use of euphemisms can become confusing for the child and may give him or her the message that the body's private parts are dirty or vulgar.

Also in the toddler to early preschool years, exploration of the child's environment will continue and will include curiosity about parents', siblings', and friends' bodies. The knowledge of their own gender and how it differs from the other is frequently discussed, at times in potentially embarrassing situations, such as in public or with new adults. This is expected, so the parents should provide simple straightforward responses that are developmentally and situationally appropriate. Touching a parent's body, particularly the mother's breast, also occurs and should prompt gentle redirection. Again a primary physician is an excellent person to educate parents about the typical and developmental nature of innocent curiosity.

Genital play often begins in the toddler to preschool years. Typical masturbation or genital exploration occurs occasionally and becomes more private as the child gets older. This type of play should not be preferred over other activities or play and involves only the external genitalia. The history or physical examination should uncover no outward signs or symptoms from such play. Abnormal findings of the genitalia should warrant further investigation. Regular masturbation, which takes the place of more typical play or occurs in an indiscreet manner, mandates further history, as this behavior would be atypical at this age.

The next stage of sexual exploration may include peers—for example, "playing doctor" or pretending to be married and showing affection. This phase, typical of the preschooler, occurs at a time when imaginative and dramatic play is at a high level. Typical sexual play at this age (a) occurs between children of the same developmental age, (b) happens infrequently, (c) comprises only a part of other pretend play, (d) takes place by mutual consent, (e) remains nonaggressive, and (f) includes age-appropriate language and knowledge. The "sexual activity" does not include any explicit actions, such as penetration or genital-genital contact. Warning signs of sexual abuse would include physical trauma, older children victimizing younger children, or greater knowledge than expected for the child's developmental age.

The younger child is also more likely to undress in public and to walk around nude. This changes over time as family socialization of the child includes the teaching of privacy, modesty, and appropriate public behaviors. Family behaviors, such as coshowering or bathing and nudity, may need to be modified over time as the child grows older to allow teaching about modesty.

Children should be taught about issues of their own safety. A young child should be allowed to say no to an "unwanted hug," even from a close relative. This autonomy will provide the child with the lesson that touch and the child's own body space is important and that it is an area in which choice is allowed. Teaching children about the private areas of their own body can explain private parts as those covered by typical underwear and, in the older girl, as the area of the body covered by a two-piece bathing suit.

Parents also need to be sensitive to behavioral cues as they relate to possible sexual abuse. These include significant behavioral change without known cause, the appearance of new fears, genital harm without explanation, or an infection with a sexually transmitted disease. At the same time, no amount of discussion with the child can protect the young child against an adult intent on harming him or her. Parents need to supervise young children and to be familiar and comfortable with any caregivers and babysitters. Establishing a comfortable relationship with children in which they can bring parents their concerns and fears and be listened to in an open manner is the best advantage and protection for the child. As children reach school age, parents need to know their friends and the households the child visits when away from home. If in doubt about a companion's home situation, the child could invite the friend to their home initially. When going about their own neighborhood, parents and children should establish mutually acceptable boundaries and routes and should discuss the location and timing of activities. Supervision of the child's exposure to the media, such as television and the Internet, is essential.

III. School-Aged Years

As children reach school age and adolescence, their need for greater and more specific knowledge about their bodies and sexuality will increase. The best source for getting answers to questions and gaining knowledge is the parents. Frequently information is simply not provided by parents because of their hesitation or embarrassment. If a parent does not provide the information, the child will still seek it, often from immature or inappropriate sources, such as older siblings, peers, or even the Internet. Some information may be available in schools, but the type of information varies from school to school. The primary care provider should approach the parents with the need for a discussion before the onset of the pubertal growth spurt so that some dialogue takes place with the child before pubertal changes occur.

Simple brochures about sexuality can be shared with the family at the 7- or 8-year-old well-child check. As children spontaneously ask questions concerning sex, body changes, and pubertal development, parents need to be prepared and able to address these. Good times to talk are difficult to orchestrate without the discussion feeling like a lecture. The parent often finds that asking open-ended questions is best and learns to listen closely for the "unasked" question and to give the information requested without overburdening the child. These discussions should not be of the "one-sex-talk" variety but should be a series of evolving discussions geared specifically to the information needed at a given time and developmental stage with the knowledge that further talks will occur. Boys and girls both require information geared to their gender and developmental needs, such as a discussion about menstruation with girls and about wet dreams with boys. A possible location for some of these discussions is the car. This setting allows for an in-depth discussion without unexpected interruptions and with only the desired participants present. Furthermore, the car allows greater limitation of eye contact, which parents and children who may be somewhat uncomfortable might find easier.

Genital play or masturbation, done privately, will continue in the school-aged child; by late adolescence, it will be more typical of adult practice. Sexual play between young school-aged children will fade as the relationship between boys and girls changes to more same-sex interest. This interest evolves again in early adolescence with attraction to the opposite sex.

IV.   Adolescence

Sexual play in adolescence can include all types of sexual activity, and primary care physicians and parents both need to discuss with teenagers the issues of premature sexual activity and intercourse, the dangers of infection, the use of contraception, and the risk of pregnancy. Knowledge promotes informed decisions and reduces risk-taking behavior on the part of the adolescent. Other chapters in this book discuss the adolescent visit and contraception. Physical sexual maturity ratings (see Appendix C) and the timing of typical sexual development (see Appendix D) are included in the appendices.

The creation of sexually well-adjusted adults is an evolving process that begins in childhood with the model provided by family relationships and parental guidance. This is affected over time by extended family, peers, the media, and societal values. Primary care providers can act as educators, coaches, and confidants and can supply needed expertise if difficulties occur.

ADDITIONAL READING

Dixon S, Stein M. *Encounters with children: pediatric behavior and development.* St. Louis: Mosby Yearbook; 1992.

Friedrich WN, Grambsch P, Broughton D, et al. Normative sexual behavior in children. *Pediatrics* 1991;88:456–464.

Haka-Ikse K, Mian M. Sexuality in children. *Pediatr Rev* 1993;14: 401–407.

Schoentjes E, Deboutte D, Friedrich W, et al. Child sexual behavior inventory: a Dutch speaking normative sample. *Pediatrics* 1999; 104:885–893.

42 ♣ Sibling Rivalry

Janet R. Schultz

***Teaching task:* To help children develop skills for expression of needs and desires, for negotiation, and for management of conflict in relationships.**

Sibling rivalry has been an almost universal issue dating back to Cain and Abel. Few families exist where the children are cooperative and caring to each other all the time. Often, mutually aggravating behavior between or among siblings is a major challenge for parents. These relationship problems may or may not represent dysfunction. More often than not, these behaviors have become habits that are maintained by their consequences, regardless of their origin.

I. Etiology

Although the most well-known formulation of the etiology of this problem is the theory of displacement from the sole or at least youngest position, children can have rivalrous feelings about older or younger siblings. In fact, the sibling still *in utero* may evoke these feelings. Most research suggests, however, that the etiology may be the change in the relationship between the parent (especially the mother) and the child after a baby is born. Even parents who try very hard not to be different with their older child(ren) have been documented to have changes in expectations, time availability, and patience (partly related to new-baby fatigue). Practically speaking, behaviors that were once acceptable, even admired (e.g., making siren noises while playing with a toy fire engine), may now be disruptive or forbidden. Things are different when a new baby arrives!

II. Preventing Sibling Rivalry

Parents can do several things to prevent sibling rivalry from occurring (proactive management) or at least from becoming a significant problem (reactive management):

A. Prepare the older children for the arrival of a new infant, through talking, children's books, and reminiscing about what they were like as infants, preferably complete with pictures of their early days. Parents should describe what a baby's behavior will be like.

B. Friends and family often bring gifts for the new baby and pay much attention to the new arrival, to the exclusion of the older children. If extended family members ignore older children, they should be encouraged to pay attention to them and perhaps to take them for a few hours to help out. Gifts brought home from the hospital "from the baby" can also help balance things. Paying attention to the older child's new status as a big brother or sister helps as well. This should include some new status symbol (e.g., staying up 15 minutes later) as well as being included in the care of the baby (e.g., getting diapers, pushing the stroller, helping to burp the baby).

C. Avoid comparing children to each other, even for "motivation."

D. Accept the feelings, even unpleasant ones, of the siblings about each other and help put them into words. Parents should establish limits on behavioral expressions of the feelings, however (e.g., the child can say that he does not like his new sister but may not hit her).

E. Parents should spend some positive time, even if not always alone, with each of the children.

F. As soon as the second sibling has verbal capabilities, try to coach verbal ways, instead of physical, for requesting things (e.g., *"May I have the train?"* instead of grabbing it). Verbal means of managing anger (e.g., *"I'm really mad at you for calling me a brat"* rather than hitting the other) and negotiating (e.g., *"I'll trade you the ball for the Barbie"*) should also be taught. Siblings are perfect practice partners for social skills relevant to children outside the home.

G. With children under 5 years of age put names on possessions in easily visible locations. In the preschool years, a printed name develops into greater proof of ownership than use. A child shares things more easily if they are indisputably marked as the child's own.

H. Not all possessions need to be shared. Special toys can be designated for one child's use only, but the child must play with them in a private place or when the other child is not present. This method often frees the child to share other, less precious toys.

I. Parents should not play favorites. The meaning is not that parents should buy each child a pair of socks because one child needs a pair. However, parents should avoid behavioral expressions of emotional favoritism, such as praising a behavior or accomplishment of one child while ignoring the same or a similar achievement in another.

J. Set limits on the expression of the rivalry or other disagreements. Parents should model these behaviors in their interactions with the children. Possible rules include no hitting, breaking things, or calling names. Follow-through with consequences for breaking these rules is necessary.

K. Parents should try to stay out of the arguments of their children, especially those of school-aged children. Children sometimes inadvertently learn that arguing is a way to engage parents. Besides, an easy solution for parents rarely exists. If the arguing annoys the parents, they can announce, *"I don't want to hear your arguing. Please solve this peacefully or find somewhere else to argue."* If they do not comply, the children can be sent outdoors or can be geographically separated. One exception follows: if an argument becomes physically aggressive, the parents should stop the fight, geographically separate the children, and treat them as equally responsible. Physical fights left without intervention tend to escalate and are often unfairly matched.

L. Like most behaviors, bickering can be addressed by the suggested general problem-solving paradigm.

Positive reinforcement for getting along and "response cost" for arguing can be effective when used together. For example, children receive points for playing cooperatively and/or getting along for specific periods of time and lose a certain number of points for arguing. The remaining points are then redeemable for a joint reward.
M.   Sometimes parents find thinking about their own positions in their families of origin helpful. Often when two parents consistently interpret situations differently and fight over conflicting views, they are reflecting their own experiences as children. Other times, one of the children reminds a parent of their own sibling, themselves, or a former spouse; and reactions lose any hint of objectivity.
N.   "Tattling," which can be a form of sibling rivalry, is a very powerful tool for siblings to "get even" with each other. A rule that "telling" is allowed only when the sibling or someone with him or her could get hurt can prevent tattling. Responses, such as "Thank you for letting me know" or "It really bugs you when he does that, doesn't it?," are equally clear messages to the child that the parent is not allowing himself or herself to be engaged in the power play.
O.   Time apart can reduce arguing and bickering between siblings.

ADDITIONAL READING

Faber A, Mazlish E. *Siblings without rivalry*. New York: WW Norton; 1987.
Schmitt B. When siblings quarrel. *Contemp Pediatr* 1991;8:74–75.

Books for Parents

Crary E. *Kids can co-operate*. Seattle: Parenting Press; 1988.
Leach P. *Your baby and child*. New York: Knopf; 1978.
Kingsley EP. *A baby sister for herry*. New York: Western Publishing; 1984.

Websites for Parents

http://www.gartland.com/phoenix/95–7/7-sibli.html
http://www.tnpc.com/parentalk/toddlers/todd4.html

43 ♣ Sleep and Bedtime Behaviors

Janet R. Schultz

Few parents understand that an element of learning exists not only in bedtime behavior but also in the sleep process itself. The behavioral factors and principles outlined in Chapter 29 are relevant insofar as both development and consequences of behavior need to be considered with regard to sleep.

I. Newborns
Teaching tasks: **To help infants differentiate wakefulness from sleep and to help them sleep more at night than during the day.**

Newborns typically sleep from 16 to 22 hours a day. Not much will make them sleep more or less. In the earliest days, babies tend to "drift" between states of alertness. To help them learn to be either completely awake or completely asleep, parents should have the child "go to bed" for sleep, rather than allowing them to be held or kept in a "pumpkin seat." The infant should then be "gotten up" when he or she is awake. This will also help strengthen the association between bed and sleep.

Similarly, at night falling asleep in their cribs is important for infants. Since rocking the baby to sleep is a pleasant ritual of parenthood, parents may find the following recommendation difficult; however, whenever possible, the sleepy infant should be placed in the crib while still somewhat awake. Doing this helps the child learn to fall asleep on his or her own and to associate bed with sleeping.

Things that improve the quality of sleep at night include making sure that the infant has been fed and burped, keeping the room warm (but not hot), darkening the room so that even if bedtime is early in the evening, the room looks different from what it does in the daytime, and swaddling the infant. There is some evidence that infants who have had more body contact during the day (e.g., in a baby carrier) sleep better at night and that, by contrast, infants who are not handled much have more difficulty sleeping. Little evidence exists to show that in the first 6 months of life, an infant can make himself stay awake.

Colic of course can complicate this scenario. In many instances, the parents move into a "making it through" mode, a totally understandable mind set. Parents need to know that colic is not a result of disease or poor parenting. Knowing that, in general, colic lasts no more than 8 weeks and is related to the infant temperament and the maturity of the infant's nervous and digestive systems is helpful to parents. Coping strategies include swaddling the child, using an infant swing (motion), and recognizing that sometimes only time will stop the crying. Parents need adequate sleep at other times of the day so that they can remain relatively calm during the episodes. Getting support and hands-on assistance from other adults is useful.

II.   Six to 18 Months
Teaching task: **To teach infants to soothe them-selves to sleep without adult help.**

Babies in the 6 to 18 months age range need to have short, simple, and predictable bedtime routines. Bedtime should be fairly consistent. Similar to younger infants, they should be put in the crib while still somewhat awake, but sleepy, to help them learn to "put themselves to sleep."

After 6 months of age, some infants can keep themselves awake, and many still need to learn to soothe themselves back to sleep when they wake up. In particular, babies who are accustomed to an adult "putting them to sleep" (i.e., falling asleep while being rocked or cuddled by an adult) or who have a history of an illness that necessitated parental involvement during the night may need to learn (or relearn) to help themselves back to sleep. When sleep lightens as part of the normal sleep cycle and infants reach a relatively wakeful state, they may require adult inter-vention to go back to sleep. The result is frequent wakenings in the night unrelated to nutritive or other needs. Parents often feel the baby who wakens in the night "must be hungry," but they must be reassured that this is not the case. Healthy 6-month-olds can meet their nutrition needs during the daytime alone. When fed repeatedly during the night, the child not only learns to asso-ciate return to sleep with feeding but also is more likely to have particularly wet diapers, which may contribute to waking.

If a bedtime routine has not been established, then one should be, preferably for a week or more before attempting to intervene further in the baby's sleep. Most babies who need help learning to put themselves back to sleep can learn to do this in less than a week **if parents are willing and committed.** First, at bedtime (after feeding), the infant should be put in the crib while still somewhat awake. The parent should not "disappear," but should putter around the room for a few minutes before leaving. The room should resemble the conditions that will be present when he wakens later in the night (degree of darkness and quiet). Favorite comfort items like a treasured toy or favorite "blankie" should be available in the crib. When the child begins to cry, the parent should wait 5 minutes (by the clock) before responding. Then the parent should briefly check the child to make sure no cause for discomfort exists and should leave again. The infant will be aware of the parent's presence when he or she checks in, but the adult must not pick up, hug, or sing to the child. A few words said to the infant or brief patting on the back should be the extent of the interaction. After the next 10 minutes (by the clock) of crying, the checking procedure should be repeated. This is then repeated every 10 minutes until the child falls asleep in the absence of the parent. On succeeding nights the waiting periods can be gradually lengthened. The usual time of wakening in the morning and the length of naps should be maintained during this learning period.

A commitment should be made to try this method for 4 to 5 days. Parents should be prepared for the first night, which is almost always the worst, because the child will keep on crying until he unlearns the old pattern of expecting a parent to put him to sleep and learns to do it himself. If the family lives in an apartment, warning the immediate neighbors that the infant may cry and why may be necessary. A supportive call from office staff or the pediatrician can be very helpful to parents, especially the first morning after implementation. On rare occasions, an infant will cry until he vomits. This should be treated with a matter-of-fact clean-up and the resumption of the process. If this pattern repeats itself, the crib can be prepared with multiple layers of crib sheet alternating with moisture-proof pads, to expedite "peel-off" change of bedding. For some parents, keeping track of when the baby awakens and for how long is a way to measure progress and to reassure them that things are in fact getting better (it also gives them "something to do"). Many parents prefer to start on a Friday night when they have no work obligations the following day and both parents can participate.

About 20% to 30% of infants, 12 to 36 months of age, have trouble sleeping throughout the night. The same basic plan can be used throughout this age range if the problem is related to frequent awakenings. Infants who are accustomed to frequent feedings during the night may also benefit from gradually decreasing night feeding before implementation of the plan. When the two habits occur concurrently (night waking and night feeding), the same plan is used, after assuring the parents that the infant's nutritional needs are fully satisfied by daytime feeding and a bedtime feeding.

III.   Toddlers and Preschoolers

Teaching tasks: **To teach child in this age group to recognize body clues of fatigue, to become comfortable with the separation of bedtime, and to go to bed and fall asleep without behavioral disruptions or unusual fears.**

A.   Resisting bedtime. As children move into the toddler and preschool years, the emphasis shifts from sleeping *per se* to getting the child to go to bed and stay there. In this age period, having a set bedtime and a well-established bedtime routine (ritual) is important for teaching the child that separating from the many interesting, exciting, and comforting elements of the waking environment is safe and even pleasant. Physical needs (e.g., *"I want a glass of water!"* and *"I gotta go potty"*) should be addressed during the bedtime routine.

Parents also need to understand that they can legislate bedtime but cannot control sleep. The goal of behavior management is to get the child to go to bed peacefully and to stay there so that the possibility of sleep is increased and encouraged. The parent can promise a fearful or reluctant child that he or she will return to check on the child 5 minutes after tucking him in. The first few times the child will stay awake to make sure the parent keeps his word, so the parent cannot be waylaid by other tasks or children. When the parent checks the child, he should be praised for staying in bed and told that the parent will check again later. Generally, after a few nights, the child falls asleep sooner and the frequency of checking can be reduced.

Often, when the problem is limit setting, the parent has trouble getting the child to go to sleep, but other adult care-takers (e.g., babysitters) do not. If the child does not fall asleep until the same time every night, regardless of the care provider present, the bedtime may be set too early (or the child may be rising too late).

B.   Not staying in bed. For "jack-in-the box" children who pop out of their beds (and usually their bedrooms) as soon as they are put to bed, parents must be consistent with man-agement; reminding them that this behavior can be hard to eliminate without consistency is imperative. The child should not be allowed "just this once" to stay up later, watch a tele-vision show, have a snack, or read another book. Calmly and quietly, the parent should take the child by the hand and walk him back to bed without reassurance or reprimanding. The child should be tucked in, and the parent should leave. **This procedure should be repeated each time the child gets out of bed.** If a few evenings of applying this procedure consistently do not solve the problem, a behavioral program involving positive consequences for staying in bed should be implemented. For example, the child should be told that the parent will come back in 5 minutes and check on the child. At that point, if the child has stayed in bed, he gets praise and a star or sticker on a chart. The parent needs to continue this, stretching out the time span, until the child is asleep. If the child remains in bed all night (except to get up to go to the bathroom), he gets a bonus in the morning, such as eating a favorite food for breakfast or watching cartoons during break-fast. Occasionally, a child still refuses to stay in his or her bed or bedroom. In this case, a safety gate may need to be installed so that the whole room becomes more or less the crib. Doing this prevents the need to close the door, which makes many parents uncomfortable and scares some children.

Inconsistency of follow-through is the primary reason that this plan does not work. Sometimes parents' motivation is mixed, because of guilt about lack of their own daytime availability to the child (working parents) or because of fears of being alone at night. Sometimes children's "popping out of bed" serves the needs of parents who are trying to prevent or avoid marital disputes.

C.   Trouble falling asleep. If the child has trouble falling asleep but stays in bed, allowing tapes, books, or other quiet activities may be helpful. However, parents need to monitor this because some children will stay awake longer just to do those things. Children who are afraid of the dark often do well when a room light, instead of just a nightlight, is left on to eliminate scary shadows. Children in the 4- to 5-year age range love flashlights, which allow them to feel some personal control over checking out fears. Many times children who have been roughhousing just before bedtime or who have had caffeinated drinks at bedtime are too "wired" to sleep. Reconsidering the evening routine and intake can reduce or eliminate these problems. If a child consistently does not fall asleep while in bed and still gets up the following morning at the necessary hour without seeming tired, bedtime may need to be readjusted.

D. Children who join their parents during the night. Parents need to evaluate their own feelings about this behavior. For a variety of reasons, some parents like it, although they may not freely admit this truth to themselves. No evidence shows that cosleeping (sharing the adult bed with children) is harmful in the absence of sexual abuse or exposure to parental sexual activity. If the parents, however, want to eliminate the child's nighttime visits, then the following plan can be implemented. When the child comes to the parents' bed during the night, a parent should get out of bed and quietly but firmly take the child back to bed. The parent should check on the child's comfort needs and simply tuck the child in, say "good-night," and go back to his or her own bed, with the promise of returning to check on the child in a few minutes. The parent needs to keep that promise. Generally this procedure will end the nighttime visiting behavior **if consistently applied.** The star chart and bonus system described earlier may also be used to provide positive consequences for the desired behaviors.

If parents say that they do not waken when the little visitor arrives and therefore cannot take the child back to bed consistently, they should hang a string of jingle bells, a couple of empty cans on a string, or another noisemaker on the door knob of the bedroom. The door to the bedroom should be kept closed or at least partially closed so that opening the door makes enough noise to waken the parent. If parents do not feel they can leave a very fearful child (which gives the child the idea that something exists that they really should be frightened of!), then the child should be kept in his or her own bed, and the parent should stay in the child's room—but not in the child's bed. The parent should sit on a chair near the bed for awhile. Then, each subsequent evening the chair the parent sits on can gradually be moved closer to (and finally out) the door.

IV. School-Aged Children
Older children tend to have a more adult pattern of having their sleep affected by daily tensions. Avoiding disciplinary confrontations at bedtime, having a slow-down time before bedtime (quiet play rather than roughhousing), maintaining a routine at bedtime, and encouraging positive quiet time with parents can all help children to relax and sleep. Fears are still common for this age group. However, while ghosts and monsters still play a role, more realistic fears regarding achievement, world events, burglars, kidnappers, and social rejection may emerge at this age.

Older children may resist going to bed. If the bedtime is appropriate for the child's school schedule or parents' needs, compliance can be improved by imposing consequences and rewarding desired behaviors. Allowing in-bed activities, such as reading or listening to the radio for awhile, can often make the transition to bed easier. Dawdling as a way of delaying bedtime can be addressed by the child having to "pay back" the time missed in bed one night by going to bed that much earlier the next night.

V.   Sleep Disruptions

A.   Sleepwalking.

Sleepwalking can occur from infancy (even sleep crawling!) through adolescence. Although one-third of children between 5 and 12 years of age have walked in their sleep at least once, persistent sleepwalking occurs in only 1% to 6% of children. Some evidence suggests that sleepwalking is more common in boys and may run in families.

1. *Typical episodes.* Sleepwalking typically begins about 90 to 120 minutes after the child goes to sleep. Episodes usually last 5 to 15 minutes and occasionally occur more than once in a night. Youngsters appear to wake up and sit up suddenly in bed with wide open eyes that are glassy or staring. Sleepwalkers seem to be able to see objects and avoid tripping, but they are pretty much unaware of their surroundings. This means that common discriminations are often lost—a child may not be able to tell the difference between the bedroom and closet doors or between the toilet and a wastebasket. Actions remain relatively simple and repetitive and are usually ones that are common during the day, such as opening doors, turning on lights, getting dressed, and so on. Speech, if any, is incoherent. Episodes are generally not recalled in the morning.

2. *Risks.* Injury prevention is the major concern, but sleepwalking is hard to anticipate except in persistent or frequent sleepwalkers. Keeping floors and hallways clear is important, and gates at the top of the stairs are important for younger sleepwalkers in particular. For children sleeping in bunk beds, the lower bunk is a safer place for a somnambulist. Occasionally, a high lock is required on outside doors to keep children from leaving the apartment or house. Firearms are also particularly risky. If the child sleepwalks persistently, a bell on the child's door or a Radio Shack–type doormat that rings a bell when stepped on can increase parents' awareness of episodes.

3. *What to do.* Parents who encounter a sleepwalking child should talk quietly and calmly to the child while directing him or her to go back to bed. If a child is agitated or seems upset, physical contact with the child may bring about frightened flailing that could hurt the parent. Sometimes children seem to want to stop to urinate in the bathroom, which should be permitted on the way back to bed. No reason exists for wakening the child, and little is gained by doing so. Older children are more likely to wake up

spontaneously. Parents should maintain a calm, matter-of-fact approach at the time and avoid teasing the next day.

A small group of parents finds sleepwalking is a very frightening event because they hold the belief that awakening a sleepwalker can result in sudden death for them. These parents, however, may not tell you that belief spontaneously, but their intense concern may be a clue. Respectful reassurance and education can be helpful.

4. *Prevention.* Prevention of sleepwalking is best done by ensuring adequate rest and a normal bedtime routine. These two things are particularly true for younger children. Reducing and talking about life stresses may be more helpful in older children. Sleepwalking diminishes spontaneously after 10 to 12 years of age.

B. Nightmares. Life events, stress, or watching scary movies or television programs (or even the news) can help trigger nighttime fears in some children. Sometimes the fears affect the child's comfort going to sleep, but they may also stimulate nightmares. Nightmares tend to occur 1 to 4 hours after the child has gone to sleep. Parental reassurance is usually all that is required for occasional nightmares. Recurrent nightmares may reflect high levels of stress or family change. These can be addressed through discussion, clear nighttime structure, and sometimes referral to a mental health professional.

C. Partial awakenings:

1. *Partial awakenings.* These are more common in younger children. Preschool children, from about 6 months of age on, may have partial awakenings, during which they cry, moan, and/or thrash about wildly for brief periods of time.

2. *Night terrors (pavor nocturnus).* In their more extreme forms, these partial awakenings are termed night terrors. Children "appear" to waken suddenly and scream, cry, and sometimes thrash about or even run around the room. During these partial awakenings, they may have their eyes open, but the eyes appear "glazed" as if they really are not seeing anything. Generally, they do not respond to comfort even though they may call out for a parent who is sitting with them. Night terrors occur most commonly in the first 3 hours of sleep and last 10 to 20 minutes, although parents may overestimate their length since "it feels like forever." Night terrors are fairly common between 3 and 5 years of age. More rarely these occur in older, school-aged children, especially boys. After 10 years of age their frequency usually diminishes.

3. *What to do.* These children are not awake during the episodes. The most important aspect of their management is to protect them from injury. Injury usually occurs most often in the children who get out of bed and run around wildly. If these episodes happen frequently and involve running, nursery monitors can help parents keep their child

safe. If the child sleeps on the second floor or higher, parents should consider installing Plexiglas or security bars across windows.

Parents can help by wiping a cool washcloth over the face of the child, not in an attempt to wake the child but in an effort to alter the child's arousal state. Parents generally should not attempt to hug or hold the child if the child does not recognize them. Asking the child what is wrong then or in the morning tends to be met with a lack of comprehension. Parents should avoid making the child feel "weird" or "different" in the morning by repeated questioning regarding the incident.

If the episodes have a major motor component, a short course of benzodiazepines at bedtime may help, but medication is not generally recommended for the treatment of this disorder except in extreme cases. Benadryl has also been found to be helpful in reducing the incidence of night terrors. If episodes persist, psychotherapy and/or stress reduction should be considered for families and/or children. This intervention is recommended even if no major psychosocial issues are obvious, but the terrors are frequent, intense, or dangerous. From middle childhood on, psychological factors are particularly likely to be relevant.

ADDITIONAL READING

Guilleminault C, ed. *Sleep and its disorders in children.* New York: Raven Press; 1987.

Kataria S, Swanson MS, Trevathan GE. Persistence of sleep disturbances in preschool children. *Behav Pediatr* 1987;110:642–646.

Books for Parents

Ferber R. *Solve your child's sleep problems.* New York: Simon and Schuster; 1985.

Leach P. *Your baby and child.* New York: Knopf; 1978.

Schaefer C, Petronko M. *Teach your baby to sleep through the night.* New York: Putnam and Sons; 1987.

Schmitt BD. *Your child's health,* rev. ed. New York: Bantam Books; 1991.

Websites for Parents

www.allkids.org/ Epstein/Articles/Sleepwalking.html (Sleepwalking)
www.drkoop.com/family/childrens.asp (Sleep)
www.drkoop.com/conditions/ency/article/00809.htm (Night terrors)

44 ♣ Speech and Language Disorders in Children

Ann W. Kummer

The ability to communicate, a critical human skill, affects the way that an individual functions in society and impacts most activities of daily living. Unfortunately, an estimated 6 million children under 18 years of age, as estimated by the National Institutes of Health, have a speech or language disorder. Boys make up about two-thirds of this population. Although some children who are identified as late or slow talkers at the age of 2 years begin to pick up communication skills, many continue to have speech and/or language problems at the age of 4 or 5.

A communication disorder can have a negative impact on the child's social and emotional development and can affect the child's ability to learn. Therefore the primary care physician should closely monitor the child's development of communication skills, particularly in the first 6 years. In addition, the provider should be prepared to answer questions of concerned parents regarding their child's development of these skills. Since in children "normal" changes with chronologic age, the physician must have a clear understanding of what is expected at each developmental stage. (For more information regarding normal developmental milestones, please see the Chapter 12, "Normal Speech and Language Development.") Table 44.1 lists populations at high risk for speech and language disorders.

The purpose of this chapter is to present an overview of the types of speech and language disorders that are commonly identified in children. This information should help the physician recognize communication disorders in children and gives the timeline for initiating a referral to a speech/language pathologist.

I. Articulation (Speech) Disorders

An articulation disorder is characterized by difficulty producing speech sounds in comparison to what is expected at the child's chronologic age. The difficulty in production typically occurs with consonants, although in severe cases, even vowel distortions can occur. When difficulties with articulation exist, the child may be forced to compensate by producing sounds in an easier way. As a result, the speech may consist of speech sound omissions, sound substitutions, or distortions. In addition, overall oral inactivity or slurring may be noted. As a result of these errors, the child's speech may be difficult to understand or even unintelligible. Poor speech intelligibility is a primary characteristic of an articulation disorder.

A. Omissions occur if the child has so much difficulty with the motor requirements for speech that he leaves out sounds in words. Omissions occur most with the medial or final sounds in words and with consonants in

**Table 44.1.   Populations at high risk
for speech and language disorders**

History of cleft palate, submucous cleft, or craniofacial anomalies
Significant dental malocclusion or macroglossia
Hearing loss or chronic middle ear effusion
Sensory or perceptual difficulties
Laryngeal or vocal fold pathology
History of traumatic brain injury
Neuromotor or neurologic disease or dysfunction
History of prematurity or traumatic birth history
History of significant feeding or swallowing difficulties
History of developmental delay
Autism or psychosis
Environmental deprivation for a variety of reasons, including long-
    term hospitalization

blends. Examples of typical patterns of sound omissions are
as follows:

I ri the bu to coo. (*I ride the bus to school.*)
Daey bo a cu. (*Daddy broke a cup.*)
My ca a do ah paying ousi. (*My cat and dog are playing outside.*)

In more severe cases, the child may omit all consonants,
and only produce vowel sounds with a grunt (glottal stop) in
place of the consonants. This causes speech to be essentially
unintelligible.
**B.   *Substitutions* are noted when an incorrect sound
is substituted for the correct one.** Most commonly, the
child will substitute a sound that is easier to produce and developed earlier for a sound that is harder to produce and therefore developed later. Some common examples of sound substitutions are as follows:

t/k: I eat tate and tooties. (*I eat cake and cookies.*)
d/g: I'm a dood dirl. (*I'm a good girl.*)
p/f: I have pive pingers. (*I have five fingers.*)
t/s: I tee the tun in the ty. (*I see the sun in the sky.*)
w/l: I wike yewow wowwepops. (*I like yellow lollipops.*)
w/r: I have a wed fiuh twuck. (*I have a red fire truck.*)

When substitution errors are noted, they usually occur
on many different sounds. In fact, the child may use only the
early developmental sounds, or babbling sounds (p, b, m, t, d,
n, k, g), as substitutions for the later-developing consonants.
In more severe cases, the child may only use one or two consonants as a substitution for all other speech sounds.
**C.   *Distortions* occur when the child is attempting to
produce the sound correctly, but an incorrect articu-
latory placement results in an altered sound.** A com-

mon distortion occurs with the production of the /r/ sound. Many children have difficulty with the motor requirements for producing this sound. If the tongue is not high enough or retracted enough, a distortion will result. Other common distortions are lisps, which occur on sibilant or "teeth sounds" (s, z, sh, ch, j). An anterior or *frontal lisp* is the result of the tongue articulating against or between the incisors during sibilant sound production. This causes a distortion that sounds almost like a /th/ sound. A *lateral lisp* occurs when the tongue tip or dorsum of the tongue articulates against the alveolar ridge or palate, stopping the anterior movement of the airstream. As a result, the airstream is redirected laterally, causing a slushy type of sound. At times, saliva can be seen bubbling at the sides of the mouth during speech.

D.   Some patients demonstrate *oral/motor dysfunction* that causes distortion of all speech sounds, particularly in connected speech. One motor speech disorder is *dysarthria*. Dysarthria is the result of neurologic dysfunction associated with cerebral palsy or acquired neurologic damage. Characterized by poor movement of all the articulators, it causes slow, slurred, and inarticulate speech. Respiration, phonation, and resonance may also be affected. As a result, dysarthric speech is usually hypernasal, and utterances can be short and choppy because of poor respiratory support.

E.   *Apraxia of speech,* also known as *verbal apraxia,* is another motor speech disorder. In this disorder, the patient has difficulty with motor planning and sequencing of movements. Although he or she may be able to move the oral structures normally for feeding and other nonspeech activities, difficulty in coordinating movements required for speech is demonstrated. As a result, the speech is characterized by many inconsistent substitutions, frequent sound omissions, sound and syllable reversals, and occasional struggle behaviors during speech production. Speech is best when producing single sounds or words but breaks down when the child is combining the sounds and words to produce the longer utterances of connected speech.

F.   The causes of articulation disorders include structural anomalies, such as a history of cleft palate or velopharyngeal dysfunction. If the velopharyngeal insufficiency causes a significant leak of air pressure into the nasal cavity during speech, inadequate air pressure in the oral cavity may prevent the normal production of sounds. Dental abnormalities, particularly anterior crossbite or class III malocclusion, often can affect speech sound production. For normal speech production, the maxillary arch should overlap the mandibular arch. If the anterior maxillary teeth are retrusive relative to the mandible or are inside the mandibular arch, they can interfere with the movement of the tongue during speech, causing faulty articulation. Hearing loss, especially a sensorineural loss, can affect speech sound perception and learning, thus affecting articulation production. Even chronic otitis media has been shown to affect speech development. Finally, **oral/motor dysfunction,** as mentioned previously, is a common cause of articulation disorders. Oral/motor dysfunction can be found as a result of neurologic damage, but it is also commonly found in patients with no other apparent neurologic problems.

G. Contrary to popular belief, *ankyloglossia,* commonly known as *tongue-tie,* usually does not interfere with speech production. Whether the lingual frenulum has an anterior attachment on the tongue tip or is unusually short, the tongue tip is usually mobile enough for adequate elevation and protrusion for speech. The tongue only needs to elevate slightly to the alveolar ridge for the /l/ sound, and must protrude only to the back of the maxillary incisors for the /th/ sound. If ankyloglossia is noted in a patient with an articulation disorder, the problem is usually just coincidental. Most speech/language pathologists agree that a frenulectomy is usually not indicated for speech purposes. It may be indicated to improve feeding abilities, however, because the restriction of the tongue affects the ability to move a bolus in the oral cavity, particularly from the lateral sulci.

H. A *phonology disorder* is much like an articulation disorder in that the patient demonstrates speech sound substitutions, omissions, and distortions, making the speech difficult to understand. The cause, however, is related not to structural or functional difficulties, but to a faulty "rule" that the child is using in producing speech patterns. For example, the child may always produce the /t/ sound as a substitution for sibilant sounds (s, z, sh, ch, j). Treatment would therefore focus not on the individual sounds but on correcting the rule for all the affected sounds.

II. Language Delays and Disorders

Verbal language requires the use of words, phrases, and sentences to convey information to the listener. In the course of normal development, various auditory, neurologic, and even environmental factors can affect the ability to acquire language normally, resulting in a language delay or disorder. A **language delay** is characterized by a normal, although unusually slow, progression of language acquisition. In contrast, a **language disorder** is characterized by deviant language skills or by language difficulties that are not typically seen during the course of normal development.

Judging the adequacy of verbal language in children can be difficult and challenging for the physician for a variety of reasons. First, considering the child's chronologic and mental age and comparing his or her skills with what is expected for that developmental level is important. Therefore basic knowledge of normal language development is crucial. Another consideration is the child's cultural and linguistic background. For example, many African-Americans use a dialect that has its roots in Africa.

This dialect has rules of syntax that are different from Standard English. In assessing language skills, the ability to distinguish language disorders from dialectical differences is important. Finally, language assessment can be difficult in view of the extremely complex nature of verbal language.

In evaluating a child's language skills, the physician must consider both receptive and expressive language. In addition, three basic components of receptive and expressive language must be developed by all children. These components are the content (semantics), the form (syntax and morphology), and the use of language (pragmatics).

A. Children with a *receptive language disorder* demonstrate difficulty understanding the speech of others. They may be unable to follow commands as easily as their peers, and they may have difficulty answering questions appropriately. Some children with receptive language disorders demonstrate *echolalia.* For example, the child is asked, "How old are you?" and he responds, "Old are you." With echolalia, the child may echo back all or part of a question or command that he does not understand but will respond appropriately when he does understand. Since children need to be able to understand language meaning and form before they are able to generate language, children with receptive language disorders also demonstrate expressive language problems.

B. Children with *expressive language disorders* may have limited vocabulary skills or may use words inappropriately. They may have difficulty formulating sentence structures. As a result, they may use short, "telegraphic" phrases and sentences or may have faulty sentence structures.

C. The content of language, called *semantics,* is the meaning of the words, phrases, and sentences that are used for communication. Children with semantic problems have difficulty categorizing words based on perceptual and functional features, and they have difficulty associating words with meaning. They may also have difficulty retrieving those words that they know and want to use from long-term memory. As a result of these problems, these children often have limited vocabulary skills, demonstrate word-finding difficulties, or frequently use words inappropriately. In comparison to their peers, their utterances contain proportionally more concrete words, such as nouns and verbs, and fewer abstract words, such as adjectives, adverbs, prepositions, articles, and conjunctions. Children with semantic problems have particular difficulty with abstract language, such as understanding concepts, figurative language, and words with multiple meanings.

D. The form of language involves syntax and morphology. *Morphology* refers to the rules that govern the structure of words. Children with morphology problems have difficulty understanding and using the rules of words for appropriate verb tense, plurals, possessives, prefixes and suffixes, and comparatives. *Syntax* refers to the structure of the sentences. Children with syntax problems may have difficulty with word order and with the use of words that have little meaning but that form the glue for the sentence. As a result, they may use improper sentence structures or omit the smaller words, such as prepositions, articles, and conjunctions. This may cause the sentences to be somewhat telegraphic. They may also use improper forms of words, such as the *be* verbs (*is, am, are*) or forms of *do* (*do, did, does*). Examples of problems with syntax and morphology include the following:

That a dog.
Him go school.
What her doing?
Mommy Daddy go work.
How him break that?

In the course of normal development, children learn the rules of syntax and morphology long before they learn the exceptions to the rules. As a result, they may make frequent errors as they apply the rules inappropriately. Examples may include errors, such as *"I got stang by a bee"* or *"I have two fishes."* Since in this case the child has learned a rule and is applying it in a novel situation, these errors actually represent very good language learning. Therefore in preschool- and early-school-aged children, regularizing irregular noun and verb forms is part of the normal developmental process and is not characteristic of a language disorder.

E. Finally, the *use* of language is referred to as *pragmatics.* Children with pragmatic disorders do not understand certain basic rules of conversation, such as the following:

* A conversation begins with a greeting.
* All of one's utterances must relate to the topic at hand.
* The speaker needs to let the listener know if he or she is changing the topic.
* All pronouns should be referenced before using them.
* A conversation is based on what the listener knows.
* Conversation and responses should be appropriate for the situation.
* A conversation is ended in a certain way, usually by saying "bye."

Children who have difficulty with pragmatics may have clear speech and normal sentence structures. However, they may not reference the topic or even pronouns in their conversations. Their comments are often off the topic or even socially inappropriate. Understanding the message that they are trying to convey may be difficult because they do not give enough (or even appropriate) information to make sense.

Children with pragmatics problems also have difficulty understanding subtle or inferred meaning or the speaker's communicative intent. For example, the sentence *"Could you please pass the salt?"* is actually a command and does not require an affirmative answer. Expressions or idioms, such as *"Two heads are better than one,"* may be interpreted literally, with no understanding of the deeper meaning.

F. Causes of language disorders include hearing loss, mental retardation, environmental deprivation, or neurologic damage or dysfunction. The term *aphasia* refers to an acquired language disorder resulting from neurologic damage.

III. Screening for Communication Disorders

Routinely screening all preschool children for speech and language problems is important, particularly for those between the ages of 2 and 5 years. An informal screening assessment can be done by the physician or nurse and can usually yield enough information to make a decision regarding the need for referral (Table 44.2). Speech and language can be screened informally by use of the following means:

- Ask the child to point to certain objects or to follow certain commands.

Table 44.2. Sentences for articulation and language screening

Have the child repeat these sentences while noting articulation and language errors.

p	Popeye plays putt putt.
b	Buy baby a bib.
m	My mommy makes lemonade.
w	Wade in the water.
y	You have a yellow yo yo.
h	He has a big horse.
t	Take teddy to town.
d	Do it for Daddy.
n	Nancy is not here.
k	I eat cake and ice cream.
g	Go get the wagon.
ng	Put the ring on her finger.
f	I have five fingers.
v	Drive a van.
l	I like lollipops.
s	I see the sun in the sky.
z	Zip up your zipper.
sh	She went shopping.
ch	I eat cherries and cheese.
j	John told a joke to Jim.
r	Randy has a red fire truck.
th	Thank you for the toothbrush.
blends	Splash, sprinkle, street

- Listen to the child's spontaneous speech while he is talking to a parent or playing.
- Elicit communication by saying such things as the following:
  What do you want to be when you grow up? Why?
  What does a (fireman) do?
  Tell me how you make a peanut butter and jelly sandwich.
  Explain the game of baseball to me.
- Have the child repeat words or sentences, such as those listed in the articulation and language-screening test noted in Table 44.2. Even in repeating, the child will use his own form of articulation and will usually revert to his own form of syntax and morphology.

Finally, the physician can screen for communication problems merely by interviewing the parents regarding their observations and concerns. The physician might ask the parents questions, such as the following:

- *Do you have any concerns regarding your child's communication abilities?*
- *Do you understand your child's speech all the time, most of the time, some of the time, or hardly at all?*
- *How well do strangers understand his or her speech?*
- *When your child is talking, how many words does he or she put together at a time?*
- *Does your child leave out words in the sentence?*
- *Is your child talking as well as other children his age?*
- *Have your child's communication skills improved in the last 3 months?*

Parents are usually very good observers of their own children and can often effectively compare their child's communication skills with those of siblings or peers. A simple rule of thumb is that if the parents are worried about their child's speech or language development, a referral for evaluation is usually appropriate.

Once screening is completed, the child's communication skills should be compared with what is expected at the child's developmental level. If the child seems delayed in development or demonstrates any of the problems noted in Table 44.3, the physician should evaluate for any medical problems that could cause or contribute to the communication disorder. Once this evaluation is complete, a referral should be made to a speech/language pathologist for complete assessment and intervention.

IV. Referral for Treatment

If a communication disorder is suspected or if the child does not have prerequisite skills for normal communication, then a referral should be made to a speech/language pathologist for evaluation and treatment. Speech/language pathologists are found in hospitals, private practice, health care agencies, home health, and school settings.

The prerequisites of speech and language development, particularly feeding skills, can be evaluated and treated in infancy. At that age, the speech/language pathologist may work directly

Table 44.3. Indications for referral

12 Months
Quiet infant who seldom cooed or babbled.
Quiet with limited vocalizations.
Infant doesn't vocalize with consonant sounds (such as *b*, *m*, *d*, and *n*).
Infant shows evidence of significant feeding problems.
Development of motor milestones appears significantly delayed.

18 Months
Uses mostly vowel sounds and gestures for communication.
Does not use any meaningful single words.
Cannot follow simple commands.
Cannot point to body parts or common objects following a verbal request.

2 Years
Does not combine words for short utterances (e.g., *"Get doggie. Go bye bye."*).
Cannot follow two compound commands (e.g., *"Go get your shoes and give them to Daddy."*).

3 Years
Child does not communicate with complete sentences.
Sentences are short, telegraphic, or incomplete.
Child echoes parts of questions or commands rather than responding appropriately.
Speech is usually hard to understand.
Many omissions of consonants in speech.

4 Years or Older
Sentence structures are noticeably defective and short.
Child frequently uses words inappropriately.
Child has difficulty expressing ideas or conveying what happened in an event.
Speech is somewhat difficult to understand, especially by strangers.

6 Years
Child has difficulty producing any speech sounds.

Any Age
Speech or language development is delayed in comparison to peers of the child's age.
Child is embarrassed by or self-conscious about his or her speech.
Abnormal number of dysfluencies are noted and have persisted over many months.
Voice is abnormal in pitch, quality, or resonance.
Child has difficulty with feeding or swallowing.

with the infant or may prescribe a treatment program for the parents to use at home. At any age, the speech/language pathologist can provide parents with developmentally appropriate activities for use in stimulating speech and language development in the home. Although begun earlier in certain cases, formal speech and language therapy is most commonly started around the age of 2 or 3 if problems persist.

V.   Timetable for Intervention

Early intervention is very important for children with communication disorders and can ultimately affect the long-term prognosis for normal communication skills. Intervention is best started during the preschool years. At this time the brain is particularly receptive to speech and language learning, which is why normal children are able to learn a foreign or second language much faster than their parents. Since this is a critical period for normal speech and language learning, intervention for communication disorders should be done at this time to take advantage of this receptivity to speech and language learning.

Early intervention is also important because of the strength of habit. Since speech and language skills are used every day, patterns of communication become strongly habituated early in development. If those patterns are faulty, they become harder to change as the child grows older due to the habit strength factor.

Finally, early intervention is important since a communication disorder can affect a child's social and emotional development and can seriously impair the child's ability to learn in school. The goal of therapy in the preschool years is to correct or to improve the communication disorder as much as possible so that the child is prepared to handle all communication, academic, and social challenges once he or she enters school.

ADDITIONAL READING

Bzoch KR, League R. *Receptive-expressive emergent language scale.* Gainesville, FL: Computer Management Resources; 1991.

Capute AJ, Accardo PJ. Linguistic and auditory milestones during the first two years of life. *Clin Pediatr* 1978;17:847–853.

Capute AJ, Shapiro BK, Palmer FB. Marking the milestones of language development. *Contemp Pediatr* 1987;4:24–41.

Coplan J. Normal speech and language development: an overview. *Pediatr Rev* 1995;16:91–100.

Emerick LL, Haynes WO. *Diagnosis and evaluation in speech pathology,* 3rd ed. Englewood Cliffs, NJ: Prentice Hall; 1986.

Glascoe FP. Can clinical judgment detect children with speech-language problems? *Pediatrics* 1991;87:317–322.

Kummer AW. Assessment of speech and language disorders. In: Cotton RT, Myer III CM, eds. *Practical pediatric otolaryngology.* New York: Lippincott Raven; 1999.

National Deafness and other Communication Disorders Advisory Board. Research in human communication. NIH Publication No. 92–3317, Bethesda, MD: National Institute on Deafness and Other Communication Disorders; 1991.

Office of Scientific and Health Reports. *Developmental speech and language disorders. Hope through research.* NIH Publication No. Pamphlet 88–2757, Bethesda, MD: National Institute of Neurological and Communicative Disorders and Stroke; 1988.

Olswang LB. Developmental speech and language disorders. *Asha* 1993;35:42–44.

Ruben RJ. Communication disorders in children: a challenge for health care. *Prevent Med* 1993;22:585–588.

Web Site

http://www.asha.org/publications (American Speech and Hearing Association Web Site)

45 ♣ Childhood Stuttering

Irving L. Wollman and Ann W. Kummer

The ability to communicate with ease, without attention to the actual mechanics of one's speaking, is something that most people do quite naturally and automatically. However, for an estimated 3 million people, this function is most unnatural. For them, communication discomfort may range from slight to severe and can have a profound impact on their social, emotional, and physical states. These feelings or perceptions of discomfort are at the heart of "stuttering" and cause many people to develop negative attitudes about themselves, their speech, and oral communication in general. For some, such feelings are not easy to resolve, even over time. What presents as a rather benign, almost inconsequential mistake of early speech learning develops into a significant problem that has the potential to continue throughout the individual's lifetime.

As children between the ages of 2 and 5 develop both motorically and linguistically, they often experience periods of disruption during speech production. These disruptions are commonly referred to as **speech dysfluencies—speech that is characterized by interruption in the forward flow of the intended message.** Dysfluencies occur in a variety of forms and are often inconsistent in young children. Some types of dysfluencies are quite normal and ultimately resolve without assistance from parents or professionals. Other types of dysfluencies, those that are considered true "stuttering" behaviors, are different and may require professional attention.

The purpose of this chapter is to describe contributing factors to the onset and development of stuttering, to differentiate characteristics of normal dysfluency versus characteristics of stuttering, and most important, to describe key characteristics to identify for making a decision on when and how to refer children to a speech/language pathologist if stuttering is suspected.

I. Causes and Contributing Factors

If many children experience dysfluencies during the early ages of language development, then what causes some children to begin stuttering while others are able to speak fluently? Unfortunately, exactly what causes stuttering to develop in some children and not in others is not known. Certain conditions have been found to coincide with the onset of stuttering; however, being exposed to these conditions does not always result in stuttering. Therefore one may safely assume that other, unknown factors may contribute to the development of stuttering.

We do know that the population of people who stutter is heterogeneous. Numerous studies have shown that children who stutter do not differ from their peers in terms of intelligence, physical development, or personality factors. Stuttering runs in families, although the exact method of genetic transmission remains unknown. Even though genes make a difference, many children whose parents stutter develop normal speech; and many children who stutter do not have a family history of stuttering. Stuttering is most likely to occur in males, but females who stutter are at greater risk of having children who stutter than are males who stutter. Furthermore, cases of sudden onset of stuttering have been known to occur under conditions that involve emotional distress (e.g., absence of one or both parents, moving to a new location, starting a new school, death or a serious illness in the family, or hospitalization of the child or of a sibling). In these cases, the likely cause is that the cumulative impact of the environmental stressors, in combination, affects the motor speech system in a manner that results in fluency breakdown.

II.   Onset and Development

As mentioned earlier, a child's speech fluency between the ages of 2.5 and 5 years is largely dependent upon his or her developing motor systems and the child's capacities to learn and organize language effectively and efficiently. Added to those variables is the function of the environment and its role in the child's life. The interaction between a child's given capacities and the nature of his or her environment has been determined to be the critical component in the onset and later development of stuttering in young children.

For some children brief periods of dysfluency may emerge, then increase and diminish in response to specific environmental factors, such as fatigue, excitement, and a rush to speak. Additionally, these dysfluencies may persist for weeks or months and then decrease significantly until a child's developing capacities are mature enough to handle those normal life stresses that precipitate speech breakdown. Typically, these children and their families do not react negatively to the speech disruptions, and they ultimately resolve. For other children the early periods of dysfluency may be similar but may occur with greater frequency and may last longer. Affected to a greater degree by environmental factors, they may begin to notice the "mistakes" in their speech and to react to them negatively. Others in their immediate environment may also respond in a like manner, reacting in ways that cause development of a negative awareness or attitude about speech. When this response occurs, the likelihood that stuttering will develop is increased.

III.   Differentiation Between "Normal" and "Abnormal" Speech

Over the years researchers and clinicians have developed a variety of behavioral classifications to distinguish stuttering from normal developmental dysfluencies. The terminology varies among researchers, academicians, and clinicians, but in general the differentiation rests largely upon the size of the fragmented speech event. According to Zebrowski, "Measuring the types of dysfluencies produced by a stuttering child can help the clinician determine the severity of stuttering as well as the likelihood that the child will require speech/language therapy." Gregory and Hill differentiate a "more typical" type of speech breakdown (non-stuttered event) from "less typical" (stuttered) speech breakdown in children and adults. Others use terminology that reflects the actual way in which a word is broken up. Conture's classification of within- and between-word breakdown provides a meaningful description of the way in which normal or developmental types of speech breakdown can be differentiated from abnormal or stuttered speech (Table 45.1).

The first category, **between-word dysfluencies,** represents large fragmentations of speech that are present in the speech of all speakers and are considered quite normal. Types of between-word dysfluencies include revisions, phrase repetitions, multisyllabic whole-word repetitions, and interjections. Revisions occur when there is a change of thought (e.g., "*He went, she went to the store*"). Repetition of phrases, such as "*I want . . . I want to get that toy,*" and multisyllabic whole-word repetitions, as in "*She can come because . . . because her mom said she could,*" are considered between-word dysfluencies. Interjections are pauses in thought filled with words, such as *um, ah,* and *uh.* An example could include the sentence "*When can I um play with that?*" The fact that children will demonstrate these speech behaviors more often than adults is merely a reflection of their developing linguistic, motor, and cognitive systems and the nature of processing in less mature speakers.

Table 45.1. Types of dysfluencies

Type	Example
Between-Word Dysfluencies*	
Revision	*He went—She went to the store.*
Phrase repetition	*I want I want to get that toy.*
Multisyllabic whole-word repetition	*She will come because because her mom said she could.*
Interjection	*When can I um play with that?*
Crossover Behaviors	
Monosyllabic whole-word repetition	*I I I want to play with that.*
Less Typical/Within-Word Dysfluencies†	
Syllable repetitions	*Mo mo mo mommy is coming soon*
Sound repetitions	*T T Tomorrow is my birthday.*
Prolongation—audible	*W—e are leaving in the morning.*
Prolongation—inaudible (Block)	*(‡We) We are leaving in the morning.*
Multicomponent dysfluency	*We w—e we will be going home soon.*

*Often found in normal speech.
† Often characteristic of stuttering.
‡ Denotes placement of the articulators for production, but without sound production.

The second category of speech breakdown, **within-word dysfluencies,** consists of smaller units of fragmentation and is considered "less typical" or less normal speech; it is more consistent with true stuttering. These dysfluencies reflect more than just processing or language interference and clearly differ from the breakdowns observed in children's normally developing speech. Within-word dysfluencies are considered the core stuttering behaviors. These speech behaviors are believed to be abnormal and reflective of the child's development of a negative reaction to the difficulty he or she is having moving through words. Types of within-word dysfluencies include syllable repetitions, sound repetitions, audible and inaudible prolongations, and multicomponent dysfluencies.

Several types of repetitions can occur in speech. As noted earlier, phrase repetition and multisyllabic whole-word repetition are considered "more typical" dysfluencies. However, sound repetitions (e.g., "*T-T-T-Tomorrow is my birthday.*") and syllable repetitions (e.g., "*Mo-mo-mo-mommy is coming soon.*") are the most common types of "less typical" or within-word dysfluencies. These smaller types of fragmentation are varied in the number and rate at which they are produced. Monosyllabic whole-word repetitions (e.g., "*I-I-I-want to play with that.*"), on the other hand, are referred to as "crossover behaviors." These can also be grouped in the within-word dysfluencies category, although differentiation should be made between those that are produced unevenly and with irregular tempo and those produced casually and with even rate (e.g., "*Can I have . . . have some juice?*"). If the rate is rapid and the tempo irregular, Gregory and Hill consider these "crossover behaviors" that may signify the emergence of stuttering.

Prolongations (audible or inaudible) of individual sounds are also observed in the speech of children who stutter. Audible prolongations occur when the speech sound is lengthened. An example is "*W–e are leaving in the morning.*" Inaudible prolongations are also referred to as "blocks" and occur when the posture of the lips, tongue, or other articulators becomes fixated in an attempt to modify the stuttering pattern but emits no sound. Such prolonged speech segments are typically viewed as a more advanced stage of the fluency disorder. Researchers agree that prolongations of either audible or inaudible type are a child's attempt to "cope with" or to hold back the repetitive mistakes in his speech, which in all likelihood appeared at an earlier stage of the disorder. According to Guitar and Conture, children who consistently demonstrate these behaviors may "begin to exhibit longer and more physically tense speech behaviors as they respond to their speech difficulty with embarrassment, fear, and frustration." The duration of these prolonged segments varies and becomes an index of severity. Therefore, both the number and the duration of repeated or prolonged elements are critical factors when determining the extent or severity of the problem.

Another factor that differentiates normal from abnormal speech is the presence of tension. As Wall and Meyers stated,

"When identifying characteristics reflective of the differentiation between normal and abnormal dysfluent events, cardinal potency seems to be associated with greater tension, greater self-awareness, and greater negative feelings associated with communication." Tension may be observable in the facial area, such as eyes, lips, jaw, or neck area. Extraneous bodily movements are also worth noting when assessing the severity or degree with which a child may be attempting to cope with an inability to move forward in his speech. Further elements that may indicate the presence of stuttering include changes in pitch and loudness, obvious signs of tremor, fear, and an effort to avoid the possibility of a stuttered event as well as the use of multicomponent dysfluent behavior. The presence of struggle or observable tension is therefore a diagnostic sign that should be considered significant. Although in some cases these behaviors are present at onset, in most they occur as the disorder begins to progress.

The presence of these observable (surface) behaviors in the speech of children who stutter can be clearly differentiated from normal nonfluent behavior. The importance of making this distinction early can have a long-term impact upon the ultimate severity of the problem and the prognosis for recovery. Differential diagnosis is the key to effective early intervention. For clinicians the ability to determine whether a child's dysfluencies are normal or abnormal is critical. Too often parents report that the pediatrician, the teacher, or family members urged them not to worry about the child's stuttering, even though the child had significant early-warning signs as early as 2.5 years of age. Parents desperately want to believe that their child is okay. When professionals ease their worries with a platitude, such as "Ignore it, he will outgrow it," many listen. Later, when the child is enrolled in stuttering therapy after many years of chronic dysfluencies, they often report feeling guilty or angry for not heeding their instincts that the stuttering was not "normal."

Certainly, the variability of speech behavior among young children will continually cloud our decision making regarding the presence or absence of incipient stuttering. In addition, the question of whether or not a particular child will spontaneously recover without treatment is not one that can be answered with any degree of accuracy. However, with attention to the danger or warning signs in a child's speech patterns, greater probability exists of minimizing the development of a chronic, long-term problem.

IV. **When to Refer**
    A. **When the child appears to be frustrated or fearful regarding the quality of his or her speech production.**
    B. **If parents express concern about their child's speaking difficulties.**
    C. **If the child exhibits any of the danger or warning signs as outlined above.**
    For additional resources, see Table 45.2.

Table 45.2.   Resources

American Speech-Language-Hearing Association
10801 Rockville Pike
Rockville, MD 20852
(301) 897-5700

National Stuttering Project
2151 Irving Street, Suite 208
San Francisco, CA 94122-1609
(415) 566-5324
(800) 364-1677

Stuttering Foundation of America
PO Box 11749
Memphis, TN 38111-0749
(800) 992-9392

ADDITIONAL READING

Conture EG. *Stuttering*, 2nd ed. Englewood Cliffs, NJ: Prentice Hall; 1990.

Gregory H, Hill D. Differential evaluation-differential therapy for stuttering children. In: Curlee R, ed.: *Stuttering and related disorders of fluency.* New York: Thieme Medical Publishers; 1993.

Guitar B, Conture E. *The child who stutters: to the pediatrician.* Stuttering Foundation of America Publication, No. 23. Memphis, TN: The Stuttering Foundation of America; 1991.

Starkweather CW, Gottwald SR, Halfond M. *Stuttering prevention: a clinical method.* Englewood Cliffs, NJ: Prentice Hall; 1990.

Van Riper C. *The nature of stuttering,* 2nd ed. Englewood Cliffs, NJ: Prentice Hall; 1982.

Wall MJ, Myers FL. Assessment of childhood stuttering. In: Wall MJ, Myers FL, eds. *Clinical management of childhood stuttering.* Austin, TX: PRO-ED; 1995.

Walton P, Wallace M. *Fun with fluency: direct therapy with the young child.* Bisbee, AZ: Imaginart International; 1998.

Zebrowski PM. Duration of the speech dysfluencies of beginning stutterers. *J Speech Hearing Res* 1991;34:483–491.

Web Site

www.mankato.msus.edu/dept/comdis/kuster (Stuttering Home Page)

46 ♣ Temper Tantrums and Breathholding Spells

Janet R. Schultz

Temper tantrums tend to occur in children between 12 months and 5 years of age, peaking between 18 and 48 months. Although not all children have the "lay-down-and-kick-and-scream" variety of tantrum, most have some angry outbursts that their parents see as tantrums. One study showed that 15% of parents report that their 1-year-olds have tantrums every day. Another suggested that children who have daily tantrums at 2 years of age are likely still to have frequent tantrums at 3 and that a third of them continue to have tantrums at 4 and 5 years of age. Boys have a slightly higher incidence, according to some studies. An estimated 5% of children who "throw fits" incorporate breathholding spells in their tantrums. The prime candidates for recurrent tantrums are those 10% of children whose temperament is sometimes described as "difficult" or, more positively, "spirited." These children often have a history of head banging and head bumping at earlier ages and tend to express desires and needs in physical ways. Delays in verbal development may increase the likelihood of tantrums by limiting more acceptable means of getting needs met.

I. Preventing Tantrums
***Teaching tasks:* To learn to manage frustration and to express anger in nonhurtful, nonviolent ways.**

In the toddler years, the goal should be to prevent tantrums rather than to figure out the best response to them. Generally, the tantrums occur when the child is particularly frustrated by limits set on his behavior, by those placed on him by his own development, or by the challenges of his environment.

Parents should begin problem solving by charting all temper tantrums for several days. They should keep track of the day, time, place, person(s) present, activity at the time of the tantrum, and the ultimate result of the tantrum. Usually patterns will emerge from these observations. Commonly, they indicate that the tantrums occur most often at a specific time of day. This time of day should be evaluated in terms of hunger, fatigue, and changes in the environment, such as a decrease in availability of the caregiver (e.g., during dinner preparation) or an increase in activity and competition for attention (e.g., older children coming home from school). The circumstances of the tantrum should also be examined for sources of frustration operating at the time (e.g., teasing or bullying by a sibling).

Whatever the pattern, it provides information as to how to prevent some of the tantrums. Snack or nap times may need to be altered, and plans for entertaining small children while the parent is otherwise occupied may need to be made. Often better environmental engineering ("baby-proofing") needs to occur to reduce the frequency of the child's frustration. Parents learn to pay attention to the pattern and, using their own observations of the child's behavior, to detect when tension is mounting. They may then be able to prevent tantrums by distracting the child to a less frustrating or safer activity. At other times, children may simply need more physical outlets for their energy. Verbal children need to be coached on how to put their desires and reactions into words; then parents must at least be willing to listen. Generally, the use of routines, warnings of approaching transitions (e.g., *"In a few minutes, we will have to stop playing and go pick up Jimmy from school."*), and use of **limited** choices (e.g., *"Do you want your bunny or your tiger to sleep with you?"* rather than *"Are you ready for nap now?"*) are helpful in preventing tantrums.

Often tantrums in public places are related to timing (e.g., trying to fit in one more errand before lunch), the situation itself (surrounded by a store full of interesting things that can't be touched), and often boredom. In stores, temper tantrums can often be prevented by not exceeding the toddler's tolerance, by interacting with the child frequently, and by providing something interesting to hold, play with, and/or eat.

II. Responding to Tantrums

When tantrums cannot be prevented, the parent should try to appear calm and businesslike. In general, unless the child is endangering himself or encroaching substantially on the rights of others (e.g., screaming and kicking in church), the best approach is to reduce the positive outcomes (attention) of tantrums and ignore the negative behavior (e.g., leaving the room in which the tantrum is occurring). This approach means not giving in to the demands of or paying attention to the child during the tantrums. If this step is necessary, the child can be moved out of the public venue (e.g., grocery or church) to a car or less busy location. In this circumstance, the parent should still keep cool and, as soon as the child is moved, resume ignoring the behavior. When the child is calm, the parent has the opportunity to talk about other ways to ask for things or to handle anger/frustration.

Children should not be allowed to hurt anyone, including the parent, during the tantrum. To prevent injury, the parent may have to hold the child and to restrict the movement of the arms and legs during the tantrum, but without positive interaction (e.g., holding the child on the parent's lap, face out, without speaking during the tantrum). The intensity of children's own feelings often scares them. When a child later realizes that he or she has done something genuinely hurtful, he or she may be more frightened. The tantrum may also undermine the child's sense of security in parents' ability to protect.

Many children respond well to positive attention, cuddling and soothing *after* the tantrum, but the attention should be restricted to following the tantrum rather than as a means for stopping the tantrum. Otherwise, the child may learn to get this special attention by throwing tantrums.

III. Breathholding Spells

Although relatively uncommon, breathholding spells are extremely effective for scaring parents, especially at the initial occurrence. Mainly they are seen in toddlers, especially those with high activity levels and poor frustration tolerance. Anything that triggers tantrums can trigger breathholding spells.

A. What they look like. Usually the child is angry and screaming, perhaps in the course of a more typical tantrum with crying. Eventually the child takes a deep breath as if to scream more but holds it. His face goes from bright red to grayish blue. At this point, in an uninterrupted spell, the child's eyes may roll up; then his whole body stiffens before he slumps unconscious. Alternatively, some children, especially in response to the precipitants of trauma or fright, develop extreme pallor and bradycardia, hold their breath, and become syncopal without becoming cyanotic. Following either type of breathholding spell, a brief period of twitching or clonic movements may occur.

B. What to do. Like other tantrum behaviors, prevention is better than response. Following the same problem-solving procedure as for regular tantrums can inform the parents of the patterns and associated states, which they can then alter before the tantrum occurs. More often, parents are so frightened that they begin "walking on eggs" with the child and avoid setting limits, denying requests, or allowing anyone else to frustrate the child. In the long run, this avoidance leads to significant behavioral problems or to the child being considered "spoiled." Diverting and redirecting the child may be one, less problematic strategy, but not all situations can be handled that way. Common parental responses, such as shaking or smacking the child or throwing cold water on him or her, are ineffective and dangerous. Parents should manage the spell by laying the child down on the floor to prevent falling and then waiting it out. When the child wakens, parents must resist fussing over the child, which provides secondary gain and encourages recurrent episodes. While breathholding spells are involuntary initially, 3- and 4-year-olds learn to use them deliberately to manipulate their parents if they get a desirable outcome in the early days.

C. Parent education. Part of treatment should include reassuring parents that children do not have breathholding attacks in the absence of precipitating events and an audience, so they can be left alone in the crib at night without danger. For reassurance many parents also need to know that the child's reflexes will save him from anoxic damage even if he passes out from the breathholding. (The gray-blue color before the child passes out almost always alarms parents.)

ADDITIONAL READING

Chess S, Thomas A. *Temperament in clinical practice.* New York: Guilford Press; 1986.

Needlman R, Howard B, Zuckerman B. Temper tantrums: when to worry. *Contemp Pediatr* 1994;6:12–34.

Parker S, Zuckerman B. *Behavioral and developmental pediatrics.* Boston: Little, Brown; 1995.

Books for Parents

Crary E: *Without spanking or spoiling: a practical approach to toddler and preschool guidance.* Seattle: Parenting Press; 1979.
Leach P. *Your growing child.* New York: Knopf; 1989.
Patterson GR. *Living with children.* Champaign, IL: Research Press; 1976.

Websites

www.parentsoup.com
www.genesishealth.com
www.healthyideas.com/children

47 ♣ Thumbsucking

Janet R. Schultz and Victoria Meier

Teaching tasks: **To help children develop the ability to soothe themselves in a variety of ways and to give up thumbsucking beyond its developmental appropriateness.**

Thumbsucking is one of the common habits of children that evokes considerable parental concern, especially for parents of children more than 3 years of age who practice this habit in public places. Thumbsucking is a normal behavior in young children, although some popular press authors have portrayed it as a sign of insecurity or of poor relationship with parents. However, the general consideration is that it is a soothing behavior, most common when the child is tired, bored, worried, or generally upset.

I. Prevalence of Thumbsucking

Thumbsucking has been observed as early as the prenatal period as evidenced in prenatal ultrasound images. After birth, it is often not seen for the first few months because of the lack of motor skill necessary to bring the hand to the mouth reliably. While reliable statistics do not exist, the estimation is that more than one-third of normal children suck their thumbs and that as many as 10% to 20% continue, at least occasionally, until after 6 years of age. A very few persist into middle or late adolescence, and some even into adulthood.

II. Developmental Peaks of Thumbsucking

The two highest intensity periods of thumbsucking behavior are at 7 to 8 months (the intensity of the behavior at this age is heard in the "popping" sound from the release of suction when the thumb is forcibly pulled out of the child's mouth) and near 18 months. These ages are not good times for intervention in the habit or for attempts to stop the behavior.

III. Risks of Thumbsucking

A. Thumbsucking is mostly harmless, especially if stopped before 5 years of age.

B. Like any hand-to-mouth behavior, thumbsucking can increase the risk of lead ingestion if the child has lead paint dust on his or her hands from environmental sources. Avoidance of environmental lead is the most effective intervention for preventing lead poisoning.

C. Like any hand-to-mouth behavior, thumbsucking can increase the risk of infection if the child's hands are not kept clean. This risk increases if toilet hygiene is not monitored by an adult or if the child plays in the dirt.

D. If thumbsucking does not end before permanent teeth erupt, an increased risk of problems with dental alignment exists. However, many children suck their thumbs past the age of 5 years without disrupting alignment, and most children who require braces were not long-term thumbsuckers.

E.   Older children face a social risk of isolation or being called a "baby" for their thumbsucking.
IV.   **A Sign of Emotional Distress?**
 A.   Yes, if it develops after 2 years of age, unless it follows the removal of access to a pacifier.
 B.   Yes, if it becomes more pronounced in frequency or in the number of settings in which it occurs.
 C.   Yes, if it emerges or returns in the face of a major life change or stress.
 V.   **Formal Intervention for Thumbsucking**
 A.   Interventions should not begin before the age of 5 years.
 B.   The child who is motivated to stop should be encouraged to quit. If the child does not want to stop, then he or she can and probably will circumvent almost anything the parent chooses to do to prevent the behavior.
VI.   **Interventions to Stop Thumbsucking, in Order of Invasiveness**
 A.   Recruiting the child into participating in any treatment is key. The child has to want to stop before success is likely.
 B.   Some children may maintain their habit because of the attention it brings. Having parents ignore thumbsucking may help discourage the behavior. For some children, getting attention when they are not sucking can be beneficial. For others the attention may backfire. Punishment should be avoided, as it increases tension, which contributes to the behavior.
 C.   Often, when efforts at reducing thumbsucking have been ineffective, a no-attention moratorium that lasts for 4 to 6 weeks is enough to give everyone a rest. If not enough to reduce sucking, the time is still useful because it may contribute to effectiveness of other interventions subsequently employed.
 D.   When behavioral interventions, such as the preceding are not effective, awareness enhancement should be the next step. The unpleasant-tasting paint-on substances can be used as a reminder, not as punishment. Another way to remind the child is a Band-Aid on the thumb. The child may help select a patterned Band-Aid or may decorate it himself with colored markers. An additional option is to wrap the Band-Aid around the child's thumb, sticking the two adhesive sections to each other so that a small tab or "flag" is formed. This too can be decorated. The tab is much more noticeable to the child who puts the thumb in the mouth. A mitten or glove can also be worn, especially to bed, if the child is willing.
 E.   The next step is parental monitoring and rewarding the child for time without thumbsucking. Charts with stickers, stars, or smiling faces can be used to make the

monitoring concrete to the child. Oppositional behavior may increase transitionally but tends to fade rather rapidly. Rewards should be small, based on sucking-free recognizable periods of time ("dinner to bedtime"); they work best when decided upon by the child in conjunction with the parent. Special time with a parent, such as playing a game that normally "takes too long," is a good alternative to other, more tangible treats.

  F.   The child can often benefit from learning an alternative behavior that is incompatible with thumbsucking. For example, when the child has the urge to suck his or her thumb or when awareness enhancement makes the child aware of sucking, he or she could make a fist with the thumb tucked inside, sit on his or her hand, or participate in an activity that requires both hands. With help from the parent, the alternative can be done earlier and earlier in the process (e.g., when the child's hand nears the mouth rather than enters it).

  G.   Another option is stimulus control, where the child is allowed to suck only under certain conditions. This works best with daytime suckers. If a child wants to suck his or her thumb during activities other than going to sleep, he or she is allowed to suck only while sitting in a designated place, such as on the stairs or on his or her bed. This place should remove the child from the main flow of household events.

  H.   At the same time deterrent strategies are employed, children with thumbsucking behaviors should be taught to comfort themselves in other ways. New relaxation strategies include imagining a favorite story, TV show, or event; talking or drawing a picture about an upsetting event; or holding on to a comforting object, such as a favorite toy.

  I.   Referral to a pediatric dentist to insert an intraoral appliance to prevent sucking may help if the child is interested but is having difficulty losing the habit despite his or her best effort.

  J.   Referral to a pediatric psychologist specializing in behavioral approaches may also help parents carry out the necessary activities.

ADDITIONAL READING

Ellingson SA, Miltenberger RG, Stricker JM, et al. Analysis and treatment of finger sucking. *J Appl Behav Anal* 2000;33:41–52.

Friman PC, Leibowitz JM. An effective and acceptable treatment alternative for chronic thumb- and finger-sucking. *J Pediatr Psychol* 1990;15:57–65.

Johnson E, Larson B. Thumb-sucking: literature review. *J Am Soc Dent Child* 1993;60:385–391.

Books for Parents

Mayer CA, Brown BE. *My thumb and I: a proven approach to stop a thumb or finger sucking habit for ages 6–10.* Glenview, IL: Chicago Spectrum Press: 1997.

Norman Van R, Van Norman RM. *Helping the thumb-sucking child: a practical guide for parents.* New York: Avery Publishing; 1999.

Websites

Thumbsucking: http://yourhealth.com

Thumbsucking: http://users.forthnet.gr/ath/abyss/dep1409.htm

48 ♣ Toilet Training

Janet R. Schultz

Teaching tasks: To teach the child to recognize his or her body's physical cues for the need to empty the bowel and bladder and to maintain continence of bowel and bladder until the potty chair or toilet can be used for evacuation.

I. Readiness

Although having the first child on the block to be toilet trained seems important for a parent's self-esteem, the ability to be toilet trained is largely dependent on the child's overall developmental level. Even the most skillful trainer cannot teach a child to initiate independent toileting reliably if the child is not ready.

Generally, a child is ready for toilet training in the 24- to 36-month age range. The child should be showing interest in the task before the training is begun in earnest as readiness depends on motor, cognitive, and emotional maturation. The following screening items are useful for determining if a child is ready for toilet training. The child should be able to accomplish at least eight out of the following 10 items:

A. Point to his or her body parts when asked. These include the following parts:
1. *Eyes.*
2. *Nose.*
3. *Mouth.*
4. *Hair.*

B. Respond appropriately to verbal instructions to do the following:
5. *Sit down in a chair.*
6. *Stand up.*
7. *Walk with the parent to a particular place* (e.g., another room).
8. *Imitate the parent in a simple task* (e.g., play pat-a-cake).
9. *Bring the parent a familiar object* (e.g., one of his toys).
10. *Place one familiar object with another* (e.g., "Put your teddy bear by the book").

II. Training Techniques.

The child should be trained for daytime dryness and cleanliness before attempting nighttime training. Many children who have regular bowel movements find it easier to master bowel control first because bowel movements are less frequent and give the parent and child more warning. Constipation complicates learning and may contribute to a child's refusal to use the toilet or potty for defecation. Children can learn to control bowels and urination in either order or together.

The training is often easier if a child-sized potty is available that the child can get used to by sitting on it fully clothed. Then it can be placed in the bathroom, where the child is encouraged to sit on it while older siblings and parents use the toilet (child can be clothed or unclothed). Once the child is comfortable with the potty, he should be told (not asked) at intervals convenient to the caregiver (45 minutes to an hour), that "it is time to go" and should be brought to sit on the potty. To facilitate bowel training, parents should capitalize on the gastrocolic reflex and have the child sit after meal(s). The parents can also add sitting times when behavioral signals of impending defecation are noted. Part of preparation for toilet training is noting behavior in children that predicts urination or defecation (e.g., becoming quiet, straining or turning red in the face, passing flatus, noticing a specific time of day or timing near an event, such as bath time).

The child should be praised for sitting and praised again if he has a result in the potty. Stickers, star charts, and small candies can help the process. If the child does not produce, he should be encouraged (*"maybe next time"*) and should not be made to sit more than a few minutes. If sitting slightly longer seems to help, then the parent should come prepared with books or toys to keep the sitting time pleasant. Parents should not punish for "accidents," since this is a skill-building time, not a struggle of the wills.

Some children virtually train themselves, given proper equipment and access; others take months to learn these skills. Children who are reluctant or very verbal often benefit from such books as Mr. Rogers' book about toileting.

Parents generally find easier to teach a boy to urinate sitting down first and then to move to standing. Child potties usually have "splashguards" to accommodate male anatomy.

III. Diapers and Training Pants

Diapers can be used during this training period, but generally the use of training pants facilitates learning. They are easier for the child to lower independently, and they give quicker feedback about wetness. Some diaper services have training pants if parents do not want to wash them themselves. Of course, disposable training pants, which have the advantage of being able to be ripped down the sides and removed like diapers if the child soils them, are available. In warm weather, allowing the child to remain naked from the waist down sometimes makes training easier, albeit messier.

Diapers can still be used at night during training, and if they are not used during the day, the child makes the discrimination between expectations relatively readily.

If the parents and children go out during training, the parents should keep sitting schedules and should vigilantly watch for nonverbal (or verbal, if they are lucky) clues that the child needs to visit a bathroom. They should come prepared with extra clothes and should react calmly to accidents. Many novices are more comfortable if their parents bring a portable potty seat along.

By 36 months of age, around 80% of children are dry reliably through the daytime. Almost all children who do not have urologic problems or major developmental delays are dry during the day in time for school. However, nighttime dryness may come later.

ADDITIONAL READING

Azrin N, Fox R. *Toilet training in less than a day*. New York: Simon and Schuster; 1974.

Brazelton TB. A child-oriented approach to toilet training. *Pediatrics* 1962;29:121–128.

Matson JL, Ollendick TH. Issues in toilet training normal children. *Behav Ther* 1977;8:549–553.

Schmitt, B. *Your child's health*, rev. ed. New York: Bantam Books; 1991.

Books for Parents/Children

Frankel A. *Once upon a potty*. Hauppage, NY: Barron's Educational Series, Inc.; 1980.

Leach P. *Your baby and child*. New York: Knopf; 1978.

Rogers F. *Going to the potty*. New York: Penguin Putnam Books for Young Readers; 1997.

Website

http://www.parentsoup.com

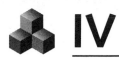

IV

Miscellaneous Topics in Pediatric Primary Care

49 ♣ Telephone Medicine in Primary Care

Raymond C. Baker

The telephone is an indispensable tool for the pediatrician and other providers of primary health care to children because it provides an instantaneous network with worried parents, hospital staff, pharmacies, and laboratories. Since telephones represent such a necessary aspect of a physician's practice, physicians, nurses, and receptionists, as health professionals and telephone users, must realize the importance of learning how to optimize their time on the telephone to the advantage of both patient and provider. Similar to the formal training medical professionals receive in the direct provision of services to patients, training in the efficient use of the telephone as part of patient care should also be an integral part of the professional's education.

I. Telephone Triage in the Primary Care Physician's Office

Because the telephone is such an integral part of any efficient primary care office, defining roles for office personnel in the management of incoming telephone calls is important. In most circumstances the receptionist or another nonmedical person takes the call initially in order to triage and redirect according to need. Nonmedical issues (e.g., appointments, billing information, travel directions, insurance issues, prior authorization) are usually handled by the receptionist, either directly or by transferring the call to another nonmedical staff member or department. Calls for medical advice are usually referred to an office nurse to answer. An alternative approach for some of the medical advice calls is providing the receptionist with written guidelines for certain straightforward medical information, which she can address with the parent. Examples of problems she could tackle include immunization and well-child visit schedules, immunization side effects and their management, and over-the-counter (OTC) medication doses.

The office nurse manages most incoming calls for medical advice, based on experience, written guidelines, such as those outlined in the telephone triage and advice books cited in the "Additional Reading" section of this chapter, and/or specific training, usually from the physician group in the office. An important part of the nurse's discussion with the caregiver is the decision regarding which patients require a physician's visit or which calls should be forwarded to the physician to handle.

Calls triaged by the nurse to the physician should occur according to a prearranged schedule. Several options exist, depending on physicians' schedules for the day, number of physicians in the group, and the season of the year. Some physicians take calls all day long between patients; others prefer to batch calls and to answer them at defined times, such as half-hour time slots, specifically written into the schedule two or three times per day.

After-hours calls are typically directed to the on-call physician via an answering service or by electronic means through specialized telephone services. A good answering service will usually provide some degree of triage and will redirect nonmedical calls to regular business hours. Medical calls, though, are usually directed to the physician. The prudent physician will develop some system for educating his patients on how (and when) to call the physician. The most effective means of doing this is to have the office staff provide written materials at enrollment in the practice and to reinforce these guidelines as part of routine anticipatory guidance during well-child care. Some physicians also recommend books to parents that address common problems and offer telephone guidelines, such as those developed by the American Academy of Pediatrics (see "Books for Parents and Caregivers" at the end of this chapter).

Recently, some urban areas of the country have begun to offer centralized, city- or regionwide after-hours call coverage for medical advice calls. These fee-for-service programs are usually staffed by nursing personnel who manage patient problems using written guidelines either from books or, more recently, from computerized algorithms. An example is the computerized system based on medical algorithms by Dr. Barton D. Schmitt at The Children's Hospital in Denver, Colorado (After Hours Care Program). These centralized programs have the advantages of consistency, individualization to specific practices, immediate notification, and reliable written documentation. In other cities, individual hospitals have contracted nursing personnel to provide this service and have opened the service up to other hospitals and practices for a fee.

II.   Elements of an Effective Telephone Encounter

Most parents are far more concerned about their child than they are about the hour of the day or about what the physician may be doing—even when the call comes after hours. Also, the parent's conception of an urgent call may be very different from that of the physician. Therefore the physician must answer each call with the same degree of empathy and interest, without being judgmental or negative. Issues regarding the appropriate use of the telephone are better addressed proactively as part of anticipatory guidance parents are given during well-child care (should be reinforced with written information).

The physician must also limit the length of the telephone encounter. A telephone encounter should rarely exceed 3 to 4 minutes. If the problem takes longer than this to resolve, an office visit is probably needed. In the real world, time availability and economic issues dictate the length of time spent on the telephone. Whether the primary care physician charges a fee for telephone advice is variable; most pediatricians do not. In most settings, given the realities of managed care, private insurance, and Medicaid, charging is rarely an option.

The elements of the effective telephone encounter are the following:

TELEPHONE ENCOUNTER FORM

Date: _____   Time: _____

Caller Name: _____   Tel: _____

Patient Name: _____

DOB: _____ Age: _____

Problem: _____

_____

_____

_____

Advice: _____

_____

_____

_____

_____ MD

Figure 49.1.   Sample telephone interview documentation form.

1. Obtaining biographic/demographic information on the patient and patient caregiver.
2. Exploring the medical problem.
3. Making a presumptive diagnosis.
4. Giving the parent medical advice.
5. Closing.

In most circumstances, all this information must be obtained to determine adequately the most appropriate disposition and treatment for the child and, at the same time, document that information for medicolegal purposes. In practices with multiple physicians, documentation is especially important to keep a running record of each child's care. In the office, the chart may be available at the time of daytime calls, so documentation can be put directly into the record. During nonbusiness hours the on-call physician often finds that having a form to carry is convenient. An example of a simple telephone documentation form is shown in Fig. 49.1. The telephone documentation form has the added advantage of prompting the care provider to discuss the necessary information. This reminder is especially important for nonphysicians and for physicians in training.

   A.   Biographic/demographic information about the child can be obtained at any time during the call,

although the parent will usually volunteer most of the information during the course of the conversation. Information not given must be asked for by the end of the encounter. Since the parent is most anxious to talk about the child's problem, the physician initially may ask only for the child's name and age and may then proceed with the problem and advice. The remainder of the information can be obtained at closure, by saying to the parent something like, "*I need a little information about your child so I can put what we've talked about this evening into his medical record.*" Biographic/demographic information needed for records includes the following:

1. *Date and time of the call.*
2. *Name and age of the child.* For documentation purposes, the first and last name of the child are required. The age of the child will influence the line of questioning that relates to the complaint.
3. *Identifying feature of the child.* To add the telephone encounter documentation to the child's medical record, at least one identifying feature of the child must be obtained. In most private offices and nonhospital clinics, the name and date of birth are adequate for this purpose. For patients who are followed in hospital clinics where a hospital medical record exists, the medical record number is the distinctive feature. Most nonprivate sources of health care provide the parent with some sort of identification card that usually has the necessary personalized information on it (if the parent can find it!).
4. *Telephone number of the parent or guardian who is placing the call.* This is necessary in case you need to recontact the parent (e.g., call back to check progress, medication instructions after speaking with the pharmacy, after speaking with consultants) at a later time.

B.   Exploring the medical problem. Evaluating the medical problem and giving appropriate advice is similar to an ill visit in the office or clinic, but shorter. The physician should begin the conversation by introducing himself or herself and asking the parent about the problem (e.g., "*Hello. This is Dr. Baker from the Primary Care Clinic. How may I help you?*"). The physician should listen while the parent explains the problem and should then become more directive by asking specific questions to clarify the illness or problem. Specific information the physician will need to determine disposition includes the following:

1. *Specific symptoms* and how long they have been present.
2. *How the child is coping with the illness* (e.g., feeding, playing, sleeping, urine output). How sick the child appears to the parent.
3. *What the parent has already done for the child;* how this has helped.

4. *Pertinent positives* to rule in the most likely diagnosis.
5. *Pertinent negatives* to rule out serious illnesses.
6. *A brief past medical history* if the child's medical record is not available. The past medical history can usually be obtained with a few brief questions:

- *Is the child on any medications right now?*
- *Does the child have any chronic illnesses?*
- *Is the child allergic to any medicines?*
- *Has the child been in the hospital recently?*
- *Has the child been exposed to any illnesses recently?*

C. Making a presumptive diagnosis. After exploring the medical problem with the caregiver by means of both the abbreviated history of the present illness and the past medical history, the physician can usually make a presumptive diagnosis, either as a specific diagnosis (e.g., viral respiratory infection, acute gastroenteritis) or as a sense of the degree or seriousness of the illness. In either case, the physician can now determine the need for a physician encounter.

D. Medical advice. The medical advice the physician gives must address three issues:

1. *The need to be seen by a medical care provider for the illness.* In general, three levels of urgency must be considered.

a. ***Immediate visit.*** For the child with a serious illness who requires an immediate evaluation, the physician must decide whether the child has

(1) **A life-threatening condition that is unstable requiring immediate transportation by lifesquad to an emergency facility** (e.g., active seizure, unresponsive patient, respiratory distress with cyanosis or altered sensorium).

(2) **A life-threatening condition that is stable requiring immediate transportation by the parents in standard transportation to an emergency facility** (e.g., asthma attack without cyanosis, broken extremity).

(3) **A potentially serious illness that can be seen in the office as an ill-add-on** (e.g., high fever).

Sometimes the decision about whether the child can be seen in the office or if he needs to go to an emergency facility is affected by the time of day (if support personnel are available in the office), the degree of laboratory and radiologic work-up that might be necessary, and the comfort level of the physician who would be seeing the child in the office as an add-on. The physician may also give the parent some first aid suggestions to do before leaving for the emergency facility or while waiting for the lifesquad. An example follows:

With the symptoms you are describing, it sounds to me like Johnny might be pretty sick. Why don't you bring

*him in right now for me to look at and see what's wrong.
Since he has such a high fever, give him a teaspoon of
acetaminophen elixir and undress him down to his
shorts. That way, by the time you get here, his fever
should be starting to come down.*

b.   ***Next-day ill add-on.*** Many illnesses require a
physician's visit for diagnostic and treatment reasons,
but the visit can be delayed until the following day. In
most situations, the physician should give the parent
some advice about the interim care of the child until
the visit. For example, the physician might say the
following:

*It sounds to me like I need to take a look at Johnny to
see if he might have an ear infection. I can see him first
thing tomorrow morning. In the meantime, I think you
can make him feel better by giving him 1 teaspoon of
ibuprofen suspension every 5 or 6 hours to keep his fever
down and to relieve his ear pain. Also make sure he
drinks plenty of fluids while he's feeling bad, even if he
doesn't feel much like eating.*

c.   ***Routine appointment.*** A routine appointment in
the next 1 to 2 weeks is usually appropriate for the child
with behavior problems, school problems, and so on,
which will require an extensive history and perhaps contact with outside agencies (such as the school). An example of how to handle this situation follows.

*Mrs. Jones, this sounds like a problem we need to sit
and talk about for awhile. Why don't you call our office
tomorrow morning and make an appointment for next
week for me to see you and Johnny? Tell the receptionist
you need a half-hour appointment. That will give us time
to figure out how to help you and Johnny with his fighting. We'll want to talk about how he is doing with his
school work too.*

2.   *Home therapy.* The second issue to be addressed, for
children who do not require a physician encounter, is management of the child at home. Most primary care physicians who have been in practice for any length of time will
have developed an armamentarium of home procedures,
home remedies, and over-the-counter (OTC) medications
that parents can use in the home. Some of these are specific medications designed to relieve symptoms; others fall
into the category of "giving the parent something to do for
the child while he recovers on his own." Chapter 54, "Symptomatic Therapy of Children," in the companion volume of
this book (*Pediatric Primary Care: Ill-Child Care*) provides
the medical care provider with several treatments that can
be given in the home.

3.   *Explanation of the illness.* The third issue that the
physician must cover with parents is a brief explanation of
the illness, including the expected course and situations

(complications) that would require recontacting the physician. For infectious illnesses, the physician should give the parent infection control suggestions to prevent spread of the illness and a time for sending the child back to school or day care.

It sounds to me like Johnny has a nasty chest cold. Chest colds are usually caused by viruses, which unfortunately don't respond to antibiotics. However, there is a medicine you can give him that will help decrease his congestion so he can sleep a little better. Do you have a pencil and paper? Pick up some Sudafed at the drugstore. It doesn't require a prescription. Give him 1 teaspoonful every 4 hours. Also you might want to check his temperature twice a day or when he feels warm. If his temperature is over 102, you can give him three chewable acetaminophen tablets every 3 to 4 hours to bring his fever down and help him feel better. He needs to stay home from preschool until his temperature has been normal for 24 hours, so he won't give his cold to the other children. If he gets an earache or a sore throat or still has a fever in 2 days, give me a call back.

E. Closure. At the conclusion of the conversation, the physician should ask if the parent has any more questions, should provide some reassurance to the parent, and should arrange a call-back time if appropriate.

I'm glad you called me about Johnny. It sounds like he isn't feeling very well right now, but if you give him the cold medicine and keep a close eye on him, he should be able to recover at home and feel better in a few days. If he's not better in 2 days or if he gets worse, give me a call back.

III. Prescribing Medications Over the Telephone

A difficult part of providing pediatric telephone advice as part of night and week-end call responsibilities is responding to pressures from caregivers to prescribe medications based on telephone consultations. In general this practice is not recommended — no telephone conversation can take the place of an actual patient encounter and physical examination to make a definitive diagnosis. However, circumstances exist in which the physician may consider prescribing medications based on a telephone conversation with the parent. This assumes follow-up for more definitive care. Access to the medical record is helpful to guard against telephone advice abuse in the patient who regularly misses or cancels appointments.

A. The most common situation in which the physician prescribes medications over the telephone is to offer symptomatic therapy for common complaints. Examples are cold preparations and nonnarcotic pain/antipyretic medications. Since some of the managed care companies pay for OTC medications if a prescription has been written, to call in prescriptions for cold preparations, acetaminophen, and ibuprofen is reasonable for the physician under these circumstances.

B. Another example is the situation in which parents can do the definitive physical examination themselves and with the help of the physician make a definitive diagnosis. Examples are head lice and perhaps monilial diaper dermatitis, oral thrush, and tinea corporis. Pediculocides, nystatin cream/suspension, and topical lotrimin may be prescribed by telephone in these circumstances if the physician is comfortable with the diagnosis.

C. Prescribing antibiotics over the telephone is usually not appropriate. However, in the circumstance where a family member has recently been diagnosed with streptococcal pharyngitis (including a documented positive throat culture or streptococcal antigen) and another child in the family develops symptoms of sore throat and fever, many physicians will prescribe appropriate antibiotics over the telephone.

D. Other situations in which a prescription by telephone may be considered are

1. *Patients known to the physician who have a chronic illness requiring chronic medications.* Examples are asthma medications, steroid cream for eczema, and prophylactic antibiotics for urinary tract infection (UTI) or otitis media.

2. *Patients as in Section II in whom a definitive diagnosis can be made over the phone, such as conjunctivitis, swimmer's ear, or acute otitis media with perforation.* This practice is not recommended routinely, but if the parent is known to the physician and is reliable, this may be considered under some circumstances.

ADDITIONAL READING

Baker RC, Schubert CJ, Kirwan KA, et al. After-hours telephone triage and advice in private and nonprivate pediatric populations. *Arch Pediatr Adolesc Med* 1999;153:292–296.

Brown JL. *Pediatric telephone medicine: principles, triage, and advice,* 2nd ed. Philadelphia: JB Lippincott; 1994.

Kempe A, Dempsey C, Poole SR. Introduction of a recorded health information line into a pediatric practice. *Arch Pediatr Adolesc Med* 1999;153:604–610.

Melzer SM, Poole SR. Computerized pediatric telephone triage and advice programs at children's hospitals. *Arch Pediatr Adolesc Med* 1999;153:858–863.

Poole SR, Schmitt BD, Carruth T, et al. After-hours telephone coverage: the application of an area-wide telephone triage and advice system for pediatric practices. *Pediatrics* 1993;92:670–679.

Schmitt BD. Calls about sick children; launching your own triage system. *Contemp Pediatr* 1998;15:49–71.

Schmitt BD. Calls about sick children: a triage system for the office. *Contemp Pediatr* 1998;15:138–152.

Schmitt BD. *Pediatric telephone advice,* 2nd ed. Philadelphia: Lippincott-Raven; 1999.

Schuman AJ. Is there a pediatric call center in your future? *Contemp Pediatr* 1998;15:75–93.

Yanovski SZ, Yanovski JA, Malley JD, et al. Telephone triage by primary care physicians. *Pediatrics* 1992;89:701–706.

Books for Parents and Caregivers

American Academy of Pediatrics Staff. *Caring for your adolescent ages 12 to 21.* Elk Grove Village, IL: American Academy of Pediatrics; 1991.

Schmitt BD. *Your child's health,* rev. ed. New York: Bantam Books; 1991.

Schor EL, ed. *Caring for your school-age child: ages 5–12.* New York: Bantam Books; 1996.

Shelov SP, Hannemann RE, eds. *Your baby's first year*, reprint ed. New York: Bantam Books; 1998.

Shelov SP, Hannemann RE, DeAngelis CD, eds. *Caring for your baby and young child: birth to age 5*, rev. ed. New York: Bantam Doubleday Dell; 1998.

50 ♣ Computers, the Internet, and the Primary Care Physician

Raymond C. Baker

If any technologic advance marked the end of the millennium, it was surely the introduction of the computer as a personal device. The personal computer industry has expanded exponentially and influenced so many areas of our everyday lives that just keeping up-to-date with computer capabilities, let alone the technology itself, is difficult. With all the medical technologic advances that have been made during the same time, that the field of medicine has been quick to take advantage of computer technology is no surprise. Although the initial computer applications in medicine were in equipment, such as CT and MRI scanners, the personal computer is now embraced by practicing physicians to help them keep up-to-date with expanding medical literature, improve communications, streamline billing and patient databases, and teach patients and physicians in training. This chapter will focus on exploring the many applications of computer technology and the internet in the primary care setting and on providing additional reading materials that expand these applications and give specific means of accessing the "information superhighway."

I. Hardware and Software

Computers and internet access have become very affordable because of the intense competition among computer manufacturers and software companies. Purchasing a state-of-the art computer system that includes the computer base with CD-ROM drive, modem, monitor, printer, and start-up software for less than $3,000 is now possible. Additional equipment needed with medical applications might include a scanner and digital camera. Internet access via the computer is available at a monthly cost of about $20 and allows instant access to medical resources far beyond the scope of most university library systems. Within the near future, another common component of the personal computer will be the digital video disk, or DVD, which can show extended video on the computer screen (e.g., lectures, procedure demonstrations, movies).

Several variables must be considered when purchasing and installing the initial system. These variables depend on how the computer will be used—the kinds of applications (or software programs) that will be run. The following features/variables can be found in affordable systems and allow optimal running of software programs and internet travel.

A. Speed, a function of the microprocessor. Speed becomes an important feature as experience on the computer increases.

B. Size of the hard drive. The hard drive provides storage space for software programs and data. Modern computers measure their hard drive size in gigabytes (1 gigabyte = 1,000 megabytes). Large hard drives are needed if large databases will be managed on the computer (e.g., research data, patient data).

C. RAM (random access memory), the memory the computer uses to run applications (software programs). A larger amount of RAM allows several programs to run simultaneously (e.g., word processing program, database management program, and internet connection).

D. Modem. The modem is the hardware that translates computer language into the digital output transmitted by telephone wire. Its speed is measured in kilobytes per second transmission rate or baud. The faster the speed, the faster data can be transmitted—an important feature if the computer's use is anticipated to be retrieving photographs or streaming video.

E. Internet service provider (ISP)—multiple ISPs are available in most communities (e.g., MSN, AOL). Choice depends on price (most are in the range of $20 per month with unlimited time, although some charge by the hour). Internet speed can be greatly enhanced by an asymmetric digital subscriber line (ADSL) at an added cost if available in the area.

Software needs are completely dependent on how the computer will be used. Most computer stores include standard software already loaded on the computer when selling the computer; standard software includes programs for word processing, database management, and internet connection. Additional software may be purchased for more specialized applications in the office setting, such as scheduling, billing, and records. Computer hookup requires only an electrical outlet, a surge protector (which usually comes with the computer) for protection of the computer's circuitry in the event of an electrical surge, and a telephone line. In most circumstances, no special expertise is necessary to set up a computer; a newly purchased computer is ready for action within 2 or 3 hours of unpacking. Most large stores dedicated to computer sales and many colleges with adult-oriented classes offer instruction in both computer and software use.

II. Use of the Computer and Internet in the Primary Care Office Setting

The computer and internet have wide applications for the primary care provider. Four areas of use are common in the office setting: communication, teaching and learning, administrative/secretarial tasks, and, perhaps most important, information access (for both physicians and patients).

A. Communication. Electronic mail, or E-mail, is communication between two or more computers. Both the internet and three types of E-mail have applications in the primary care setting:

1. *One-to-one E-mail with communication between two users.* Examples are appointment reminders to patients

from a receptionist, relaying results of blood work from a physician to a patient, or receiving results from a laboratory (physician).

2. *Group E-mail with communication between one user and a group of others on a mailing list.* An example is a regular meeting reminder to the membership of a physician's society from the president.

3. *List server.* In this variation on group E-mail, the group leader, designated the list server, sends messages to the group as above. An added feature is that any member of the group can post a message to the mailing list and the message is distributed to all members of the group. An example of a list server is a group of physicians serving on an Injury Prevention subsection of the state medical society where the chairman of the group develops the list server.

4. *Internet communication.* Synchronous (real-time chat room) and asynchronous (bulletin board) communication is a function of the internet that has application for the primary care physician. An example would be an internet site for parents to ask questions of a physician (e.g., http://www.kidsdoctor.com/) or a site where physicians participate in discussions on-line (e.g., International Pediatric Chat at http://www.pedschat.org).

B. Teaching and learning. Many applications in software or on the internet exist for teaching and learning (for both physicians and parents):

1. *Software applications.* One example is the Pediatric Advisor by Dr. Barton D. Schmitt, which prints handouts for parents about a wide range of pediatric topics. Handouts can be customized and modified.

2. *Interactive instructional compact discs (CDs).* An example is an interactive patient case simulator.

3. *Streaming audio and video via the internet.* Examples are viewing grand rounds from the local medical center or attending a lecture as part of a distance-based college course.

C. Administrative/secretarial functions. The personal computer has multiple applications for administrative and secretarial functions in the primary care office, ranging from billing to creating a newsletter for the practice's parents. All these functions can be performed on the personal computer systems described earlier with appropriate software, which is readily available commercially.

1. *Appointments.*

2. *Registration of patients* (demographics, insurance information).

3. *Patient billing.*

4. *Letter communications.*

5. *Patient information databases.*

6. *Customer satisfaction surveys.*

7. *Practice newsletter.*

D. Information access.

1. *Internet web sites with current medical information for physicians.* The lists that follow are neither comprehensive nor necessarily superior, but they are examples of some of the many informational web sites currently available. Although most are free to the user, some require subscription or registration to access them.

a. ***Comprehensive general pediatrics sites*** with textbooks, journals, patient education materials, policy statements and clinical practice guidelines, evidence-based medicine resources, case studies, professional organizations, internet directories, and search engines.

- [http://www.generalpediatrics.com]—pediatric
- [http://www.mdconsult.com]—adult and pediatric
- [http://www.medmatrix.org]—adult and pediatric
- [http://www.jhu.edu/peds/neonatology]—pediatric
- [http://www.uab.edu/pedinfo]
- [http://www.aap.org/bpi]

b. ***Subspecialty information***

- ADHD [http://www.oneaddplace.com/]
- Adolescent [http://www.education.indiana.edu/cas/adol/adol.html]
- Allergies/asthma [http://allergy.mcg.edu/] and [http://www.aaaai.org/]
- Asthma [http://www.ama-assn.org/special/asthma/] and [http://www.nhlbi.nih.gov/nhlbi/lung/asthma/prof/asthgdln.htm]
- Consumer Product Safety Commission [http://cpsc.gov/]
- Derm Atlas [http://www.derma.med.uni-erlangen.de/index_e.htm]
- Genetic Conditions [http://www3.ncbi.nlm.nih.gov/omim/]
- Growth/Development [http://www.odc.com/anthro/deskref/desktoc/html]
- HIV Infection [http://www.pedhivaids.org/]
- Infectious Diseases [http://www.cdc.gov/] and [http://www.immunofacts.com/]
- Intensive Care [http://PedsCCM.wustl.edu/]
- Metabolic Diseases [http://www.SSIEM.org.uk/]
- Neonatology [http://neonatal.peds.washington.edu/]
- Neurology [http://www.aan.com/]
- Oncology [http://www.oncolink.upenn.edu/specialty/ped_onc/]
- Ophthalmology [http://.med-aapos.bu.edu]
- Pharmacology [http://www.pdr.net]
- Sports Medicine [http://www.physsportsmed.com/journal.htm]

c. ***Professional organizations***

- American Academy of Pediatrics [http://www.aap.org]
- Ambulatory Pediatrics Association [http://www.amb-peds.org/]
- American Academy of Pediatric Dentistry [http://www.aapd.org/topics.html]
- American Board of Pediatrics [http://www.abp.org/]
- Communicable Disease Center [http://www.cdc.gov]

d. ***Medical Literature Searches***

- National Library of Medicine (including Medline) [http://igm.nlm.nih.gov/]
- The Cochrane Library—Evidence Based Medicine database [http://www.cochranelibrary.com/clibhome/clib.htm]

e. ***Addresses and Telephone Numbers***

- [http://www.anywho.com/resq.html] Tel. no. from name
- [http://www.anywho.com/telq.html] Address from tel. no.

f. ***Locating a Physician***

- [http://www.ama-assn.org/aps/amahg/htm]

g. ***Medical News***

- [http://www.cnn.com]
- [http://www.businesswire.com]
- [http://www.yahoo.com]
- [http://www.infoseek.com]

h. ***Alternative Medicine***

- [http://cpmcnet.columbia.edu/dept/rosenthal/Data-bases.html]

2. *Internet web sites with current medical information for parents / patients:*

- General [http://www.ama-assn.org/KidsHealth] and [http://www.mayohealth.org/mayo/common/htm/preg pg2.htm]
- Asthma [http://www.ama-assn.org/special/asthma/]
- Ophthalmology [http://.med-aapos.bu.edu]
- Diabetes [http://www.childrenwithdiabetes.com]
- Down Syndrome [http://www.ds-health.com]
- Infectious Disease (ID) [http://www.health.state.ny.us/nysdoh/consumer/commun.htm]
- HIV/AIDS [http://www.pedaids.org/]
- Immunizations [http://www.immunize.org/]
- Consumer Product Safety Commission [http://cpsc.gov/]

ADDITIONAL READING

Hunt DL, Jaeschke R, McKibbon KA. Users' guides to the medical literature: using electronic health information resources in evidence-based practice. *JAMA* 2000;283:1875–1879.

Izenberg N, Lieberman DA. The web, communication trends, and children's health. Part I: Development and technology of the internet and web. *Clin Pediatr* March 1998:153–157.

Izenberg N, Lieberman DA. The web, communication trends, and children's health. Part II: The web and the practice of pediatrics. *Clin Pediatr* April 1998:215–221.

Izenberg N, Lieberman DA. The web, communication trends, and children's health. Part III: The web and health consumers. *Clin Pediatr* May 1998:275–285.

Johnson KB, Feldman MJ. Medical informatics and pediatrics. *Arch Pediatr Adolesc Med* 1995;149:1371–1380.

Johnson KB, Lehmann CU. Extend your clinical reach with the internet. *Contemp Pediatr* 1999;16:67–85.

Pusic MV. Pediatric residents: Are they ready to use computer-aided instruction? *Arch Pediatr Adolesc Med* 1998;152:494–498.

Saneto RP. The information highway for the pediatrician: an understanding of the internet for the clinician. *Clin Pediatr* September 1997:505–512.

Schuman AJ. Pediatricians in cyberspace: an internet update. *Contemp Pediatr* 1996;13:65–78.

Spooner SA, Anderson KR. The internet for pediatricians. *Pediatr Rev* 1999;20:399–409.

Spooner SA. On-line resources for pediatricians. *Arch Pediatr Adolesc Med* 1995;149:1160–1168.

Spooner SA. The pediatric internet. *Pediatrics* 1996;98:1185–1192.

51 ♣ Ethical Issues in Pediatric Primary Care

Christine L. McHenry

Ethics is a systematic reflection of right character and/or right conduct in a given situation. Ethics uses principles, rules, virtues, and values as guides in this systematic reflection. When these principles, rules, virtues, or values conflict, an ethical dilemma exists.

Recognizing ethical dilemmas is fairly easy in areas where medical technology is used, such as the newborn intensive care unit or the pediatric intensive care unit, and where questions about withholding or withdrawing life-sustaining treatment arise. In primary care pediatrics practicioners tend not to confront ethical dilemmas as frequently. Nevertheless, ethical dilemmas do exist in this area, and primary care providers must be sensitive to the possibility that they will arise. The following points address several issues that are commonly seen in both the inpatient and outpatient arenas of pediatric primary care.

I. Informed Consent

The concept of informed consent is based on the ethical principle of respect for persons and, more specifically, of respect for autonomy. Respect for autonomy asserts that all individuals with decisional capacity have the right to make their own decisions. Everyone has the right to informed consent.

A. The process of informed consent consists of the following components:

1. *An individual with decisional capacity.*
2. *Disclosure of information to this individual, including:*
   a. ***The individual's condition*** (diagnosis and prognosis).
   b. ***Nature and purpose of the proposed treatment.***
   c. ***Risks and benefits of the proposed treatment.***
   d. ***Alternative treatments.***
   e. ***Consequences if the proposed treatment is not accepted.***
   f. ***Names of the health professionals who are to perform any procedure.***
3. *Assessment of the individual's understanding of the information.*
4. *Assessment of the individual's appreciation of the information* (i.e., what does the information mean in relation to the individual's life plan?).
5. *The individual's voluntary agreement to treatment or nontreatment.*
6. *The individual's authorization to proceed with treatment.*

B. Exemptions to informed consent. The following are exemptions to informed consent:

1. *Emergencies. Example:* A patient comes to the Emergency Department in an unconscious state and in need of medical treatment.

2. *Waivers. Example:* The individual with decision-making capacity specifically says that he or she does not want to know.

3. *Therapeutic privilege. Example:* The physician intentionally withholds information from a patient with cancer because the physician thinks the information may harm the patient. This exception is controversial and should not be used frivolously.

II. Informed Permission

Only an individual with decision-making capacity may consent to medical care for himself or herself. In pediatrics, physicians commonly turn to the parents (or the legal guardian) of their patients for permission to treat. Informed permission also is based on the principle of respect for persons but, even more specifically, on protection of the vulnerable. In general, society believes that parents are in the best position to determine what is in the best interest of their child. The "best interest" concept involves the principles of beneficence and nonmaleficence; that is, balancing the benefits and risks of a proposed medical intervention with the hope of promoting the welfare of the child. The informed permission process is the same as the informed consent process.

III. Religious Exemptions

The First Amendment of the Constitution grants us religious freedom. This religious freedom gives freedom of belief and of practice as long as the practice does not infringe upon the rights of or potentially harm an innocent third party. In general, adult patients with decision-making capacity have the right to reject recommended treatment based on religious or other convictions. A dilemma arises, however, when parents reject recommended treatment for their children based on their religious convictions. Parents are required to provide "adequate" medical care for their children; if they do not, they face potential criminal charges under state child abuse and neglect statutes. How the term *adequate* is defined varies from situation to situation.

A. Religious exemptions for treatment. When parents refuse medical treatment for their child based on religious conviction, the conflict for the physician is between wanting to respect the parents' wishes to raise their child according to their religious beliefs and doing what the health care provider believes is in the best medical interest of the child. How this conflict is resolved depends upon the nature of the illness (minor versus life-threatening), the prognosis with and without recommended treatment, and the nature of the recommended treatment (conventional versus experimental).

B. Religious exemptions for immunizations. When parents bring their healthy child to a physician for well-child care and refuse immunizations based on religious convictions, preservation of the relationship with the parents should take precedence over trying to coerce them into agreeing to the immunizations. The physician should use this time to educate the parents about the recommended immunizations. If this is done in a nonthreatening manner, the parents are more likely to bring their child back for medical care. If, on the other hand, an epidemic of a preventable childhood disease is spreading and other children have been seriously ill or died, then serving the child's best interest might require the doctor to obtain a court order to immunize the child. A frequently asked question in the outpatient setting is, "What about immunizations for school?" The requirements vary from state to state; therefore the physician must familiarize himself or herself with the state's statute regarding religious exemptions for immunizations and admission to public school.

IV. Confidentiality

Confidentiality is based on the ethical principle and rule of respect for autonomy and fidelity. To treat illness more appropriately and to promote the health of their patients, physicians need access to personal, sometimes intimate information. Patients or parents will be more likely to share such information if they know it will be kept confidential. Confidentiality can be violated by deliberately disclosing this confidential information to another without the person's permission or by handling carelessly the information.

A. Justified infringements to confidentiality. The following areas are justified infringements to maintaining confidentiality:

1. *Obligation to obey the law.*
    a. **Reporting child abuse, elder abuse, gunshot wounds, stab wounds, sexually transmitted diseases.**
    b. **Emergencies.**
    c. **Certain legal proceedings**, such as a malpractice claim.
2. *Obligation to protect the welfare of the community.* (Confidentiality may be breached to protect an innocent third party if the individual who may be harmed is identifiable, the harm to be averted is serious, and disclosure is the necessary minimum for protecting the third party.)
3. *Obligation to protect the individual.* (In this case, the individual must present a clear danger to himself or herself.)

B. Areas of heightened confidentiality. Areas of heightened confidentiality are usually specified by state statute. Examples include the following:

1. *Drug and alcohol rehabilitation.*
2. *Psychiatric treatment.*
3. *Minors seeking birth control and abortion* (in some states).
4. *HIV infection.*

V. Children and Decision Making

Frequently asked questions about children and decision making are the following:

- How much say should a minor patient have in controlling his or her health care?
- What should be done if the child and the parents disagree?

Obviously, the amount of participation and decision making by the child varies, depending on the nature of the decision and on the cognitive, moral, and personality development of the child. Ideally, as the child matures, he or she assumes more decision-making responsibility. Physicians should familiarize themselves with the concepts of the mature minor and the emancipated minor.

A. Mature minors are individuals 14 years of age or older who have decision-making capacity. That is, they are capable of understanding their diagnosis and prognosis, the risks and benefits of proposed treatment, and the consequences if they refuse treatment. Mature minors are capable of giving informed consent to the same degree as an adult. If the treatment does not involve serious risk (e.g., treatment for a streptococcal pharyngitis), then the mature minor has the right to consent to such treatment without parental permission. A mature minor would not, however, have the right to consent to treatment that involves serious risk (e.g., cosmetic surgery or organ transplantation) without the permission of the parent or guardian.

B. Emancipated minors are individuals under the age of 18 years who are living on their own without parental support and who are not subject to parental control. Historically, certain groups of individuals have been considered emancipated. They include minors in the military, married minors, and, in some states, minors who are pregnant or have a child. In addition, college students living on their own may be considered emancipated even if they are dependent on their parents to pay the bills. Emancipated minors are considered adults in the medical arena, and therefore parental permission is not required for treatment.

V. Gifts from Industry Representatives

The moment someone enters the medical profession he or she is confronted with the question of whether or not to accept gifts from industry representatives. These gifts range from a free pen to a free trip at a vacation resort, the cost of which is passed on to the patient. Obviously, industry representatives would not present health care professionals with gifts if this practice were not profitable on a larger scale. Such gifts have been shown to influence prescribing habits of physicians. The conflict is clear—industry's interest in earning a profit versus the physician's interest in promoting what is best for the patient. The question for all health care professionals is whether any gifts from industry should be accepted, even something as minor as a pen or a notepad. Or are certain gifts, such as drug samples for patients, acceptable? Health care providers must choose for themselves how they will answer this question. Asking themselves "Would you want your arrangements with an industry representative generally known to your colleagues and to your patients?" may help some doctors trying to make this decision.

ADDITIONAL READING

American Academy of Pediatrics, Committee on Bioethics. Informed consent, parental permission, and assent in pediatric practice. *Pediatrics* 1995;95:314–317.

American Academy of Pediatrics, Committee on Bioethics. Religious objections to medical care. *Pediatrics* 1997;99:279–281.

American Medical Association, Council on Ethical and Judicial Affairs. Code of Medical Ethics. *Current Opinions with Annotations* 1998–1999 edition. Chicago, IL: American Medical Association; 1998.

American Medical Association, Council on Scientific Affairs. Confidential health services for adolescents. *JAMA* 1993;269:1420–1424.

Beauchamp TL, Childress JF. *Principles of biomedical ethics,* 3rd ed. New York: Oxford University Press; 1989.

Chren MM, Landefeld S, Murray TH. Doctors, drug companies, and gifts. *JAMA* 1989;262:3448–3451.

Etkind P, Lett SM, Macdonald PD, Silva E, Peppe J. Pertussis outbreaks in groups claiming religious exemptions to vaccinations. *Am J Dis Child* 1992;146:173–176.

Holder AR. *Legal issues in pediatrics and adolescent medicine,* 2nd ed. New Haven: Yale University Press; 1985.

Holder AR. Minors' rights to consent to medical care. *JAMA* 1987;257: 3400–3402.

King NMP, Cross AW. Children as decision makers: guidelines for pediatricians. *J Pediatr* 1989;115:10–16.

Landwirth J. Religious exemptions in child abuse law. *Inf Dis Child* December 1989:14–15.

Margolis LH. The ethics of accepting gifts from pharmaceutical companies. *Pediatrics* 1991;88:1233–1237.

Midwest Bioethics Center Task Force on Health Care Rights for Minors. Health care treatment decision-making guidelines for minors 1995;11:A1–A16.

Ross LF, Aspinwall TJ. Religious exemptions to the inmmunization statutes: balancing public health and religious freedom. *J Law Med Ethics* 1997;25:202–209.

Sigman GS, O'Connor C. Exploration for physicians of the mature minor doctrine. *J Pediatr* 1991;119:520–525.

Wazana A. Physicians and the pharmaceutical industry. Is a gift ever just a gift? *JAMA* 2000;283:373–380.

52 ♣ Enhancing the Child/Parent/Provider Relationship in Primary Care Pediatrics

Lisa M. Vaughn

Primary care pediatricians must form an alliance with parents and children for the mutual goal of caring for children. Working together in a cooperative relationship will yield optimal results for all involved and will ultimately increase the health and well-being of children. In pediatrics primary care providers are often in a unique position as the only regular professional contact for a family. The changes in the health care system have brought a greater focus on financial issues and on increasing patient volume for physicians. This emphasis has led to concerns that patient care is in danger of being compromised. In pediatrics the relationship with the family takes on added significance because of the dependent role of children and the resources required to address the parent/child constellation, which can often involve extended family members, peers, and teachers.

The power of a pediatrician's caring, sensitive, positive relationship with parent and child can influence the family, making its members more likely to accept a practitioner's treatment and advice. The research literature suggests that if physicians build positive relationships with their patients, positive outcomes, such as improved patient satisfaction and compliance and fewer appointment cancellations, occur. In the current milieu of health care, individual autonomy and costs of care have become increasingly important. To quote Balint, these changes "must be based on mutual understanding in an evolving, caring, and dynamic relationship that must include the family. . . . Educated patient autonomy and responsibility supported by beneficence, trust, and some degree of guidance consistent with the educational and advocative roles of the physician will be necessary features of this partnership." According to a survey of the patient/physician relationship in America by Moise (1999), patients believe that the three most important things their providers can do to establish a positive working relationship are (a) provide fast and efficient medical treatment, (b) establish a friendly rapport, and (c) show compassion. Moise describes the biggest barriers to the establishment of a positive relationship between provider and family as (a) red tape (e.g., referrals, forms), (b) decreased personal attention and closeness with the provider due to the structure of the health care setting, (c) scheduling delays, (d) accessibility to the provider (e.g., parking, confusion in setting layout), and (e)reaching providers during an emergency (e.g., confusing phone systems). Patients generally report that their biggest complaints about their health care providers relate to personal interactions with and the interpersonal skills of their providers, not to their clinical abilities.

Creating the best possible patient/doctor relationship requires many skills, especially in the pediatric setting, where it is necessary to take into account the relationship with both the child and family. Building the relationship requires much more than merely diagnosing a condition and prescribing effective medication. Although much of the skill in building effective relationships with children and parents is based on interpersonal intuition and effective social skills, the pediatric provider can emphasize the following four main areas to strengthen the child/patient/provider relationship: (a) communication skills, (b) interpersonal qualities, (c) partnership mentality, and (d) awareness of external factors.

I. Communication Skills

Research on communication suggests that doctors are not as effective at communication as they think they are and that many "transmission errors" occur during the communication process. Building effective communication skills is one of the best ways to enhance the child/parent/provider relationship and at the same time to influence positively family satisfaction and health outcomes (e.g., by medication compliance). The skills of directness, candor, tact, and authenticity must be practiced and applied so that the end result is clear, open, and candid communication. Patients who rate communications with their health care providers as excellent consistently report that they receive better health care than those who give their providers lower communications ratings.

A number of useful and basic strategies can enhance communication skills in the pediatric setting:

A. Child and parent-centered interviewing. This approach to interviewing considers both the child's and parents' concerns as important as the provider's diagnosis; the child and parent(s) are viewed as the experts about the child. Child- and parent-centered interviewing requires that providers focus on the strengths of the family and attempt to increase the family's perceived sense of control in the medical process. This approach requires that providers use active listening and judicious, open-ended questioning to facilitate dialogue and that they provide, through effective verbal and nonverbal messages, an atmosphere not dominated by the physician.

B. Active listening. The goal of active listening is to search for meaning and understanding behind the child's/parent's words. Positive body language with eye contact, nodding, and leaning toward the person talking helps convey an attitude of sincerely listening. Active listening is one of the most effective ways to make the parent and child feel heard and validated. Paraphrasing is another essential part of active listening. Providers should use paraphrasing to reflect back, in their own words, the ideas and feelings they have heard from the child/parent. Providers often assume that they have understood what a child/parent is saying when, in fact, they may not have; paraphrasing offers an opportunity to make certain that the other person's message is understood.

C. Facilitation of the dialogue. Providers can facilitate the dialogue through using open-ended questions and asking for clarification and by providing structure for the visit. Using comments, such as *"Tell me more," "I see what you mean,"* and *"That must be difficult,"* can help elicit the story from the child or parent. The provider should avoid interrupting, changing the subject, making judgmental comments, and giving advice prematurely. Plain old niceness can go a long way in facilitating communication; it eases the defenses of the other person and begins the trust-building process. Providers should set an agenda for the visit to give the child/parent a framework in which to get concerns met. By allowing the parent and child to express all their concerns initially rather than focusing on any one symptom or issue, providers can avoid the "Oh, by the way, my child has been experiencing" phenomenon at the end of the visit.

D. Verbal message. Providers must be able to articulate diagnoses and treatment plans clearly and to discuss sensitive issues with children and parents in a comprehendible manner. They can accomplish this by limiting use of medical jargon and abbreviations, which may be confusing or unclear to lay people. Open, honest, direct messages that are organized clearly facilitate the understanding in the child/parent. Providers may want to use the child's/parent's own words in communicating their verbal message. They should also communicate directly with both the child and the parent to get the most detailed picture possible.

E. Nonverbal message. Research has shown that leaning forward, smiling, nodding, and high levels of eye contact affect ratings of a provider's interpersonal skills and rapport. The provider should consider the message sent to families if he or she chooses to stand up versus sit down during the visit. Research has demonstrated that if the provider's verbal messages do not match his or her nonverbal cues, most people believe the nonverbal message.

II. Interpersonal Qualities

Beyond effective communication skills, a provider's interpersonal qualities are important for building the relationship among child, parent, and provider. A provider who behaves in a brusque manner is perceived as uninterested or rushed. One who maintains total control of the interaction discourages children and parents from sharing concerns openly and honestly. Several strategies can increase the effectiveness of the provider's interpersonal nature:

A. Empathy. Using a flexible, empathetic, and compassionate approach with children and parents enhances the child/parent/provider relationship by providing support and validation to the family. Providers demonstrate empathy through both empathic understanding and empathic response.

Empathic understanding means one attempts to "be in another's shoes" by genuinely comprehending the thoughts and
feelings expressed by the child/parent; empathic responses
means commenting in a way that reflects that deep understanding of the child's/parent's concerns. Empathy is as much
an attitude as it is a skill. Providers can practice using
empathic understanding and responses, but first they must
believe that empathy toward children and parents is valuable.

B.   Approachable style. Providers should exhibit a warm,
friendly approach that respects both the child and the parent. Such an approach establishes rapport and opens the
lines of communication among the triad of child, parent, and
provider. Playing with the child, using the child as a reference point, and recognizing the child's successes and behaviors not only give positive attention to the child but also reinforce the parents' efforts at parenting, which in turn affects
positive perceptions of the provider's style.

C.   A manner that honors and appreciates diversity.
In this age of alternative medicine and holistic health practices, providers have to be sensitive to differences among
their patient populations. Providers should inquire in a nonjudgmental manner about family practices outside of traditional medicine with an attempt to understand the basis of
such beliefs/practices (religious, cultural, etc.). With a variety of health-related information easily accessible on the
internet and from literature, providers should be amenable
to learning from their families and their traditional family
medical lore. Such an open stance increases trust and open-
ness with the provider. Providers also must be culturally sensitive with respect to different family racial/ethnic backgrounds and practices in the area of health and medicine.

D.   Support and reassurance. Pediatric primary care
providers are sometimes the only regular professional contact for families. If providers are positive and hopeful with
children and parent(s) and affirm a family's strengths instead
of only focusing on their deficits/problems, families feel validated and empowered. Parents especially may require
provider support and reassurance since the provider/parent
encounter typically occurs at a time of stress for the parent
with an ill child.

E.   Personal awareness. The key to good interpersonal
qualities is the essential ability of a provider to recognize his
or her own feelings and behaviors that impede physician/
patient communication. A provider's lack of personal awareness about his or her own biases, values, beliefs, culture,
history, and attitudes influences interactions with and recommendations for families. Pediatric providers must recognize the importance of reflecting on and becoming aware of
potential triggers, such as gender, race/ethnicity, anger, difficult parents, dying patients, personal family issues, and
stress.

III. Partnership Mentality
For pediatric providers to treat and to advise their children and parents effectively, they need to understand the "world" of the family and to obtain detailed information from the family about their circumstances and concerns. To understand families, providers must believe that forming a positive alliance with both child and parent(s) is important; this forms the essence of a partnership mentality and provides a philosophical framework for child- and parent-centered interviewing as discussed earlier. Several strategies can contribute to the development of a partnership mentality:

A. A collaborative relationship. Parents generally know their children better than you do. For pediatric providers setting the framework for mutual feelings that provider and parent are "in this together" with the ultimate goal of caring for a common interest—the child—is crucial. From the first meeting, pediatric providers should sensitize themselves to parents' concerns and should initiate a relationship that establishes the parent as a lead partner in caring for the child. To invite parents into this collaboration, providers must define their own role and expectations for the child/parent/ provider relationship, thus setting the appropriate tone for working together.

B. Negotiation. Part of a partnership mentality is allowing parents and children to be involved in the negotiation phase of care. If families participate in the decision-making and problem-solving processes, they are more likely to follow through with optimal care for their child.

C. Continuity. Without the development of a long-lasting partnership among child, parent, and provider, developing a deep and understanding relationship can be difficult. Continuity of care has been shown to promote behavioral change in patients, and patients are much more likely to follow the advice of a provider given within the context of an ongoing, trusting relationship. Given high patient volumes and strict time constraints, providers might need to give themselves memory cues that aid in seamless continuity of care (e.g., noting a child's interests or hobbies in his or her chart and bringing them up during a visit, making special notes about uniqueness of a family, siblings, nicknames, etc.).

D. User-friendly education. To communicate a partnership mentality, the pediatric provider's provision of effective but efficient education to children and families is important. Research literature suggests that parents prefer information and education that addresses specific concerns about their child rather than regular, written information of a general nature. For easily understood, concrete problems and issues, verbal advice and information are adequate (e.g., medication directions). However, for more complex problems, written information is needed to supplement and to support the verbal discussion (e.g., toilet training in the resistant child). Other educational approaches, such as showing videos in the waiting room, giving handouts and/or directing to internet sites, and role playing, are demonstrated, effective methods for parent education, depending on the intended educational outcome and financial restrictions of the setting.

IV. Awareness of External Factors

Other considerations, external to the pediatric primary care provider, affect the development of a positive relationship among child, parent, and provider. These include the provider's demographics and the medical environment.

A. Demographics of provider: gender, dress style, race/ethnicity, religion. Some research suggests that families/patients prefer to see a health care provider who is similar in demographic profile—gender, race/ethnicity, and religion (e.g., women prefer to see women providers, African-Americans prefer to see African-American providers, etc.). Demographics may become an even greater concern as the pediatric patient approaches adolescence. In general, dress style has not been shown to affect the patient/provider relationship significantly—most patients report that what their providers wear makes no difference. However, patient comfort with the provider is sometimes enhanced if the provider looks to the social work model of dressing in ways that are compatible and appropriate for the population being served (rather than always wearing the traditional "white coat"). Such an approach can "level the playing field" between provider and families and helps create a more comfortable exchange devoid of superficial comparisons. Regarding religion, especially if religious beliefs dictate medical practices, patients generally prefer a like-minded provider for themselves and their children. This obviously is not always possible, which makes maintaining sensitivity to these issues even more important for the provider.

B. Medical environment. The three key descriptors for a positive environment, which encourages the child/parent/provider relationship, are *accessible, friendly,* and *pleasant.* Having an easily accessible and comfortable waiting area regardless of setting is important. The waiting area should be welcoming and reasonably comfortable with plenty of seats and magazines and should reflect the philosophy of the providers (e.g., a multicultural patient population appreciates pictures and decorations reflecting different cultures). To communicate a child-friendly environment, providers might hang pictures drawn by their patients or photographs of their patients. Pleasant greetings from a receptionist, examination rooms that have places for caregivers to sit and that maintain appropriate temperatures for undressing, a patient friendly billing system, business hours that meet the needs of the population served, and regular telephone hours all contribute to a pleasing environment.

V. The Touchpoints Model

In his book *Touchpoints: your child's emotional and behavioral development,* Brazelton describes an approach to families with children that emphasizes the importance of interpersonal relationships in a pediatric setting—the **Touchpoints Model**. This information grew out of his experience working with parents in his pediatric practice and at the Child Development Unit at Boston Children's Hospital. The model, unique to pediatric settings, recognizes the importance of both the child and the parent(s) in the system of care provided by pediatric practitioners. The Touchpoints Model includes many of the important relationship-enhancing areas mentioned earlier but places them within the context of a medical interaction. The crux of the Touchpoints Model is a conceptual framework that emphasizes both the development of the child and the relationship with the child and family. The developmental aspect of the model emphasizes the "touchpoints" themselves, which are the predictable times and events in a child's developmental progression where the child's behavior regresses, becoming difficult to manage. Touchpoints typically precede a spurt in development. For example, a child beginning to walk may have periodic night awakenings that are frustrating for parents who have enjoyed their child sleeping through the night previous to this transition.

The Touchpoints Model suggests that practitioners understand and anticipate these times of behavioral disorganization as an opportunity to intervene and to collaborate with parents about strategies to reduce or to prevent some of the negative consequences associated with these developmental changes. To collaborate with parents effectively, relationship building is emphasized in the Touchpoints Model. To build an effective alliance with the parents about their child, practitioners should value and understand the "passion" of parents (the powerful emotions associated with parenting that can sometimes be negative) through support of and collaboration with parents. Practitioners should view the parent as the expert on his or her child and should recognize their own biases and contributions to the relationship with child and family. The Touchpoints Model provides a shift from traditional deficit, prescriptive models emphasizing linear development and objective involvement to a more strength-based model emphasizing collaboration, multidimensional development, and empathetic involvement.

Pediatric providers must always remember the powerful therapeutic value of a positive child/parent/provider relationship amid the increasing technological, financial, and legal demands both in and on the medical system. Effectively partnering with children and parents can optimize and enhance the health care outcomes in primary care pediatrics.

ADDITIONAL READING

Aldrich C. *The medical interview: gateway to the doctor-patient relationship,* 2nd ed. New York: Parthenon; 1999.

Balint J, Shelton W. Regaining the initiative: forging a new model of the patient-physician relationship. *JAMA* 1996;275:887–891.

Brazelton TB. *Touchpoints: your child's emotional and behavioral development.* Reading, MA: Addison-Wesley; 1992.

Brock C, Salinsky JV. Empathy: an essential skill for understanding the physician-patient relationship in clinical practice. *Educ Res Methods* 1993;25:245–248.

Brody H. The physician-patient relationship: models and criticisms. *Theor Med Bioeth* 1987;8:205–220.

Cohen W. Establishing effective parent/patient communication. In: King M, Novik L, Citrenbaum C, eds. *Irresistible communication: creative skills for the health professionals.* Philadelphia: WB Saunders; 1983.

Emanuel E, Dubler NN. Preserving the physician-patient relationship in the era of managed care. *JAMA* 1995;273:323–329.

Emanuel EJ, Emanuel LL. Four models of the physician-patient relationship. *JAMA* 1992;267:2221–2226.

King M, Novik L, Citrenbaum C, eds. *Irresistible communication: creative skills for the health professionals.* Philadelphia: WB Saunders; 1983.

Leigh H, Reiser MF. *The patient: biological, psychological and social dimensions of medical practice,* 2nd ed. New York: Plenum; 1985.

Ley P. *Communicating with patients: improving communication, satisfaction and compliance.* New York: Croom Helm; 1988.

Moise H. *Physician-patient relations: a guide to improving satisfaction.* Chicago, IL: American Medical Association; 1999.

Schmuck RA, Runkel PJ. *The handbook of organization development in schools and colleges,* 4th ed. Prospect Heights, IL: Waveland Press; 1994.

Smith TC, Thompson TL. The inherent, powerful therapeutic value of a good physician-patient relationship. *Psychosomatics* 1993;34:166–170.

53 ♣ Teaching and Learning in the Primary Care Setting

Lisa M. Vaughn

Good teaching is an act of generosity, a whim of wanton muse, a craft that may grow with practice, and always risky business.

—Parker Palmer

It is curious that so many of our most important responsibilities are undertaken without significant preparation. Marriage and parenthood are probably the most ubiquitous illustrations, and there is little reason to expect that these states will ever evolve rationally. The task of medical teaching, on the other hand, is accepted deliberately and dispassionately, yet the preparation for that influential role is equally frail.

—George Miller

Good teachers are made, not born.

—Neal Whitman

Teaching is one of the most important and rewarding yet complex roles that a primary care pediatrician can play. Teaching is important because of the skill required to be an effective teacher, the enormous influence a teacher can have on learners, and the time and effort spent on teaching. Clinical teaching and precepting in a primary care setting differs from other medical settings and from the classroom. The types of patients dictate to some extent the learning situation, and the setting requires sharing important goals of caring for patients, managing the practice, and teaching learners. In addition, clinical teaching and precepting involve different skills from teaching in the classroom setting. They require expertise in content, supervisory skills, communication, human interaction, motivation, and group dynamics. The clinical teacher must balance both the needs of the learner and the needs of the patient while being both clinically efficient and educationally effective.

Excellent and effective clinical teachers have been described as positive role models and supervisors. Effective teachers are viewed as dynamic and supportive individuals who, in general, exhibit professional competence, a positive relationship with learners, and personal attributes affecting positive teaching (e.g., humor, patience, enthusiasm). Good teachers are also aware of the basic educational literature available and of the principles of effective teaching. (See Brown, Irby et al., Kotzabassaki et al., Lowman, and Wright for additional reading on effective teaching in the medical setting.)

I. The Basics of Effective Teaching

Most primary care pediatricians have had little formal training in educational theory and technique, yet frequently they are expected to function in the teacher/preceptor role. Despite this lack of training, the educational process in medicine is still largely successful, which accounts for its persistence in modern medical educational systems. This success is probably due in part to some preceptors who possess an innate gift of teaching, but more likely it is due to the learners, who by virtue of their selection of medical careers learn successfully on their own regardless of their teachers. Teaching in medicine has remained largely traditional despite the changes in the medical field. Teaching by the primary care preceptors usually relies on one of two strategies—either teaching the way they were taught or teaching to a reflected image of themselves and their own learning preferences. Neither of these methods is incorrect. However, having some basic framework for teaching when thinking about educational encounters with learners is helpful as these strategies can be expanded to include other types of learners.

   A. Adult learning theory. Adult learning theory principles are an important basis for teaching residents and medical students. Research suggests that learners tend to conform to the expectations of their teachers; thus if teachers expect that they are teaching dependent learners by using traditional pedagogic principles (e.g., typical of elementary, junior, and high school), then the learners will exhibit more dependent behaviors in the learning process. On the other hand, if learners are treated as "adults," then they exhibit more adult, responsible, independent behaviors in the learning process. Knowles has described the principles of adult learning as follows:
      1. *Adults have increased autonomy, which they exercise in learning situations.* Their self-concepts directly affect their learning behaviors and desire to learn.
      2. *Adults need to know that what they are asked to learn is relevant to their needs.*
      3. *Adults have a broad base of experience upon which to draw and to share with others.*
      4. *Adults seek to learn what they identify as important rather than what others have identified as such.*
      5. *Adults pursue learning that can be applied immediately.*
      6. *Adult learning is problem centered rather than subject centered.*

   B. Learner motivation. Learning is most effective when residents/medical students are motivated and involved in defining what they need to know. In the medical education arena, Mann suggests nine principles to enhance learners' motivation:
      1. *Attention to and awareness of learning context.*
      2. *Consideration of learners' experiences with the curriculum and their perceptions of its rewards and values.*
      3. *Attending to the hidden curriculum and its messages.*
      4. *Clarifying goals,* both institutional and personal.
      5. *Matching assessment and rewards with goals.*

6. *Providing regular feedback on progress.*
7. *Encouraging self-efficacy.*
8. *Making learning enjoyable and rewarding.*
9. *Using teaching and learning strategies that are intrinsically motivating.*

C. **Learning style preferences and diverse talents.** Learners have preferred learning styles and a diversity of talents that are based on past learning experiences, teaching styles to which they have been exposed, and their own strengths and optimal methods of receiving, processing, storing, and expressing information. As in all aspects of teaching and learning, some learners have innate learning skills that allow for considerable adaptability and utilize many styles with ease. Others are locked into a predominant style and have difficulty with the learning process when exposed to new teaching methods. These styles and talents range from dependent to independent in terms of reliance on the teacher.

D. **Teaching styles.** Teachers have preferred teaching styles with which they are comfortable and to which they revert in chaotic situations. These styles range from more learner-centered styles to more teacher-centered styles. Teaching styles include particular teaching roles and particular attitudes and behaviors. Adaptability to multiple teaching styles is an important tool that prepares preceptors for a variety of teaching conditions and different learners.

E. **Teacher/learner relationship.** The teacher/learner relationship in medicine is important because the teacher acts as a "relationship role model" representing aspects of the interpersonal relationship essential for the learner to emulate in the physician/patient relationship. Educational leaders have contended that the development of an interpersonal connection/relationship with learners increases their quality of learning (e.g., greater conceptual understanding, self-esteem, flexible use of knowledge, learning at different levels—affective, cognitive, skills) and their motivation to learn. These areas improve because the positive relationship stimulates learners' enthusiasm, sense of involvement, security, personal worth, and self-esteem. Collaborating with learners through mutual identification of needs, goals, and outcomes enhances that relationship.

F. **Teaching methods.** Some clinical teachers complain that they don't know about alternative teaching methods to the "tried and true" lecture and small-group discussion. Having a repertoire of teaching methods in the teacher's bag of tricks gives preceptors the tools necessary for stretching both their own teaching styles and, at the same time, their learners' learning styles. Certain methods will be more applicable to particular settings (e.g., the classroom versus bedside), and some are more appropriate to certain group sizes. Utilizing innovative teaching methods and techniques maximizes learning and makes it more fun for both teacher and learner.

In addition, teachers who attempt different teaching methodologies may become more likely to explore their own beliefs about their knowledge and the teaching/learning process.

II.   Beyond the Basics: Tips for Enhancing Teaching

A.   Have fun in the clinical teaching role. Learning increases when both teacher and learner are having fun.

B.   Use variety and creativity in teaching by taking risks, "thinking out of the box," and using multiple teaching methods and styles.

C.   Enhance understanding and refresh skills in teaching through educational development opportunities rather than by just "winging it."

D.   Recognize the importance of teaching as a professional role and realize that teaching occurs even when you don't realize it (e.g., role modeling).

ADDITIONAL READING

Bibace R, Catlin RJO, Quirk ME, Beattie KA, Slabaugh RC. Teaching styles in the faculty-resident relationship. *J Fam Pract* 1981;13:895–900.

Bland CJ, Schmitz CC, Stritter FT, Henry RC, Aluise JJ. *Successful faculty in academic medicine: essential skills and how to acquire them.* New York: Springer; 1990.

Brown ST. Faculty and student perceptions of effective clinical teachers. *J Nurs Educ* 1981;20:4–15.

DaRosa DA, Dunnington GL, Stearns J, Ferenchick G, Bowen JL, Simpson DE. Ambulatory teaching "lite": less clinic time, more educationally fulfilling. *Acad Med* 1997;72:358–361.

Deci E, Vallerand RJ, Pelletier LG, Ryan RM. Motivation and education: the self-determination perspective. *Educ Psychol* 1991;26:325–346.

Ferenchick G, Simpson D, Blackman J, DaRosa D, Dunnington G. Strategies for efficient and effective teaching in the ambulatory care setting. *Acad Med* 1997;72:277–280.

Gardner, H. *Intelligence reframed: multiple intelligences for the 21st century.* New York: Basic Books; 1999.

Grasha AF. *Teaching with style: enhancing learning by understanding teaching and learning styles.* Pittsburgh, PA: Alliance Publishers; 1996.

Griffith JW, Bakanauskas AJ. Student-instructor relationships in nursing education. *J Nurs Educ* 1983;22:104–107.

Handfield-Jones R, Nasmith L, Steinert Y, Lawn N. Creativity in medical education: the use of innovative techniques in clinical teaching. *Med Teach* 1993;15:3–10.

Hekelman FP, Snyder CW, Alemagno S, Hull AL, Vanek EP. Humanistic teaching attributes of primary care physicians. *Teach Learn Med* 1995;7:29–36.

Irby D, Ramsey P, Gillmore G, Schaad D. Characteristics of effective clinical teachers of ambulatory medicine. *Acad Med* 1991;66:54–55.

Knowles, M. *The adult learner: a neglected species,* 4th ed. Houston: Gulf Publishing Company; 1990.

Kotzabassaki S, Panou M, Dimou F, Karabagli A, Koutsopoulou B, Ikonomou U. Nursing students' and faculty's perceptions of the characteristics of "best" and "worst" clinical teachers: a replication study. *J Adv Nurs* 1997;26:817–824.

Lowman J. *Mastering the techniques of teaching,* 3rd ed. San Francisco: Jossey Bass; 1995.

Lowman J. Professors as performers and motivators. *Coll Teach* 1994;42:137–141.

Mann KV, Motivation in medical education: how theory can inform our practice. *Acad Med* 1999;74:237–239.

Montauk SL, Grasha AF, *Adult HIV outpatient care: a handbook for clinical teaching.* Cincinnati, OH: University of Cincinnati Department of Family Medicine; 1993.

Pike RW. *Creative training techniques handbook: tips, tactics, and how-to's for delivering effective training,* 2nd ed. Minneapolis, MN: Lakewood Books; 1994.

Skeff KM, Bowen JL, Irby DM. Protecting time for teaching in the ambulatory care setting, *Acad Med* 1997;72:694–697.

Vaughn LM, Baker RC. Microburst teaching and learning. *Medicl Teacher* 2001;23:36–40.

Whitman, N. *Creative medical teaching.* Salt Lake City, UT: Department of Family and Preventive Medicine, University of Utah School of Medicine; 1990.

Woolliscroft JO, Schwenk TL. Teaching and learning in the ambulatory setting, *Acad Med* 1989;64:644–648.

Wright SM, Kern DE, Kolodner, K, Howard DM, Brancati FL. Attributes of excellent attending-physician role models. *N Engl J Med* 1998;339:1986–1993.

54 ♣ Cultural Sensitivity and Competency in the Primary Care Setting

Lisa M. Lewis

Given the increase in cultural and ethnic diversity within the United States today, the health care provider's awareness of and sensitivity to patients from diverse backgrounds is central to primary care. For example, the 1993 U.S. Bureau of the Census estimated that by the year 2050 the U.S. population will be composed of people from the following groups in the following percentages: 22.5% Hispanic, 14.4% African-American, 9.7% Asian-American, and 0.9% Native American. Delivering effective primary care to families and children requires an awareness of one's own cultural values, assumptions, and beliefs. At the same time, awareness of each family's sociocultural background is necessary for delivering medical care in a culturally sensitive manner because families' cultures influence their perceptions of child development, family environment, and gender. This chapter provides guidelines for learning how to provide culturally sensitive and competent care to patients.

I. Cultural Competence

Cultural competence in the medical setting may be defined as "the ability to function effectively in the cultural context of a patient." Some educators in the area of cultural competency view it as a continuum ranging from cultural destructiveness (setting out to destroy different cultures) to advanced competence (fully integrating culture into one's way of thinking). Five elements of cultural competence are identified below and include (a) awareness and acceptance of difference, (b) awareness of one's own cultural values, (c) understanding the dynamics of difference, (d) development of cultural knowledge, and (e) ability to adapt practice skills to fit the cultural context of the client's values structure.

II. Awareness

To provide culturally sensitive and competent care, one must be aware that one reason people differ is the effect of culture; one must also accept those differences. Differences in cultural values and norms may impact primary care providers' comfort level when communicating with families. Awareness of personal biases, stereotypes, and prejudices relevant to diverse populations, however, eases providers' feelings and enables them to work more effectively in culturally diverse situations. In addition to awareness of cultural differences, health care providers must have an awareness of their own cultural values and identities and their impact on the provider's professional functioning. Such awareness helps providers recognize situations where they impose their own values and perceptions on patients.

III. Knowledge

In addition to awareness, the provider must possess knowledge of different cultures. Important areas for understanding include patterns of nonverbal communication and language usage, perceptions of health problems and healing, ways health is experienced and identified, and views of parenting and family issues. When information is not available, asking questions related to the patient's experience with health care behaviors helps increase knowledge of the family's cultural experiences. Examples of such questions are *"How is health and illness talked about, defined, or understood in your family/community/culture?"* and *"Who takes care of your child when he or she is sick?"* Other helpful questions are listed in Table 54.1. The knowledge obtained from assessing a family's cultural experiences clarifies family behaviors and responses that otherwise might be interpreted as noncompliance. Other ways to obtain cultural knowledge are to review the sociocultural literature and to consult colleagues from similar cultural backgrounds as the families to whom the primary care provider provides professional services.

**Table 54.1 Questions to learn about
a family's cultural experience and background**

When your child is ill, at what point to you call your doctor?

Do you feel that our medical staff listens and understands your concerns?

How is our medical practice different from what you and your family previously have used?

Are we doing anything that makes you or anyone in your family feel uncomfortable?

How is health and illness talked about and understood in your family?

To provide better medical care, what information do we need to know about your family traditions?

Who usually takes care of your child when he is sick?

Do you try to prevent your child from getting sick by giving him special foods, herbs, spices, diets, or food supplements, such as vitamins?

Do you use any special treatments, such as teas, herbs, honeys, steam, heat, or ice packs, when your child is sick?

Do you have any trouble having prescriptions filled?

Do you have any worries about reading or understanding the instructions that come on the medicine container (when English is a second language or the parent has stated concerns about understanding medical terms)?

Do you and your family ask for medical advice from religious or community leaders or anyone other than a medical doctor?

IV. Skills

A crucial aspect of cultural competence is having the skills to communicate genuinely, nondefensively, and effectively with culturally diverse families. Providers must recognize when their personal views and cultural values become barriers to working interculturally and/or hamper their abilitiy to demonstrate respect for their patients' values, beliefs, behaviors, and world views. Increased levels of awareness and knowledge usually enhance the provider's actual skills for communicating and interacting effectively with patients. For example, knowledge of the cultural preference of African-Americans for fried foods helps decrease the provider's frustration when discussing diet adherence with patients who have hypercholesterolemia. The provider's effectiveness in communicating information increases by recognizing that nonadherence to the suggested diet stems from cultural preferences and not blatant noncompliance.

Culture affects perceptions, communication, and medical treatment planning. Health care providers have individual cultural norms that impact their beliefs. Awareness of one's own cultural differences, the knowledge of other cultures, and cultivation of skills for interacting interculturally leads to a trusting patient/provider relationship that facilitates better adherence to treatment suggestions and improved family satisfaction with the health care experience.

ADDITIONAL READING

American Medical Association. *Culturally competent health care for adolescents: a guide for primary care providers.* Chicago: Department of Adolescent Health, AMA; 1994.

Barker JC. Cultural diversity—changing the context of medical practice, In *Cross-cultural medicine—a decade later* [Special Issue]. *West J Med* 1992;157:248–254.

Mac Kune-Karrer B, Taylor, EH. Toward multiculturality: implications for the pediatrician. *Pediatr Clin North Am* 1995;42:21–30.

Olness K. Cultural issues in primary pediatric care. In: Hoekelman RA, ed. *Primary pediatric care,* 3rd ed. St. Louis, MO: Mosby; 1997:128.

55 ♣ Contraception

Julie A. Jaskiewicz

Adolescent sexual activity is increasing in the United States. Today more than half of all adolescents between 15 and 19 years of age are sexually active. Unfortunately, many teenagers do not seek contraception until they have been coitally active for many months; they then often use contraception inconsistently and ineffectively. The adolescent's primary care physician should make counseling sexually active adolescents about prevention of unplanned pregnancies and sexually transmitted diseases (STDs) a priority.

I. The Primary Care Physician's Role
The physician must identify adolescents at risk for beginning sexual activity, counsel them about sexual behaviors, educate them about suitable contraceptive methods and protection against STDs, and provide access to contraception if requested. Discussing sexual interest, attitudes, and behaviors with an adolescent in an open and nonjudgmental way is best, preferably before the young person has initiated sexual intercourse. The benefits of delaying coital activity should be stressed, and reasons for the adolescent's desire to begin sexual activity (e.g., peer pressure, expectations) should be discussed. The physician can then help the adolescent identify his or her own goals for safe sexual behavior and can emphasize that taking responsibility for sexual decisions is part of overall adult, responsible behavior. Encouraging sexually active teens to involve their partners in decisions regarding coital activity and contraception and to consider the effects of their sexual activity on their relationships with partners and family is also crucial. For the adolescent who has already begun coital activity, the physician should provide appropriate reproductive health care and health care education, including information about contraceptive methods and prevention of STDs.

II. Evaluation
Evaluating the adolescent for birth control requires a careful history and physical examination to determine if the adolescent is at risk of pregnancy and/or STDs and if he or she wants to prevent them. The physician should also determine if he or she can understand and accept responsibility for appropriate contraceptive methods.

A. History. Adolescents and parents should be informed at the beginning of the office visit that the adolescent has a right to confidentiality except in life-threatening circumstances. The sexual history should help the physician determine the adolescent's sexual interest, knowledge about pregnancy, contraception, and STDs, current sexual behaviors, and use of contraception. The physician can help the adolescent choose the best birth control option by identifying risk factors associated with available contraceptive methods. The sexual history should include the following:
1. *General sexual history.*
   a. *Age.*
   b. *Reason for the visit.*

    c.   *Current sexual behaviors.*

    d.   *Reasons for wanting contraception* (desire to prevent pregnancy/STDs).

    e.   *Partners and family*—involvement of partners in contraceptive decisions; parental/guardian involvement; values about sexuality/sexual activity.

    f.   *Past and present use of contraception*—type, perceived benefits, problems.

    g.   *Knowledge about contraceptive choices*—concerns, perceived negative effects.

    h.   *Type of contraceptive desired*—perceived willingness of partner to use contraceptive method.

    i.   *Ability to comply with contraceptive method.*

  2.   *Medical/gynecologic history.*

    a.   *Menstrual history*—menarche, frequency and duration of menses, dysfunctional bleeding, dysmenorrhea, date of last menstrual period, date of last pelvic examination, history of abnormal Papanicolaou smear.

    b.   *Prior history of pregnancy, abortion, STDs and treatment of partners.*

    c.   *Psychosocial problems,* including depression, alcohol, and drug use.

  3.   *Review of systems should focus on the following when considering oral contraceptives:*

    a.   *Absolute and relative contraindications* (Table 55.1).

    b.   *Conditions influenced by use of oral contraceptives* (acne, contact lenses).

    c.   *Medications and drug allergies.*

Table 55.1.   Contraindications for oral contraceptive use

Absolute	*Relative*
Pregnancy	Hypertension
Coronary artery disease	Vascular or migraine headache
Cerebrovascular disease	Sickle cell disease
Thrombophlebitis/thrombotic disease	Hyperlipidemia
Breast/uterine cancer	Collagen vascular disease
Active liver disease	Lactation
Benign or malignant liver tumor	
Previous cholestasis with pregnancy	
Undiagnosed uterine bleeding	

Adapted from Jaskiewicz JA, McAnarney ER. Pregnancy during adolescence. *Pediatr Rev* 1994;15:32–38.

d. *Cardiovascular risk factors* (familial hyperlipidemia, family history of early heart disease, smoking, obesity).

e. *Psychiatric problems,* including depression, alcohol, and drug use.

4. *Psychosocial development and maturity* (see Appendices C and D).

B. Physical examination. A careful physical examination should be performed with special attention given to abnormalities that may limit contraceptive choices:

1. *General.*

a. *Height and weight.*

b. *Thyroid.*

c. *Breast examination.*

d. *Cardiovascular*—edema, pulses, cardiac.

e. *Gastrointestinal*—liver size, tenderness, evidence of chronic disease.

f. *Skin*—acne, xanthomata.

g. *Tanner stage of sexual maturity.*

2. *Pelvic (female).*

a. External and internal bimanual, speculum examinations.

b. Specimen for Papanicolaou smear.

c. Cultures of specimens for *Neisseria gonorrhea, Chlamydia trachomatis,* others as appropriate.

3. *Genital (male)*

a. Testicular and penile examination.

b. Cultures of specimens for STDs as above.

C. Laboratory. All females should have a pregnancy test before a birth control method is prescribed. Additional laboratory tests should be done on an individual basis. Some tests to consider include urinalysis, complete blood count, lipid screen, liver function, sickle cell screen, and serologic test for syphilis.

III. Contraceptive Methods

The best contraceptive method for an adolescent is one that he or she and partners will accept and use consistently. Physicians should familiarize themselves with contraceptive methods suitable for adolescents and should be prepared to help the adolescent make an informed choice for his or her situation. Contraceptive needs and preferences change over time, so the physician should provide follow-up and make adjustments as necessary. Table 55.2 lists, in order of decreasing efficacy, the most frequently chosen birth control methods of adolescents.

A. Abstinence. Any discussion of contraception with an adolescent should start with abstinence, the most effective and safe form of birth control available. Adolescents can be encouraged to choose abstinence, but the provider must be ready to discuss alternative contraceptive methods with the teenager who desires to be sexually active.

1. *Advantages.* The only 100% safe and effective birth control method; no side effects; best protection against STDs.

**Table 55.2.   Common contraceptive
methods in order of decreasing efficacy**

Abstinence
Levonorgestrel implants (Norplant)
Medroxyprogesterone acetate injection (Depo-Provera)
Oral contraceptives (combined form)
Vaginal spermicides with condom
Condom
Diaphragm
Cervical cap
Vaginal spermicides alone
Coitus interruptus (withdrawal)
Rhythm method

Adapted from Stevens-Simon C. Providing effective reproductive health care and prescribing contraceptives for adolescents. *Pediatr Rev* 1998; 19:411.

    2. *Disadvantages.* None unless the adolescent initiates sexual activity; no contraindications.
  B. Oral contraceptives. Oral contraceptive pills are the contraception method most frequently chosen by adolescents. Three types of oral contraceptives are available: (a) fixed-dose combination, with each pill containing the same dose of estrogen and progestin; (b) phasic dose, with triphasic and biphasic pills containing varying amounts of estrogen and progestin throughout the menstrual cycle; and (c) mini-pill, containing only progestin. The most recent birth control pills contain a low dose (20 to 35 μg) of estrogen and new forms of progestin. The 28-day pack of pills, containing 21 hormone pills and seven placebo pills, continues to be used successfully by many teens and is preferable to the 21-day pack because it enhances daily compliance. Adolescents who are motivated to take a daily pill and who prefer regular menstrual cycles are best suited for oral contraceptive pills. Explaining to teen-age females using oral contraceptives that their partner must also use a condom to protect against STDs is of imperative importance.
    1. *Advantages.* Highly effective when used correctly; safe; reversible; decreased menstrual blood flow; decreased risk of ovarian/endometrial cancer; decreased incidence of fibrocystic breast disease and ovarian cysts; decreased incidence of dysmenorrhea; some protection against salpingitis.
    2. *Disadvantages.* Requires compliance with daily pill; does not protect against STDs; common side effects (often reduced after a few cycles) include nausea, weight gain, breast tenderness, leg cramps, fluid retention, depression, breakthrough bleeding, headache, acne; rare side effects include corneal edema (contact lens wearers), thrombo-

embolic events, stroke, hypertension. Table 55.1 lists contraindications for using oral contraceptives.

C. Mini-pill (progestin-only pill). The mini-pill is similar to the combined oral contraceptive pill but contains progestin only. Side effects and reduced efficacy limit its use in adolescents, but this method could be considered in situations in which estrogen is contraindicated.

  1. *Advantages.* Fewer estrogen-related side effects, including reduced risk of thromboembolic events and hypertension; lactation not a contraindication.

  2. *Disadvantages.* Increased failure rate; higher incidence of breakthrough bleeding, amenorrhea, and hirsuitism; no protection against STDs.

D. Condoms. The condom is a mechanical barrier that covers the penis during sexual intercourse. Only latex condoms should be recommended, as natural membrane condoms do not afford protection against STDs. When used with a spermicide (e.g., nonoxynol-9), protection against pregnancy is close to that of oral contraceptives. Proper use of condoms should be discussed with the adolescent, including using only water-based lubricants and not using torn, damaged, or previously used condoms.

  1. *Advantages.* Easily accessible; inexpensive; no prescription necessary; few side effects; male method; best method after abstinence for protecting against STDs.

  2. *Disadvantages.* Requires male participation in contraception; requires planning for sexual activity in advance; occasional latex allergy.

E. Vaginal spermicides. Vaginal spermicides are chemical contraceptives available in a variety of forms, such as creams, gels, foams, tablets, and suppositories. Spermacides contain nonoxynol-9 and octoxynol-9. This method is most effective when used with barrier contraceptives.

  1. *Advantages.* Easily accessible; inexpensive; no prescription necessary; few side effects.

  2. *Disadvantages.* Efficacy limited when used alone; no absolute contraindications.

F. Diaphragm/cervical cap. The diaphragm is a rubber cap with a metal spring in the rim designed to fit over the cervix to provide a physical barrier to sperm entering the cervix. The cervical cap is a small, flexible latex cap that uses suction to fit over the cervix. Both methods are used with a vaginal spermicide. These methods are most successfully used by older adolescents.

  1. *Advantages.* Effective; spermicide available over the counter; offers some protection against STDs; used only when needed; few side effects.

  2. *Disadvantages.* Proper fit required; must feel comfortable inserting device herself; requires planning for sexual activity in advance; increased risk of urinary tract infection; occasional vaginal malodor and discharge; contraindications

are severely retro- or anteverted uterus, allergy to latex (cervical cap), history of toxic shock syndrome.

G. Medroxyprogesterone acetate injection (Depo-Provera). Depo-Provera is the only injectable hormonal contraceptive available in the United States. It is a long-acting progestin that can suppress ovulation for up to 12 to 14 weeks when given as a single 150-mg intramuscular injection. This method is useful for adolescents with chronic illness or for those at risk for complications from estrogen. Despite early data showing an increase in breast cancer in laboratory animals given medroxyprogesterone acetate, no evidence suggests that this progestin causes human breast cancer to develop *de novo*. Medroxyprogesterone acetate use is associated with a delay in return to fertility upon its discontinuation. With prolonged use of this hormone, some women have evidence of decreased bone mineralization, but no pathologic fractures have been reported. Teens using this contraceptive method must also use a condom to prevent STD transmission.

1. *Advantages.* Effective; does not require daily medication; lack of estrogen-related side effects; protection against endometrial cancer and iron deficiency anemia.

2. *Disadvantages.* Menstrual irregularities; side effects, including weight gain, headaches, bloating, depression, mood changes; does not protect against STDs.

H. Levonorgestrel implants (Norplant). Norplant is a long-acting, subdermal, progestin-only implant that provides continuous contraception for up to 5 years. Six Silastic capsules that release 30 μg of levonorgestrel per day are inserted in the upper arm under local anesthesia.

1. *Advantages.* Highly effective; no estrogen side effects; effectiveness does not depend upon compliance; fertility returns quickly after removal.

2. *Disadvantages.* High initial cost; no protection against STDs; side effects include irregular menstrual bleeding, weight gain, headaches; requires experienced health professional for removal.

I. Other methods. Two methods commonly used by adolescents are coitus interruptus (male partner withdrawal before ejaculation) and the rhythm method (periodic abstinence around the time of anticipated ovulation). Neither method is indicated for pregnancy prevention in adolescents. Adolescents do not use these methods consistently or correctly, and failure rates can be high (Table 55.2). Most importantly, neither method provides protection against STDs. Adolescents who desire to be sexually active should be advised to use other forms of birth control.

ADDITIONAL READING

American Academy of Pediatrics Committee on Adolescence. Contraception and adolescents. *Pediatrics* 1999;104:1161–1166.

Braverman PK, Strasburger VC. Contraception—adolescent sexuality: part 2. *Clin Pediatr* 1992;32:725–734.

Greydanus DE, Patel DR. Contraception. In: McAnarney ER, ed. *Textbook of adolescent medicine.* Philadelphia: WB Saunders; 1992.

Jaskiewicz JA, McAnarney ER. Pregnancy during adolescence. *Pediatr Rev* 1994;15:32–38.

Jenkins RR, Raine T. Helping adolescents prevent unintended pregnancy. *Contemp Pediatr* 2000;17:75–99.

Neinstein LS. *Adolescent health care: a practical guide,* 3rd ed. Baltimore, MD: Williams & Wilkins; 1996.

Stevens-Simon C. Providing effective reproductive health care and prescribing contraceptives for adolescents. *Pediatr Rev* 1998;19: 409–417.

Woods ER. Contraceptive choices for adolescents. *Pediatr Ann* 1991; 20:313–321.

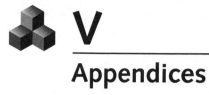

Appendices

Appendix A 🔹 Infant Formula Composition

Table A.1.   Infant formula composition—standard formulas

| Formula Name | Caloric Density (kcal/oz) | Protein | | | Carbohydrate Source | Fat Source |
		Source	Density (g/L)	Whey/Casein (%/%)		
Human milk	20	Human milk	10.5	70/30	Lactose	Human milk fat
Cow's milk	20	Cow's milk	33	18/82	Lactose	Medium chain and long chain triglycerides
Enfamil	20	Cow's milk	14.2	60/40	Lactose	Palm olein, soy, coconut, high-oleic sunflower
Similac	20	Cow's milk	14.5	18/82	Lactose	Soy, coconut
Good Start	20	Cow's milk	16.2	100/0	Lactose	Palm olein, soy, coconut, high-oleic sunflower oils
Gerber	20	Cow's milk	15	18/82	Lactose	Palm olein, soy, coconut, high-oleic sunflower oils
ProSobee	20	Soy protein	20	NA	Corn syrup solids	Palm olein, soy, coconut, high-oleic sunflower oils
Isomil	20	Soy protein	17	NA	Corn syrup, sucrose	Soy, coconut oils

Adapted from Kleinman RE, ed. *Pediatric nutrition handbook*, 4th ed. Elk Grove Village, IL: American Academy of Pediatrics; 1998.

Table A.2.   Infant formula composition—specialized formulas

Formula Name	Caloric Density (kcal/oz)	Density (g/L)	Protein Source	Carbohydrate Source	Fat Source
Nutramigen	20	19	Casein hydrolysate, L-cystine, L-tyrosine, L-tryptophan, taurine	Corn syrup solids, modified corn starch	Palm olein, soy, coconut, high-oleic sunflowers oils
Pregestimil	20	19	Casein hydrolysate, L-cystine, L-tyrosine, L-tryptophan, taurine	Corn syrup solids, modified corn starch, dextrose	Medium-chain triglycerides, corn, soy, and high-oleic safflower oils
Alimentum	20	19	Casein hydrolysate, L-cystine, L-tyrosine, L-tryptophan	Sucrose, modified tapioca starch	Medium-chain triglycerides, soy, and safflower oils
Similac Special Care 24	24	22	Nonfat milk, whey protein concentrate	Lactose, glucose polymers	Medium-chain triglycerides, soy, coconut oils
Enfamil Premature 24	24	24	Nonfat milk, whey protein concentrate	Glucose polymers, lactose	Medium-chain triglycerides, soy, coconut oils
PM-60-40	20	15	Milk whey, casein	Lactose	Coconut, corn, and soy oils
Lacto-Free	20	15	Milk protein isolate	Corn syrup solids	Palm olein, soy, coconut, and sunflower oils
Protagen	20	22	Sodium caseinate, taurine	Corn syrup solids, sucrose	Medium-chain triglyceride and corn oils

Adapted from Kleinman RE, ed. *Pediatric nutrition handbook*, 4th ed. Elk Grove Village, IL: American Academy of Pediatrics; 1998.

Appendix B ♣ Blood Pressure Norms

Table B.1. Blood pressure norms, girls

Age (yr)	% ile	Systolic BP (mm Hg) by Percentile of Height							Diastolic BP (DBP5) (mm Hg) by Percentile of Height						
		5%	10%	25%	50%	75%	90%	95%	5%	10%	25%	50%	75%	90%	95%
1	90th	94	95	97	99	101	102	103	49	49	50	51	52	53	54
	95th	98	99	101	103	105	106	107	54	54	55	56	57	58	58
2	90th	98	99	101	103	104	106	107	54	54	55	56	57	58	58
	95th	102	103	105	107	108	110	110	58	59	60	61	62	63	63
3	90th	101	102	103	105	107	109	109	59	59	60	61	62	63	63
	95th	105	106	107	109	111	112	113	63	63	64	65	66	67	68
4	90th	103	104	105	107	109	110	111	63	63	64	65	66	67	67
	95th	107	108	109	111	113	114	115	67	68	68	69	70	71	72
5	90th	104	105	107	109	111	112	113	66	67	68	69	69	70	71
	95th	108	109	111	113	114	116	117	71	71	72	73	74	75	76
6	90th	105	106	108	110	112	113	114	70	70	71	72	73	74	74
	95th	109	110	112	114	116	117	118	74	75	75	76	77	78	79
7	90th	106	107	109	111	113	114	115	72	72	73	74	75	76	77
	95th	110	111	113	115	117	118	119	77	77	78	79	80	81	81
8	90th	108	109	110	112	114	116	116	74	75	75	76	77	78	79
	95th	112	113	114	116	118	119	120	79	79	80	81	82	83	83
9	90th	109	110	112	114	116	117	118	76	76	77	78	79	80	80
	95th	113	114	116	118	119	121	122	80	81	81	82	83	84	85

(continued)

Table B.1. *Continued*

Age (yr)	% ile	Systolic BP (mm Hg) by Percentile of Height							Diastolic BP (DBP5) (mm Hg) by Percentile of Height						
		5%	10%	25%	50%	75%	90%	95%	5%	10%	25%	50%	75%	90%	95%
10	90th	111	112	113	115	117	119	119	77	77	78	79	80	81	81
	95th	115	116	117	119	121	123	123	81	82	83	83	84	85	86
11	90th	113	114	115	117	119	121	121	77	78	79	80	81	81	82
	95th	117	118	119	121	123	125	125	82	82	83	84	85	86	87
12	90th	115	116	118	120	121	123	124	78	78	79	80	81	82	83
	95th	119	120	122	124	125	127	128	83	83	84	85	86	87	87
13	90th	118	119	120	122	124	125	126	78	79	80	81	81	82	83
	95th	121	122	124	126	128	129	130	83	83	84	85	86	87	88
14	90th	120	121	123	125	127	128	129	79	79	80	81	82	83	83
	95th	124	125	127	129	131	132	133	83	84	85	86	87	87	88
15	90th	123	124	126	128	130	131	132	80	80	81	82	83	84	84
	95th	127	128	130	132	133	135	136	84	85	86	86	87	88	89
16	90th	126	127	129	131	132	134	134	81	82	82	83	84	85	86
	95th	130	131	133	134	136	138	138	86	86	87	88	89	90	90
17	90th	128	129	131	133	135	136	137	83	84	85	86	87	87	88
	95th	132	133	135	137	139	140	141	88	88	89	90	91	92	93

Source: Rosner B, Prineas RJ, Loggie JMH, et al. Blood pressure nomograms for children and adolescents, by height, sex, and age, in the United States. *J Pediatr* 1993;123:871. Reproduced with permission.

Table B.2. Blood pressure norms, boys

Age (yr)	% ile	Systolic BP (mm Hg) by Percentile of Height							Diastolic BP (DBP5) (mm Hg) by Percentile of Height						
		5%	10%	25%	50%	75%	90%	95%	5%	10%	25%	50%	75%	90%	95%
1	90th	98	98	99	101	102	103	104	52	52	53	53	54	55	55
	95th	101	102	103	104	106	107	108	56	56	57	58	58	59	60
2	90th	99	99	101	102	103	104	105	57	57	58	58	59	60	60
	95th	103	103	104	106	107	108	109	61	61	62	62	63	64	64
3	90th	100	101	102	103	104	105	106	61	61	61	62	63	64	64
	95th	104	104	106	107	108	109	110	65	65	66	66	67	68	68
4	90th	101	102	103	104	106	107	108	64	64	65	65	66	67	67
	95th	105	106	107	108	109	111	111	68	68	69	69	70	71	71
5	90th	103	103	105	106	107	108	109	66	67	67	68	69	69	70
	95th	107	107	108	110	111	112	113	71	71	71	72	73	74	74
6	90th	104	105	106	107	109	110	111	69	69	69	70	71	72	72
	95th	108	109	110	111	113	114	114	73	73	74	74	75	76	76
7	90th	106	107	108	109	110	112	112	71	71	71	72	73	74	74
	95th	110	111	112	113	114	115	116	75	75	75	76	77	78	78
8	90th	108	109	110	111	112	114	114	72	72	73	74	74	75	76
	95th	112	113	114	115	116	117	118	76	77	77	78	79	79	80
9	90th	110	111	112	113	114	116	116	74	74	74	75	76	77	77
	95th	114	115	116	117	118	119	120	78	78	79	79	80	81	81

(continued)

Table B.2. Continued

Age (yr)	% ile	Systolic BP (mm Hg) by Percentile of Height							Diastolic BP (DBP5) (mm Hg) by Percentile of Height						
		5%	10%	25%	50%	75%	90%	95%	5%	10%	25%	50%	75%	90%	95%
10	90th	112	113	114	115	116	118	118	75	75	76	77	77	78	78
	95th	116	117	118	119	120	122	122	79	79	80	81	81	82	83
11	90th	114	115	116	117	119	120	120	76	77	77	78	79	79	80
	95th	118	119	120	121	122	124	124	81	81	81	82	83	83	84
12	90th	116	117	118	119	121	122	123	78	78	78	79	80	81	81
	95th	120	121	122	123	125	126	126	82	82	82	83	84	85	85
13	90th	118	119	120	121	123	124	124	79	79	79	80	81	82	82
	95th	122	123	124	125	126	128	128	83	83	84	84	85	86	86
14	90th	120	121	122	123	124	125	126	80	80	80	81	82	83	83
	95th	124	125	126	127	128	129	130	84	84	85	85	86	87	87
15	90th	121	122	123	124	126	127	128	80	81	81	82	83	83	84
	95th	125	126	127	128	130	131	131	85	85	85	86	87	88	88
16	90th	122	123	124	125	127	128	129	81	81	82	82	83	84	84
	95th	126	127	128	129	130	132	132	85	85	86	87	87	88	88
17	90th	123	123	124	126	127	128	129	81	81	82	83	83	84	85
	95th	127	127	128	130	131	132	133	85	86	86	87	88	88	89

Source: Rosner B, Prineas RJ, Loggie JMH, et al. Blood pressure nomograms for children and adolescents, by height, sex, and age, in the United States. *J Pediatr* 1993;123:871. Reproduced with permission.

Appendix C ♣ Clinical Stages of Pubertal Development

Table C.1.   Clinical stages of pubertal development (Tanner stages)

Tanner Stage	Girls (Breast)	Boys (Genitalia)	Both Sexes (Pubic Hair)
I	None	Prepubertal penis (<7 cm) Testes <2.5 cm long	None
II	Budding less than diameter of areola	Prepubertal penis (<7 cm) Scrotal thinning Testes >2.5 cm long (4–6 mL in volume)	Few dark, thick hairs over labia, mons, or both, or scrotum, base of penis, or both
III	Breast greater than diameter of areola	Enlarging penis >7 cm Testes 3–4 cm long (6–10 mL in volume)	Visible dark hairs over mons and labia or base of penis and scrotum
IV	Puffy areola	Larger penis with developed testes 4–5 cm long (10–15 mL in volume)	Thick hair distribution over wider area
V	Adult	Adult	Adult

Adapted from Marshall WA, Tanner JM. Variations in the patterns of pubertal changes in boys. *Arch Dis Child* 1970;45:13; and Sizonenko PC. Normal sexual maturation. *Pediatrician* 1987;14:191.

Appendix D ♣ Sequence of Sexual Maturity

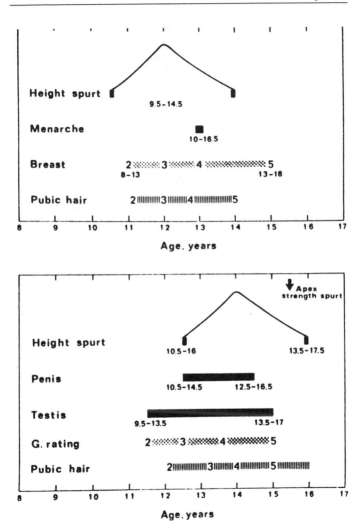

Figure D.1 Sequence of sexual maturity.
Source: Marshall WA, Tanner JM. Variations in the patterns of pubertal changes in boys. *Arch Dis Child* 1970;45:22. Reproduced with permission.

Appendix E ⚜ Denver Developmental Screening Test—II

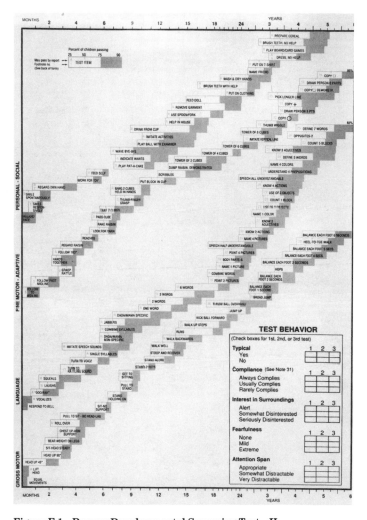

Figure E.1 Denver Developmental Screening Test—II
Source: Frankenberg WK, Dodds J, Archer P, et al. The Denver II: a major revision and restandardization of the Denver Developmental Screening Test. *Pediatrics* 1992;89:91. Reproduced with permission.

Appendix F ⚛ Early Language Milestone Scale

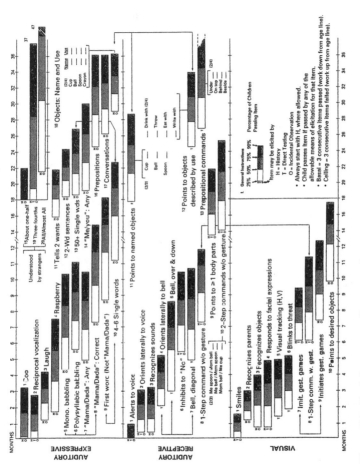

Figure F.1 Early language milestone scale

Source: Coplan J. Early Language Milestone Scale. PRO-ED, Inc; 1987. Reproduced with permission.

Appendix G ♣ Preschool Children's Behavior Checklist

Table G.1. Preschool children's behavior checklist (2–5 Years)

Child's Name: _____ Birth Date: _____

Your relationship to the child: _____

Note: This list will not be included in your child's permanent record. It will be discarded after the visit.

Are you concerned about any of these behaviors your child may have? (Circle *Yes or No.*)

Bed wetting	Yes	No
Wetting during the day	Yes	No
Trouble sleeping; restless at night	Yes	No
Getting him/her to go to sleep at night	Yes	No
Thumb sucking	Yes	No
Nervous habits	Yes	No
Being easily upset	Yes	No
Being overactive	Yes	No
Being shy	Yes	No
Getting feelings hurt too easily	Yes	No
Demanding attention all the time	Yes	No
Contrary or stubborn	Yes	No
Won't mind; disobedient	Yes	No
Discipline problems	Yes	No
Selfish, not wanting to share	Yes	No
Fighting with other children	Yes	No
Destroying things on purpose	Yes	No
Appetite (too much or too little)	Yes	No
Problems at mealtime	Yes	No
Hearing problems	Yes	No
Speech problems	Yes	No
Poor attention span	Yes	No
Frequent stomachaches or headaches	Yes	No
Temper tantrums	Yes	No
Problems with toilet training	Yes	No

(continued)

Table G.1. *Continued.*

Below are listed some situations often troubling to many families. Circle those that are of concern to you.

Day care, babysitter, or preschool	Yes	No
Divorce, separation, or other marital problems	Yes	No
Violence in the home or neighborhood	Yes	No
Death or illness of family member	Yes	No
Adjustment to a new brother or sister	Yes	No
Not enough money for family's needs	Yes	No
Effects of television and movies	Yes	No
Effects of a new job	Yes	No

Other problems (e.g., drugs, alcohol)

(_____)
(_____)
(_____)
(_____)

Adapted from Willoughby JA, Haggerty RJ. A simple behavior questionnaire for preschool children. *Pediatrics* 1964;34:798–806.

Appendix H ♣ Pediatric Symptom Checklist for School-Age Children

Table H.1. Pediatric symptom checklist for school-age children (6–12 Years)

Child's Name: _____ Birth Date: _____

Your relationship to the child: _____

Note: This list will not be included in your child's permanent record. It will be discarded after the visit.

Please check the heading that best fits your child:

	Never	Sometimes	Often
Complains of aches or pains	____	____	____
Spends of lot of time alone	____	____	____
Gets tired easily; doesn't have much energy	____	____	____
Fidgety; unable to sit still	____	____	____
Has trouble with a teacher	____	____	____
Not very interested in school	____	____	____
Acts as if driven by a motor	____	____	____
Daydreams too much	____	____	____
Distracted easily	____	____	____
Is afraid of new situations	____	____	____
Feels sad, unhappy a lot of the time	____	____	____
Is irritable or angry a lot	____	____	____
Feels hopeless a lot	____	____	____
Has trouble concentrating	____	____	____
Doesn't have much interest in friends	____	____	____
Fights with other children	____	____	____
Has missed a lot of school	____	____	____
School grades are dropping	____	____	____
Is down on himself or herself	____	____	____
Frequent visits to the doctor for minor complaints	____	____	____
Has trouble sleeping; wakens a lot at night	____	____	____
Worries a lot	____	____	____

(continued)

Table H.1.   *Continued.*

	Never	Sometimes	Often
Tends to be clingy with you	___	___	___
Feels he or she is "bad"	___	___	___
Takes unnecessary risks	___	___	___
Gets hurt frequently	___	___	___
Doesn't seem to have much fun	___	___	___
Acts younger than other children his or her age	___	___	___
Does not listen to rules	___	___	___
Does not show feelings	___	___	___
Does not understand other people's feelings	___	___	___
Teases other children	___	___	___
Blames others for his or her troubles	___	___	___
Steals things	___	___	___
Refuses to share	___	___	___

Adapted from Jellinek MS, Murphy JM, Robinson J, et al. Pediatric symptom checklist: screening school-age children for psychosocial dysfunction. *J Pediatr* 1988;112:201–209.

Appendix I ♣ Adolescent Previsit Questionnaire

Table I.1. Adolescent previsit questionnaire (13–21 Years)

Child's Name: _____

Age: _____ School Grade: _____

Remember: Our discussions with you are private. We hope you will feel free to talk openly with us. Information is not shared with other people without your permission unless we are concerned that someone is in danger. This list will not be included in your medical record. You can throw it away or take it home after your visit.

These are some health problems young people sometimes have.

Circle *Yes* or *No* for each item:

I have trouble sleeping	Yes	No
I feel tired all the time	Yes	No
I sometimes wet the bed	Yes	No
I worry about my health	Yes	No
I worry about what I can eat	Yes	No
I have headaches	Yes	No
I have stomachaches	Yes	No
I have leg pains	Yes	No
I have pains elsewhere	Yes	No

Sexual feelings are a normal part of growing up, but lots of young people have worries and questions about sex. Do you wonder about:

How do I know when sex is right for me?	Yes	No
How do I keep from becoming a parent too soon?	Yes	No
Sexually transmitted diseases	Yes	No
AIDS and HIV infection	Yes	No
Being gay or lesbian	Yes	No

Some young people don't like the way they look. Do you think you are:

_____ Too short

_____ Too fat   _____ Too thin

_____ Too tall   _____ I don't look right

Are you worried about:

_____ Acne/pimples?

_____ Breasts?

_____ Genitals?

_____ Other things: _____

(continued)

Table I.1. *Continued.*

Some young people have been forced into sex against their will. Has this ever happened to you or a friend?

_____ Yes   _____ No

Some young people have been physically abused or injured by someone on purpose. Has this ever happened to you or a friend?

_____ Yes   _____ No

I am worried about my parents' relationship with each other.

_____ Yes   _____ No

My relationship with my mother would be better if: _____

_____

_____

_____

My relationship with my father would be better if: _____

_____

_____

_____

I have a friend I can talk to about anything at all.	Yes	No
I worry a lot about school and my grades.	Yes	No
I worry about my future.	Yes	No

I often feel:

_____ Lonely.

_____ Like I might want to hurt myself.

_____ Like I don't get any fun out of life.

Adapted from Prazar GE, Friedman SB. An office-based approach to adolescent psychosocial issues. *Contemp Pediatr* 1997;14:59–76.

Appendix J ♦ Body Mass Indices

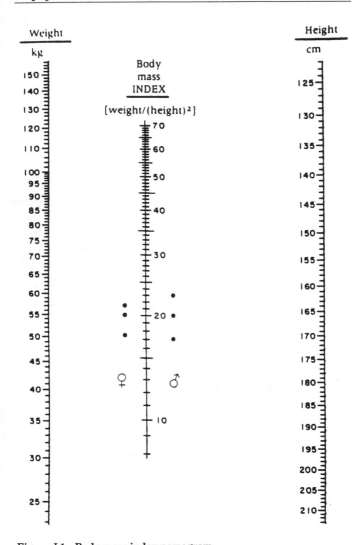

Figure J.1   Body mass index nomogram
Source: McArney ER, Kreipe RE, Orr DP, Comerci GD. *Textbook of adolescent medicine*. Philadelphia: WB Saunders; 1992. Reproduced with permission.

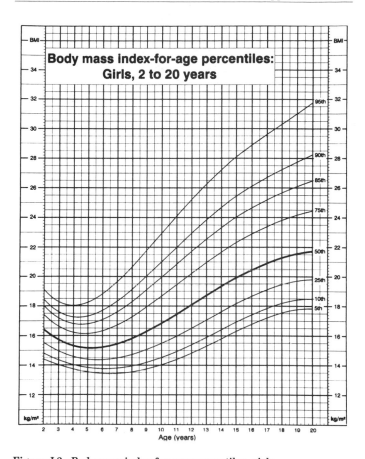

Figure J.2   Body mass index-for-age percentiles, girls
Source: Centers for Disease Control and Prevention, National Health Center for Statistics. *CDC growth charts*. Atlanta, GA: Centers for Disease Control and Prevention; 2000.

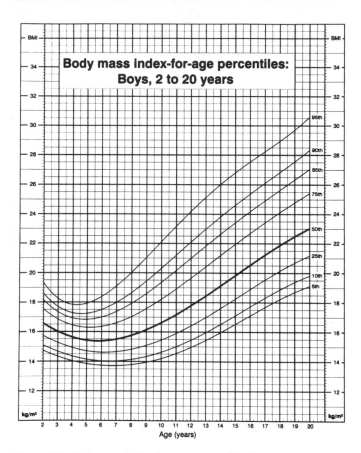

Figure J.3   Body mass index-for-age percentiles, boys
Source: Centers for Disease Control and Prevention, National Health Center
for Statistics. *CDC growth charts*. Atlanta, GA: Centers for Disease Control and
Prevention; 2000.

Appendix K Developmental Norms According to Gender

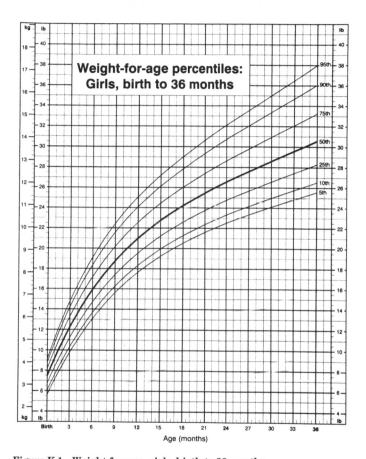

Weight-for-age percentiles: Girls, birth to 36 months

Age (months)

Figure K.1 Weight for age, girls, birth to 36 months.
Source: Centers for Disease Control and Prevention, National Health Center for Statistics. *CDC growth charts*. Atlanta, GA: Centers for Disease Control and Prevention; 2000.

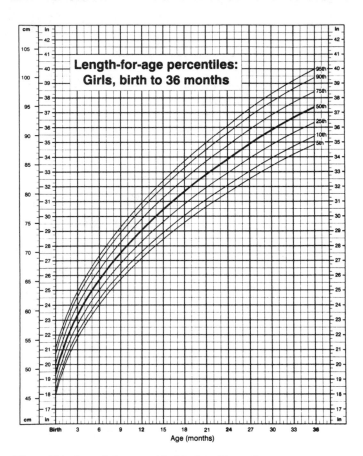

Figure K.2   Length for age, girls, birth to 36 months.
Source: Centers for Disease Control and Prevention, National Health Center
for Statistics. *CDC growth charts.* Atlanta, GA: Centers for Disease Control and
Prevention; 2000.

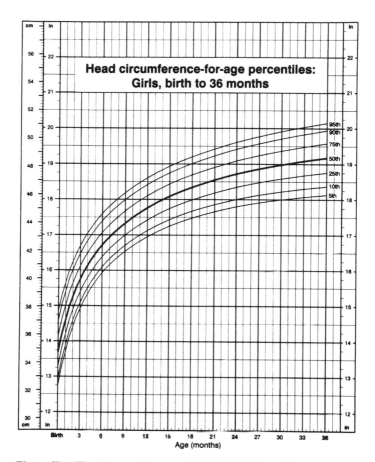

Figure K.3 Head circumference, girls, birth to 36 months.
Source: Centers for Disease Control and Prevention, National Health Center for Statistics. *CDC growth charts*. Atlanta, GA: Centers for Disease Control and Prevention; 2000.

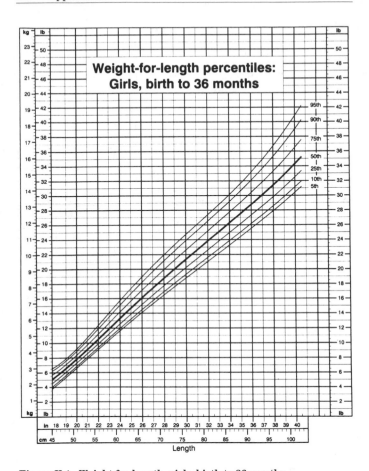

Figure K.4   Weight for length, girls, birth to 36 months.
Source: Centers for Disease Control and Prevention, National Health Center
for Statistics. *CDC growth charts*. Atlanta, GA: Centers for Disease Control and
Prevention; 2000.

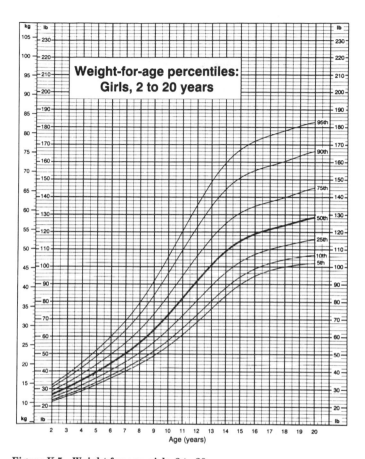

Figure K.5   Weight for age, girls, 2 to 20 years.
Source: Centers for Disease Control and Prevention, National Health Center
for Statistics. *CDC growth charts*. Atlanta, GA: Centers for Disease Control and
Prevention; 2000.

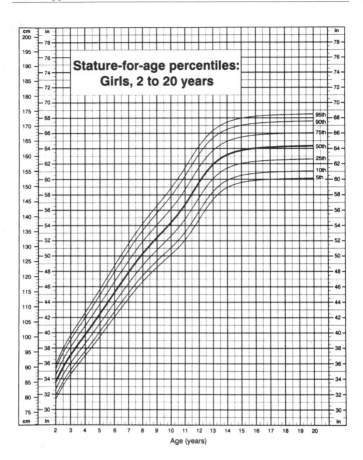

Figure K.6   Stature for age, girls, 2 to 20 years.
Source: Centers for Disease Control and Prevention, National Health Center for Statistics. *CDC growth charts*. Atlanta, GA: Centers for Disease Control and Prevention; 2000.

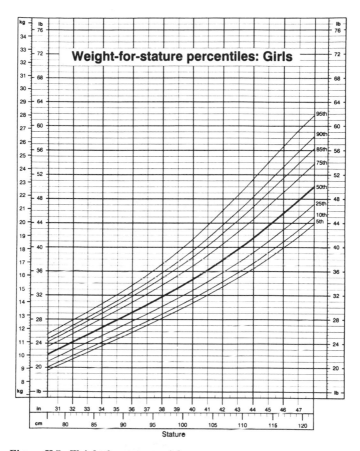

Figure K.7   Weight for stature, girls.
Source: Centers for Disease Control and Prevention, National Health Center
for Statistics. *CDC growth charts*. Atlanta, GA: Centers for Disease Control and
Prevention; 2000.

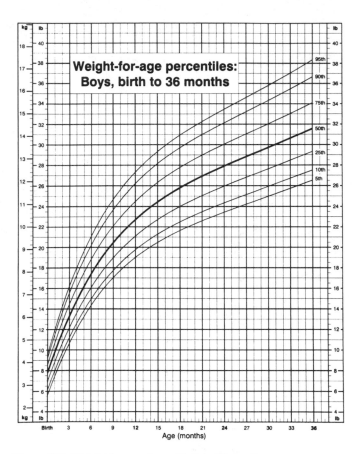

Figure K.8   Weight for age, boys, birth to 36 months.
Source: Centers for Disease Control and Prevention, National Health Center
for Statistics. *CDC growth charts*. Atlanta, GA: Centers for Disease Control and
Prevention; 2000.

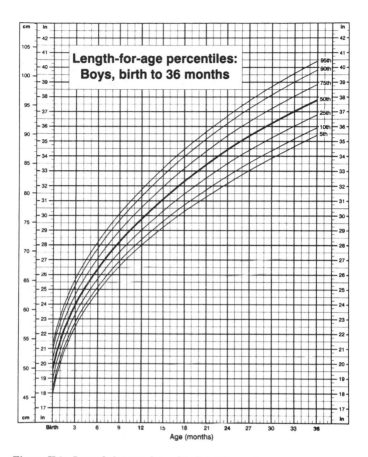

Figure K.9   Length for age, boys, birth to 36 months.
Source: Centers for Disease Control and Prevention, National Health Center for Statistics. *CDC growth charts*. Atlanta, GA: Centers for Disease Control and Prevention; 2000.

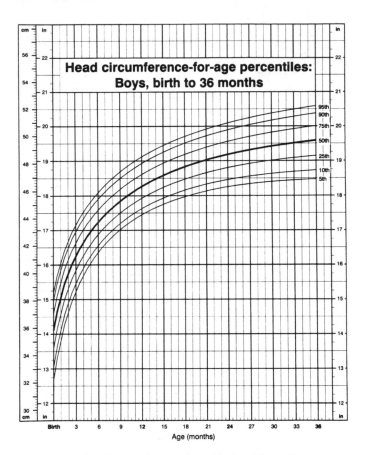

Figure K.10   Head circumference, boys, birth to 36 months.
Source: Centers for Disease Control and Prevention, National Health Center for Statistics. *CDC growth charts*. Atlanta, GA: Centers for Disease Control and Prevention; 2000.

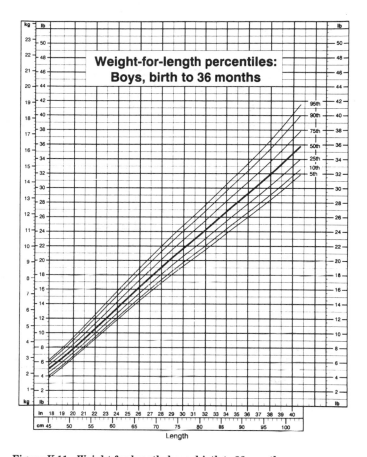

Figure K.11   Weight for length, boys, birth to 36 months.
Source: Centers for Disease Control and Prevention, National Health Center
for Statistics. *CDC growth charts*. Atlanta, GA: Centers for Disease Control and
Prevention; 2000.

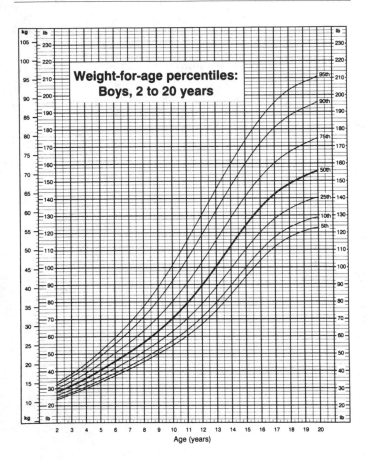

Figure K.12   Weight for age, boys, 2 to 20 years.
Source: Centers for Disease Control and Prevention, National Health Center for Statistics. *CDC growth charts*. Atlanta, GA: Centers for Disease Control and Prevention; 2000.

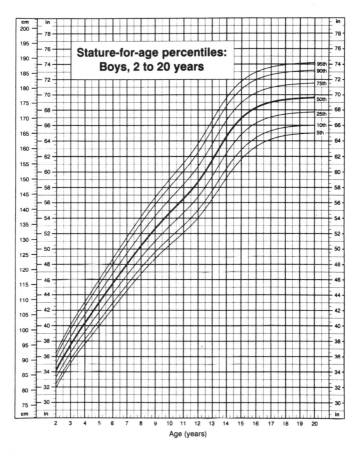

Figure K.13   Stature for age, boys, 2 to 20 years.
Source: Centers for Disease Control and Prevention, National Health Center for Statistics. *CDC growth charts*. Atlanta, GA: Centers for Disease Control and Prevention; 2000.

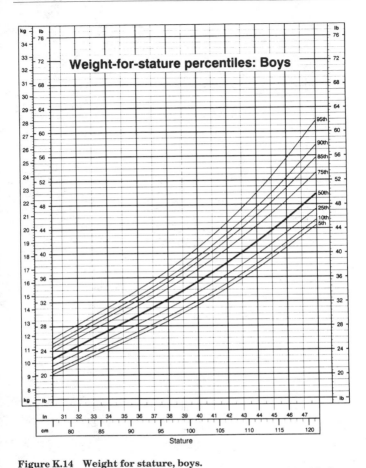

Figure K.14 Weight for stature, boys.
Source: Centers for Disease Control and Prevention, National Health Center
for Statistics. *CDC growth charts.* Atlanta, GA: Centers for Disease Control and
Prevention; 2000.

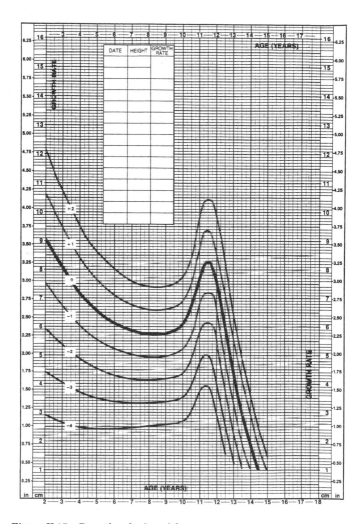

Figure K.15   Growth velocity, girls.
Source: Genetech, Inc., 1988. Reproduced with permission.

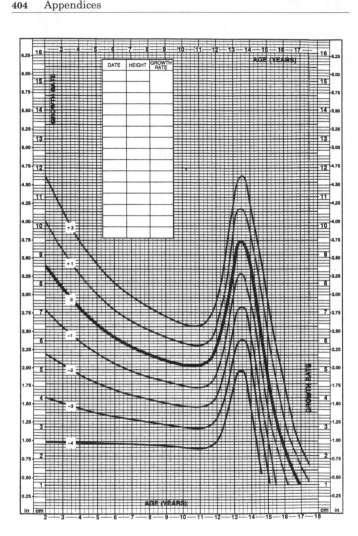

Figure K.16 Growth velocity, boys.
Source: Genetech, Inc., 1988. Reproduced with permission.

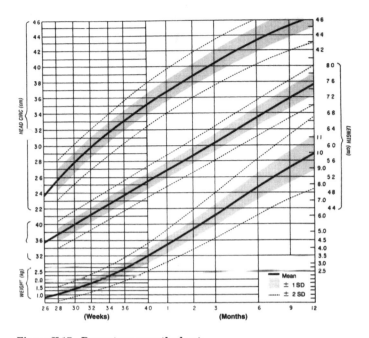

Figure K.17   Premature growth chart.
Source: Babson SG, Benda GI. Growth graphs for the clinical assessment of infants of varying gestational age. *J Pediatr* 1976;89:814. Reproduced with permission.

Appendix L ♣ Recommended Routine Childhood Immunization Schedule

Age → Vaccine ↓	Birth	2m	4m	6m	12m	15m	18m	4-6y	11-12y	14-16y
Hepatitis B[1]	HBV	HBV		HBV					HBV Catch-up	
H.influenzae type b[2]		HIB	HIB	HIB	HIB Booster					
DTaP[3]		DTaP	DTaP	DTaP			DTaP	DTaP		Td
Poliomyelitis[4]		IPV	IPV	IPV				IPV		
MMR					MMR			MMR	MMR Catch-up	
Varicella[5]						VAR			VAR Catch-up	
S.pneumoniae[6]		SPN	SPN	SPN	SPN Booster					

(Adapted from: Pickering LK, ed. *2000 Red Book: Report of the Committee on Infectious Diseases.* 25th ed. Elk Grove Village, IL: American Academy of Pediatrics, 2000.)

1 Minimum interval between 1st and 2nd, 1mo; between 2nd & 3rd, 2 mos; between 1st and 3rd, 4 mos; 3rd dose at ≥ 6 mos. of age.
2 If PRP-OMP (PedVaxHib or ComVax, Merck) used, 6 mo. dose not needed.
3 Booster DTaP may be given at 12 mos. of age if at least 6 mos. since third dose of primary series. Td booster must be at least 5 years after last dose of DTaP.
4 Inactivated vaccine is recommended for all doses.
5 If VAR given at age 13 yrs. or older, two doses at least 4 wks. apart should be given.
6 Heptavalent conjugate pneumococcal vaccine

Figure L.1.   Recommended routine childhood immunization schedule.

🏵 Subject Index

Note: Page numbers followed by *f* indicate figures; those followed by *t* indicate tables.